Recent Advances in Liver Diseases and Surgery
http://dx.doi.org/10.5772/59737
Edited by Hesham Abdeldayem, Ahmed El-Shaarawy and Tary Salman

Contributors

Hanan Mesfer Alghamdi, Zeno Sparchez, Tudor Mocan, Pompilia Radu, Alessandro Uzzau, Serena Bertozzi, Ambrogio P Londero, Stefano Bacchetti, Enricomaria Pasqual, Andrea Risaliti, Hesham Abdeldayem, Ahmed Elshaarawy, Tary Salman, Mirela Patricia Sîrbu Boeți, Mirela Boros, Amalia Petrisor, Irinel Popescu, Vlad Herlea, Ilze Strumfa, Andrejs Vanags, Ervins Vasko, Janis Gardovskis, Zane Simtniece, Peteris Trapencieris, Abdullah Saeed Gozai Al-Ghamdi, Ayman Zaki Azzam, Ahmed Abu-Zaid, Rou Li Zhou, Jing An Rui, Pasquale Pierimarchi, Giuseppe Nicotera, Gianluca Sferrazza, Federica Andreola, Paolo Daniele Siviero, Annalucia Serafino, Eric Hilgenfeldt

Published by InTech

Janeza Trdine 9, 51000 Rijeka, Croatia

Publishing Process Manager Iva Simcic

Technical Editor InTech DTP team

Cover InTech Design team

First published October, 2015

Printed in Croatia

Additional hard copies can be obtained from orders@intechopen.com

Recent Advances in Liver Diseases and Surgery, Edited by Hesham Abdeldayem, Ahmed El-Shaarawy and Tary Salman

p. cm.

ISBN 978-953-51-2193-0

Meet the editors

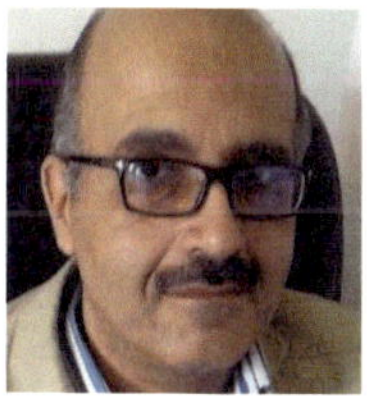

Hesham Abdeldayem, Professor of Surgery and Vice Dean of Postgraduate Studies and Research at the National Liver Institute, Menoufia University, Egypt. He has graduated from Kasr Elaini School of Medicine in 1987, where he was appointed as a resident of General Surgery and Assistant Lecturer of Microbiology. Prof. Abdeldayem joined the National Liver Institute in 1993. He has several publications in the field of hepato-pancreato-biliary surgery and liver transplantation. He was appointed as a Member of InTech's Editorial Advisory Board, and Associate Editor of Frontiers in Surgery.

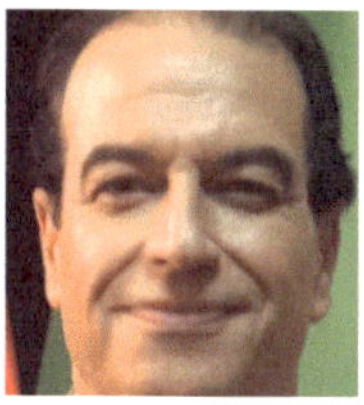

Ahmed Elshaarawy, Professor of Clinical Pathology and Dean of the National Liver Institute, Menoufia University, Egypt. He has graduated from the School of Medicine, Benha University in 1981, where he was appointed as a resident of Clinical Pathology, after which he moved to the National Liver Institute in 1988 as an Assistant Lecturer in Clinical Pathology. There he was promoted to a position of Lecturer, Assistant Professor and lastly, to Professor of Clinical Pathology. Prof. Elshaarawy has contributed to many research projects and publications in the field of clinical pathology, liver diseases, liver transplantation and stem cells.

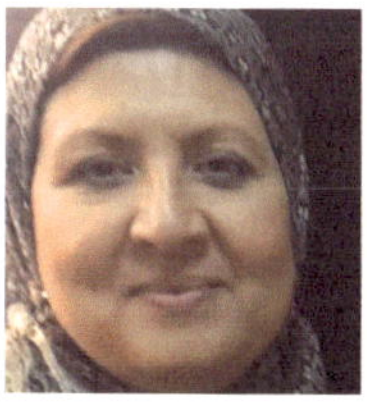

Tary Salman, Professor of Hepatology and Vice Dean for Community and Environmental Service, National Liver Institute, Menoufia University, Egypt.
She has graduated from the School of Medicine, Alexandria University in 1985, where she was appointed as a resident of Tropical Medicine, after which she moved to the National Liver Institute in 1990 as an assistant Lecturer in Hepatology. There Prof. Salman was promoted to a position of Lecturer, Assistant Professor and lastly, to Professor of Hepatology. She contributed in many research projects and publications in the field of liver diseases and transplantation.

Contents

Preface

The outstanding advances, new discoveries, and observations in hepatobiliary sciences have resulted in remarkable changes in the approach to the diagnosis and management of many liver diseases. The editors, being the dean and vice deans of the National Liver Institute, Menoufia University, Egypt, a leading center in liver diseases in the Middle East, intended to capture and present these advances in this publication. Leading experts in this super-subspecialty from North America, Europe, Asia, and Africa have participated in this book. In other words, the book team reflects an international *dream team* of expert clinicians and investigators in the field of liver diseases.

The current book contains the most recent advances in the hepatobiliary sciences, including the remarkable advances in the therapy for Hepatitis C, primary and secondary malignant liver tumors, liver injuries, as well as liver cysts, liver resections, liver transplantation, and preoperative management of patients with liver diseases. This book is addressed to researchers in the field of liver diseases, practicing gastroenterologists, hepatologists, and HPB surgeons as well as medical students, residents, and fellows.

We wish to thank all our distinguished authors for their cooperation and desire to share their precious experience with the medical community. On their behalf, we wish to express hope that this publication will facilitate access to the latest scientific achievements in the field of liver diseases all over the world. We are particularly thankful to Ana Pantar and Iva Simcic and their colleagues at InTech®, the publisher of one of the largest multidisciplinary open access collections of books covering the fields of science, for their expertise and support in bringing this edition to completion. We wish to extend our appreciation to all of our colleagues at the National Liver Institute, Menoufia University, for their tremendous support.

Prof. Hesham Abdeldayem, Prof. Ahmed El-Shaarawy and Prof. Tary Salman
National Liver Institute
Menoufia University
Egypt

Chapter 1

Preoperative Evaluation and Management of Patients with Liver Disease

Hesham Abdeldayem, Ahmed El Shaarawy, Tary Salman and Essam Salah Hammad

Additional information is available at the end of the chapter

http://dx.doi.org/10.5772/60999

Abstract

Patients with liver disease who undergo surgery have an increased risk of morbidity and mortality. Impairment of the liver functions increases the risks of surgery and anesthesia.The risk depends on the severity of liver disease, nature of the surgery and comorbid conditions. Patients with compensated cirrhosis and normal synthetic function have a low risk. Elective surgery should be postponed in patients with abnormal liver tests. All patients should have thorough preoperative evaluation, and their conditions are to be optimized before elective surgery. Thorough history and physical examination usually provide important informatation. Elective surgery can be rescheduled or cancelled once the severity of underlying liver disease is assessed. When surgery is mandatory, meticulous perioperative management is required, including hemodynamic stability, broad-spectrum antibiotics, correction of coagulopathy, improvement of nutritional status, avoidance of nephrotoxins and sedatives that could precipitate hepatic encephalopathy, and intensive care unit admission if needed.

Keywords: Liver, Liver failure, liver surgery, Liver tests, Liver functions, preoperative preparation

1. Introduction

Patients with liver disease who undergo surgery have an increased risk of morbidity and mortality [1-3].

The optimal management of such patients requires the following:

1. Diagnosis of the underlying liver disease
2. Assessment and stratification of the risk of surgery
3. Estimation of functional hepatic reserve
4. Correction of underlying conditions if feasible
5. Hepatic hemodynamic evaluation and identification of the site of upper gastrointestinal hemorrhage, if present

Impairment of the liver functions increases the risks of surgery and anesthesia in several ways, including the following [4-6]:

1. Bleeding risk may increase because of coagulopathy
2. Susceptibility to infection is increased due to altered functions of the hepatic reticuloendothelial cells and changes in the immune system and portal hypertension
3. Reduced hepatic blood flow
4. Altered drug metabolism

1.1. Factors contributing decreased liver blood flow and hypoxia [7, 8]

1. Hyperdynamic circulation with increased cardiac output and decreased systemic vascular resistance
2. Systemic and splanchnic vasodilation, with subsequent activation of the sympathetic nervous system and neurohormonal axis in an attempt to maintain arterial perfusion pressure
3. Alterations in the systemic circulation due to arteriovenous shunting and reduced splanchnic inflow
4. Anesthetic agents may reduce hepatic blood flow
5. The compensatory inotropic and chronotropic response to pharmacologic and physiologic stress, including surgery, is blunted

Induction of anesthesia hypotension, intermittent positive-pressure ventilation, pneumoperitoneum during laparoscopic surgery, traction on abdominal viscera, hemorrhage, hypoxemia, vasoactive drugs, surgical maneuver, and even positioning of the patient may all result in intraoperative and perioperative hepatic hypoxemia and further increase in the hepatic dysfunction. Risk factors for hepatic hypoxemia include ascites, hepatic hydrothorax, and hepatopulmonary syndrome [7, 17]

1.2. Altered drug metabolism

The duration of action of many drugs can be increased as a result of [10]

1. altered metabolism by cytochrome P450 enzymes,

2. decreased concentration of plasma-binding proteins,
3. decreased biliary excretion.

Hepatic dysfunction can significantly impair the metabolism of certain medications. Examples are as follows [10, 11]:

1. The volume of distribution of nondepolarizing muscle relaxants is increased, and larger doses may be required to achieve adequate neuromuscular block.
2. Sedatives, narcotics, and intravenous induction agents must be used with caution, as they may result in prolonged depression of consciousness and may lead to hepatic encephalopathy. The perioperative use of opioids as morphine should be avoided, as their bioavailability is increased.
3. Benzodiazepines should be avoided, and, if necessary, remifentanil and oxazepam are the preferred narcotic and sedative because their metabolism is not affected by liver disease.
4. Isoflurane is the recommended volatile anesthetic because it does not impair hepatic blood flow and undergoes the least amount of hepatic metabolism.

2. Preoperative assessment

If liver dysfunction is suspected, elective surgery should be deferred until extensive evaluation is made. Evaluation will include the following items [12].

2.1. History and physical examination [1-3, 13]

Thorough history and physical examination usually provide important informatation.

1. History of previous blood transfusions, drug abuse, or excessive alcohol intake.
2. Family history of jaundice, anemia, hereditary liver disease, and prior adverse reactions to anesthesia.
3. Medication history includes the use of analgesics and alternative medications.
4. Physical examination may identify signs of underlying liver disease, as temporal wasting, jaundice, palmar erythema, spider nevi, ascites, or hepatosplenomegaly.

2.2. Laboratory tests [1-18])

The term "liver function tests" is a misnomer and can be misleading. Because of the complexity of liver functions, the ideal liver function test has not been invented yet. A successful liver function test, to assist with preoperative assessment of liver function, should be safe, reproducible, and easily performed.

The aims of the tests are as follows:

1. To determine the presence or absence of hepatic injury
2. To decide whether the injury is cell necrosis or cholestasis
3. To specify the particular disease
4. To determine its severity
    - Markers of hepatocellular injury include aminotransferases and lactate dehydrogenase
    - Markers of cholestasis include alkaline phosphatase, gamma glutamyl transpeptidase, 5′-nucleotidase, and bilirubin
    - Markers of synthetic functions of the liver are prothrombin time and albumin

2.3. Aminotransferases

Alanine aminotransferase (ALT) (normal range: 10-55 U/L)

Aspartate aminotransferase (AST) (normal range: 10-40 U/L)

- Serum level rises as a result of leakage from damaged tissue
- Mild to moderate elevations occur in many types of liver disease
- Marked elevations occur in hepatitis (viral, toxic, autoimmune, and ischemic)
- AST/ALT >2 suggests alcoholic liver disease or cirrhosis of any etiology
- ALT is more specific than AST for hepatic injury
- AST is nonspecific and can originate from skeletal muscle, red blood cell, kidney, pancreas, brain, and myocardium

2.4. Alkaline phosphatase (AP)

- Normal range 45-115 U/L
- Serum level rises as a result of increased production and leaks into the serum
- Moderate rises occur in many liver diseases
- Marked rises occur in extra- and intrahepatic cholestasis, diffuse infiltrating disease (e.g., liver neoplasms), and rarely alcoholic cirrhosis
- Considerable rises occur in bone diseases (e.g., tumor, fracture, Paget's disease)
- It also originates from the intestine, placenta, and some neoplasms

2.5. Gamma Glutamyl Transpeptidase (GGTP)

- Normal range: 0-30 U/L
- Serum level rises as a result of overproduction and leakage into serum, as for AP; induced by ethanol and drugs

- GGTP/AP >2.5 suggests alcoholic liver disease
- Kidney, spleen, pancreas, heart, lung, and brain are other sources

2.6. 5′-Nucleotidase

- Normal range:: 0-11 U/L
- Serum level rises as a result of overproduction and leakage into serum, as for AP
- Found in many tissues, but serum elevation is relatively specific for liver disease

2.7. Bilirubin

- Normal range::0.0-1.0 mg/dL
- Unconjugated hyperbilirubinemia

The mechanisms that result in elevation of serum unconjugated bilirubin levels include increased production (increased breakdown of hemoglobin (resulting from hemolysis, disordered erythropoiesis, and resorption of hematoma) or myoglobin (resulting from muscle injury)) and defects in hepatic uptake or conjugation.

- Conjugated hyperbilirubinemia

The mechanisms that result in the elevation of serum-conjugated bilirubin levels are hepatobiliary diseases, including extrahepatic and intrahepatic bile duct obstruction, viral, alcoholic or drug-induced hepatitis, and inherited hyperbilirubinemia.

2.8. Prothrombin Time (PT) (10.9-12.5 s), International Normalized Ratio [INR]: (0.9-1.2)

- All clotting factors except factor VIII are synthesized by hepatocytes; factor VIII is produced by vascular endothelium and reticuloendothelial cells.
- Serum values rise as a result of the following:
  1. Decreased synthetic capacity as in acute or chronic liver failure (prolonged PT unresponsive to vitamin K)
  2. Biliary obstruction (prolonged PT usually responsive to vitamin K administration)
  3. Vitamin K deficiency (secondary to malabsorption, malnutrition, and antibiotics) and consumptive coagulopathy

2.9. Albumin

- Normal range: 3.5-5.0 g/dL
- Serum level decreases as a result of decreased synthesis; or increased loss as in
  1. chronic liver failure
  2. nephrotic syndrome, protein-losing enteropathy, and vascular leak

2.10. Markers of viral hepatitis

2.10.1. Hepatitis A

Acute infection is confirmed by detection of IgM anti-hepatitis A antibody (IgM HAV), which appears early in the course of infection and has high sensitivity and specificity. IgG anti-HAV predominates in convalescence and persists throughout life.

2.10.2. Hepatitis B

- Acute infection is associated with the presence of hepatitis B surface antigen (HBsAg).
- Detection of HBsAg precedes serum aminotransferase elevations.
- HBsAg becomes undetectable 1-3 months after jaundice.
- Some time after HBsAg disappears; HBsAg antibody (anti-HBs) appears and persists for life.
- In the interval between disappearance of HBsAg and appearance of anti-HBs, hepatitis core antigen antibody (anti-HBc) is present and helps as a marker for current or recent HBV infection.
- Anti-HBc may remain for years after infection longer than anti-HBs.
- IgM anti-HBc distinguishes recent from remote infection

2.10.3. Hepatitis C

- Hepatitis C antibodies are detected relatively late in the course of the HCV infection.
- False-positive test is a problem.
- Reverse transcriptase polymerase chain reaction and branched amplification assays are the most sensitive and specific.

2.11. Liver function quantitative tests

These tests offer attractive means to assess the liver functions. However, they have limitations, including expense, availability, invasiveness, and lack of validity.

2.11.1. Indocyanine green clearance

This dye is taken up almost exclusively by hepatocytes and excreted unchanged into the bile. It is measured photometrically in blood samples taken at regular intervals after a bolus intravenous injection (0.5 mg/kg). Clearance of the dye decreases with loss of hepatocyte mass.

2.11.2. *Aminopyrine breath test*

Radioactivity ($14CO_2$) is measured in breath at 15-min intervals for 2 h after oral or intravenous administration of 14C-labeled methyl aminopyrine. It may predict death and histology in chronic hepatitis.

2.11.3. *Monoethylglycinexylidide (MEGX)*

This lidocaine metabolite is measured in blood samples 15 min after intravenous administration of lidocaine (1 mg/kg). It may predict death and complications before and after liver transplantation

2.12. Ultrasound

Ultrasound is useful for assessing liver size, spleen size, intra- and extrahepatic biliary tree, and the presence of liver masses. It can also detect ascites in its earliest stages (≥100 mL). Doppler ultrasonography is helpful in assessment of portal venous patency, direction of portal flow.

3. Risk estimation [10-30]

The risk of surgery in patients with impairment of liver functions depends on the severity of liver disease, nature of the surgery, and comorbid conditions. Patients with compensated cirrhosis and normal synthetic function have a low risk. The risk increases for patients with decompensated liver cirrhosis. Patients with advanced liver disease may benefit from non-surgical therapy when appropriate.

3.1. Contraindications to elective surgery

1. **Acute hepatitis:** Patients with acute hepatitis of any cause have an increased operative risk.
2. **Alcoholic hepatitis:** Alcoholic hepatitis greatly increases perioperative mortality.
3. **Acute liver failure:** For acute liver failure (the development of jaundice, coagulopathy, and hepatic encephalopathy within 2-6 weeks without preexisting liver disease), all surgery other than liver transplantation is contraindicated.
4. **Decompensated cirrhosis.** Elective surgery is contraindicated in patients with Child's class C cirrhosis; these patients should be considered for surgery only in life-threatening situations, such as an incarcerated hernia, gangrenous cholecystitis, or bowel infarction.

Elective surgery should be postponed in patients with abnormal liver tests. All patients should have thorough preoperative evaluation, and their conditions are to be optimized before elective surgery. Elective surgery can be rescheduled or cancelled once the severity of underlying liver disease is assessed.

When surgery is mandatory, meticulous perioperative management is required, including hemodynamic stability, broad-spectrum antibiotics, correction of coagulopathy, improvement of nutritional status, avoidance of nephrotoxins and sedatives that could precipitate hepatic encephalopathy, and intensive care unit admission if needed.

4. Assessment of the risk factors

4.1. Severity and nature of the underlying liver disease

Operative risks are markedly influenced by the severity and nature of the underlying liver disease.

Obstructive jaundice: Obstructive jaundice markedly increases perioperative mortality.

Acute hepatitis: Acute hepatitis is associated with increased morbidity and mortality associated with surgery.

Cirrhosis: The perioperative risk is influenced by the degree of hepatic dysfunction, portal hypertension, and its complications as ascites, intra-abdominal varices, renal impairment, and portopulmonary hypertension.

The amount of perioperative risks is related to the degree of liver decompensation. An accurate assessment of the degree of liver decompensation is important for determination of the perioperative risk.

4.2. Child's classification and its modifications

This is based on the patient's serum bilirubin and albumin levels, prothrombin time, and severity of encephalopathy and ascites.

Child–Pugh scoring system

Points	1	2	3
Ascites	None	Small or diuretic controlled	Tense
Encephalopathy	Absent	States I–II	States III–IV
Albumin (g/L)	>3.5	2.8–3.5	<2.8
Bilirubin (mg/dL)	<2	2–3	>3
PT(sec above control), or INR	<4 <1.7	4–6 1.7–2.3	>6 >2.3

In general, elective surgery is well tolerated in patients with Child class A, permitted with careful preoperative preparation in patients with Child class B, and contraindicated in patients with Child class C.

Score	Child–Turcotte-Pugh Class
5–6	A
7–9	B
10–15	C

Other factors can also increase the perioperative risk beyond the Child classification. The perioperative risk is increased if there is portal hypertension. Emergency surgery is associated with a higher mortality rates.

Child score for estimating the perioperative risks has been shown to be quite variable. This may be explained by the following:

1. Patients with class A may have ascites, hyperbilirubinemia, and portal hypertension.

2. The variables (ascites and hepatic encephalopathy are graded subjectively) are operator dependent.

3. It is unable to stratify patients with severely decompensated liver disease.

For this reason, alternative systems have been sought

4.3. Model for end-stage liver disease (MELD) score

The MELD score is a linear regression model based on a patient's serum bilirubin and creatinine levels and international normalized ratio (INR).

4.3.1. MELD scoring equation

MELD score for TIPS = 0.957 × loge (creatinine [mg/dL]) + 0.378 × loge (bilirubin [mg/dL]) + 1.120 × loge (INR) + 0.643 (cause of liver disease)

MELD score for liver transplantation = 0.957 × loge(creatinine [mg/dL]) + 0.378 × loge(bilirubin [mg/dL]) + 1.120 × loge(INR) + 0.643

It was created to predict mortality after TIPS, then to stratify the risks in patients awaiting liver transplant, and recently used to predict perioperative mortality. It has several distinct advantages over the Child classification, being objective, and does not rely on cutoff values.

The general guidelines are as follows:

- Patient with an MELD score below 10 can undergo elective surgery.

- Patient with an MELD score of 10-15 should be managed with caution.

- In patients with an MELD score above 15, elective surgery should be avoided and the patient should be considered for liver transplantation.

These guidelines should be modified for specific circumstances.

4.4. Type of surgery

The operative risk is higher with certain types of surgery, such as hepatic resection, biliary surgery, gastric surgery, colectomy, and cardiac surgery.

Emergency surgery carries higher mortality in hepatic patients than patients with normal hepatic function.

Abdominal surgery as cholecystectomy, gastric bypass, biliary procedures, peptic ulcers, and colon resection is associated with increased morbidity and mortality risks in patients with cirrhosis.

Biliary tract surgery: Patients with obstructive jaundice have increased risk of infections, disseminated intravascular coagulation, gastrointestinal bleeding, delayed wound healing, wound dehiscence, incisional hernias, and renal failure. Patients with cirrhosis are at increased risk of gallstones and their complications. For Child class C patients, cholecystostomy, rather than cholecystectomy, is considered. For patients with obstructive jaundice, nonsurgical approaches to decompression via endoscopic retrograde cholangiopancreatography or percutaneous transhepatic cholangiography are preferred.

Cardiac Surgery: Procedures that require cardiopulmonary bypass are associated with greater mortality in patients with cirrhosis.

Hepatic Resection: Hepatectomies in cirrhotic patients are associated with increased risks. The extent of hepatectomy is a predictor of mortality.

5. Preoperative care of patients with liver disease [28-48]

5.1. Aims

1. Prophylactic measures to prevent complications
2. Early recognition and treatment of complications

5.2. Complications of liver diseases

1. Refractory ascites
2. Spontaneous bacterial peritonitis (SBP)
3. Fluid and electrolyte disturbances
4. Hepatorenal syndrome (HRS)
5. Portal hypertensive bleedings
6. Hepatic encephalopathy (HE)
7. Hepatocellular carcinoma (HCC)

8. Malnutrition
9. Progress of other medical diseases

5.3. Tests to assess the complications of liver disease

1. Liver imaging and AFP, CA19-9 to exclude neoplasms
2. Doppler ultrasound: to exclude portal vein thrombosis
3. Upper GI endoscopy: to assess portal hypertension
4. Bone densitometry: in selected patients
5. Neuropsychologic testing: selected patients
6. ABG: to exclude hypoxemia-hepatopulmonary syndrome

Particular attention needs to be paid to the management of common complications of advanced liver disease, as coagulopathy, thrombocytopenia, ascites, renal insufficiency, encephalopathy, and malnutrition, as well as to disease-specific factors.

5.4. Coagulopathy

The cause of coagulopathy is multifactorial. It may result from poor absorption of vitamin K due to cholestasis or impaired synthesis of coagulation factors.

- Parenteral vitamin K and transfusions of fresh frozen plasma can be used before surgery.
- Intravenous cryoprecipitate may be infused with a minimal volume load. It contains large amounts of fibrinogen and von Willebrand factor together with clotting factors.
- Intravenous recombinant factor VIIa is a safe and effective in correcting coagulopathy and normalizing the INR.
- For patients with thrombocytopenia, platelet transfusion of may be recommended.
- Prolonged bleeding time can be corrected bydesmopressin acetate.

5.5. Ascites

Grades of ascites:

Grade 1: ascites only detected by ultrasound

Grade 2: moderate with symmetrical distention of the abdomen

Grade 3: large or tense with marked abdominal distension

- Fluid restriction is not necessary in most patients.
- Due to hyperkalemia, spironolactone as a single agent is recommended only in minimal fluid overload.

- The usual regimen is a single morning dose of 100 mg spironolactone and 40 mg furosemide. The dose can be increased every 3-5 days, if weight loss is not satisfactory. Maximum doses are 600 mg/day spironolactone and 200 mg/day furosemide.
- Side effects include volume depletion, which may precipitate encephalopathy, or renal failure.
- Weekly monitoring of electrolytes and weight must be undertaken when initiating or changing therapy.
- Encephalopathy, serum Na <125 mmol/L, creatinine >1.7mg/dL, should lead to cessation of diuretic use.

Refractory ascites is that which is unresponsive to high-dose diuretics and a Na-restricted diet and tends to rapidly recur following paracentesis. Prior to labeling a patient as having refractory ascites, an in-hospital trial of dietary management and diuretic therapy should be attempted.

Treatment options include the following:

1. Paracentesis with albumin replacement remains the first treatment option for patients on the waiting list and are likely to undergo LT within a few months.

   - For large volume paracentesis, an albumin infusion of 8-10 g/L of fluid removed should be considered.
   - Paracentesis increases the risk of peritonitis.

2. TIPS is considered for the following:

   - Cases where the frequency of paracentesis is >3 times/month
   - Patients not tolerating large-volume paracentesis
   - Large-volume paracentesis is ineffective due to multiple adhesions or loculated ascites
   - Refractory hepatic hydrothorax

The major disadvantages are shunt stenosis and HE.

3. Peritoneovenous shunt: for historical interest only

4. Surgical shunts are rarely indicated

5.6. Spontaneous bacterial peritonitis

Definition: infection of the ascitic fluid in the absence of any known intra-abdominal source.

Diagnosis: positive ascites culture and/or polymorphonuclear cell count ≥25 0 cells/mm^3.

Its prevalence justifies diagnostic paracentesis in cirrhotics with ascites admitted to the hospital. Norfloxacin (400 mg/day) significantly reduces the probability of SBP.

Secondary long-term prophylaxis is recommended for all patients with a history of SBP. Antibiotic prophylaxis is recommended in patients with an upper GI bleed irrespective of the presence or absence of ascites.

5.7. Renal impairment

Patients with ESLD are at increased risk to develop renal failure (RF), either spontaneously (hepatorenal syndrome [HRS]) or iatrogenically (diuretics, nephrotoxic drugs). Preoperative renal function significantly affects postoperative survival.

HRS can only be diagnosed after other causes of renal failure are excluded: obstruction, volume depletion, ATN, and drug-induced nephrotoxicity. All diuretics should be stopped. Fluid challenge with 1.5 L of isotonic saline should be administered to exclude volume depletion.

5.7.1. Types of HRS

Type I HRS: rapidly progressive renal failure with an increase in the serum creatinine to more than 2.5 mg/dL within 14 days and marked oliguria.

Type II HRS: stable or slowly progressive impairment in renal function in patients with refractory ascites.

Management:

1. Combination of

   - vasoconstrictor drugs, such as vasopressin analogues, noradrenalin, and the combination of midodrine and octreotide together,

   - plasma volume expansion with albumin (1 g/kg intravenously on day 1, 20-40 daily thereafter).

Hemodialysis as a bridge to liver transplant might be useful in patients who fail to respond to medical treatment.

Nephrotoxic drugs should be used with cautious, and overtreatment with diuretics should be avoided. It is recommended to stop diuretics if serum creatinine is >1.7 mg/dL.

5.8. Dilutional hyponatremia

Definition: Serum sodium <130 mmol/L.

Cause: impaired free water clearance by the kidneys due to nonosmotic hypersecretion of ADH.

- It represents a late event and indicates poor prognosis. Occurs months after the onset of Na retention.

- It has been proposed to incorporate serum Na concentration in the MELD score; however, this remains controversial.

Management

- As long as the serum Na remains >125 mmol/L, no specific measures are required.
- If the serum Na level is <125 mmol/L, the following should be considered:
  1. Diuretics should be stopped.
  2. Infusion of albumin (100 g/24 h) or red blood cells is instituted attempting at expanding the effective circulating blood volume.

     Na level will increase as a result of turning off ADH secretion by the increased blood volume. Once the serum sodium starts to rise, the albumin infusion is tapered.
  3. Free water restriction.
- Attempts to rapid correction with hypertonic saline can lead to more complications.

5.9. Hepatic Encephalopathy (HE)

HE is a diagnosis of exclusion. Other etiologies as space-occupying lesions, vascular events, metabolic disorders, and infectious diseases should be excluded.

Stages of hepatic encephalopathy

1. Slowing of consciousness
2. Drowsiness
3. Confusion, reactive only to vocal stimuli
4. Coma

Precipitating factors

1. Renal and electrolyte abnormalities
2. Gastrointestinal bleeding
3. Infection
4. Constipation
5. Benzodiazepines, narcotics, or other sedatives
6. Excessive dietary protein intake
7. Worsening liver function, e.g., portal vein thrombosis
8. Noncompliance with medications, especially lactulose

Therapy

1. The mainstay is correcting the precipitating event.
2. Intubation has to be considered to prevent aspiration, depending on the level of consciousness.

3. Nasogastric tube should be placed.

4. Nonabsorbable disaccharides such as lactulose: The usual starting dose is 20 mL, 3-4 times daily with the aim of achieving 2-4 soft bowel movements per day.

5. Neomycin 3-6 g/day in divided doses might be added. Alternatively, metronidazole can be used.

6. Low-protein diet (minimum 30 g/day).

7. Gluconeogenesis is a significant source of production of endogenous ammonia and may result in worsening of the encephalopathy. Patients should be provided with at least of 400 calories daily in the form of IV glucose to reduce gluconeogenesis.

- Once the patient recovers, a moderate amount of protein (40 g/day) is given and increased to the maximum tolerated dose within few days.
- It is important to avoid protein restriction for a long time to prevent worsening of the nutritional state.
- The role of ornithine-aspartate, sodium benzoate, and branched-chain amino acids is questioned.
- Ammonia level is a poor predictor of the degree of encephalopathy. Changes in ammonia levels should not be considered an indicator of therapeutic benefit; improvement in mental status is the therapeutic end point.

5.10. Portopulmonary Hypertension (PPHTN)

Definition: portal hypertension (clinical diagnosis), mean pulmonary artery pressure (MPAP) >25 mm Hg, pulmonary artery occlusion pressure (PAOP) 15< mm Hg, pulmonary vascular resistance (PVR) >240 dyne/s/cm^{-5}.

The detection of PPHTN is crucial as it increases the perioperative and long-term risks.

The most common presenting symptom is progressive dyspnea on excretion; however, patients with even severe PPHTN can be completely asymptomatic. Echocardiography is the screening method of choice. A systolic right ventricular pressure (RVsys) of >50 mm Hg as a cutoff is used. Only these patients need to undergo right heart catheterization to characterize pulmonary hemodynamics.

5.11. Hepatopulmonary syndrome

This is defined as a triad of the following:

1. Chronic liver disease

2. Hypoxemia (PaO_2 <70 mm Hg or alveolar to arterial oxygen gradient >20 mm Hg)

3. Intrapulmonary arteriovenous dilatation or shunts as detected by contrast echocardiography, lung perfusion scanning, or pulmonary angiography

Hypoxemia at rest is the prerequisite for the diagnosis. Medical management is disappointing, and liver transplant is advocated as the treatment of choice.

5.12. Malnutrition

Malnutrition is common with liver impairment and is a risk factor for mortality following LT. Nutritional supplementation has not been proven to affect outcome. The total amount of calories provided should be at least 30-35 kcal/kg/day. Adults can receive daily 1-2 g protein/kg of dry body weight. Patients should take daily multivitamin and other supplements as needed. Specific fat-soluble vitamin supplements are provided if a deficiency is present.

5.13. Psychosocial stress

The preoperative period can be extremely stressful. Declining health, uncertainty about the results, and inability to continue working and participating in daily activities may increase the risk of depression and/or anxiety. Patients with chronic HCV have a greater incidence of depression and anxiety. Patients who experience significant psychological distress have increased complications.

6. Preoperative checklist

The preoperative evaluation concludes with a review of all pertinent studies and information obtained from investigative tests.

1. Informed consent after discussion with the patient and family members regarding the indication for the anticipated surgical procedure, as well as its risks and proposed benefits

2. Review the need for β-blockade, DVT prophylaxis

3. Antibiotic prophylaxis: The appropriate antibiotic is chosen before surgery and administered before the skin incision is made

4. Preoperative mechanical bowel cleansing, whenever indicated

5. Revision of medications

    - Careful review of the patient's medications is important.

    - The aim is to judiciously give medications that control the patient's illnesses and at the same time minimizing the risk associated with anesthetic and other drugs interactions.

    - In general, patients taking cardiac drugs, pulmonary drugs or anticonvulsants, antihypertensives, or psychiatric drugs are advised to take their medications with sips of water on the morning of operation.

    - Parenteral medications are used if the patient remains NPO for any significant period postoperatively.

- It is important to restitute patients to their usual medications as soon as possible.
- Drugs affecting platelet function are withheld for variable time: aspirin and clopidogrel (Plavix) are withheld for 7-10 days, while NSAIDs are withheld depending on the drug's half-life between 1 day (ibuprofen and indomethacin) and 3 days (naproxen and sulindac).

6. Preoperative fasting

7. Postoperative monitoring

- The patients are monitored for signs of hepatic decompensation, such as ascites, worsening jaundice encephalopathy, coagulopathy, and renal impairment.
- If any of these occur, supportive therapy is started immediately.
- Prothrombin time is the single best indicator of the synthetic function of the liver.
- Elevated serum bilirubin level may result from worsening of the liver function and also may be elevated because of other conditions, as blood transfusions, blood extravasation, or infection.
- Renal function must be monitored closely. If renal impairment occurs, the cause should be suspected and treatment started.
- In cases of severe impairment of the liver functions, hypoglycemia may occur as a result of depletion of liver glycogen stores and impaired gluconeogenesis. Serum levels of glucose should be monitored closely if postoperative liver failure is suspected.
- Careful attention should be paid to the IV fluid infusions.

Intravascular volume maintenance minimizes the risk of hepatic and renal underperfusion.

At the same time, crystalloid overinfusion results in liver congestion, venous oozing and pulmonary congestion and edema, ascites, peripheral edema, and wound disruption.

8. Bottom lines

- Accurate preoperative identification of patients with liver disease allows their treatment plans to be adjusted.
- In patients with acute liver disease, elective surgery should be postponed until symptoms resolve.
- Elective surgery should be avoided in patients with acute liver diseases such as acute viral hepatitis or alcoholic hepatitis, if there is evidence of ongoing hepatic injury.

- In cases of chronic liver diseases, it is mandatory to assess the severity of underlying disease before deciding whether to proceed with surgery.
- MELD and CTP scores can be used to stratify the risks of surgery for patients with chronic liver disease.
- Optimal preoperative management can reduce the risk of postoperative morbidity and mortality.
- Preoperative management of complications related to patients' underlying liver disease is essential to optimize their outcomes.

Author details

Hesham Abdeldayem, Ahmed El Shaarawy, Tary Salman and Essam Salah Hammad

National Liver Institute, Menoufia University, Egypt

References

[1] Wu CC, Yeh DC, Lin MC, Liu TJ, P'Eng FK. Improving operative safety for cirrhotic liver resection. Br J Surg. 2001 Feb;88(2):210-5.

[2] Chung SW, Greig PD, Cattral MS, Taylor BR, Sheiner PA, Wanless I, Cameron R, Phillips MJ, Blendis LM, Langer B, Levy GA. Evaluation of liver transplantation for high-risk indications. Br J Surg. 1997 Feb;84(2):189-95.

[3] Donovan CL, Marcovitz PA, Punch JD, Bach DS, Brown KA, Lucey MR, Armstrong WF. Two-dimensional and dobutamine stress echocardiography in the preoperative assessment of patients with end-stage liver disease prior to orthotopic liver transplantation. Transplantation. 1996 Apr 27;61(8):1180-8.

[4] Chiang PP. Perioperative management of the alcohol-dependent patient. Am Fam Physician. 1995 Dec;52(8):2267-73.

[5] Nagawa H, Kobori O, Muto T. Prediction of pulmonary complications after transthoracic oesophagectomy. Br J Surg. 1994 Jun;81(6):860-2.

[6] Shimada M, Matsumata T, Taketomi A, Nishizaki T, Itasaka H, Sugimachi K. Major hepatic resection in patients with a prosthetic heart valve receiving anticoagulation treatment. Hepatogastroenterology. 1994 Jun;41(3):290-3.

[7] Takeda J, Hashimoto K, Tanaka T, Koufuji K, Kakegawa T. Review of operative indication and prognosis in gastric cancer with hepatic cirrhosis. Hepatogastroenterology. 1992 Oct;39(5):433-6.

[8] Gholson CF, Provenza JM, Bacon BR. Hepatologic considerations in patients with parenchymal liver disease undergoing surgery. Am J Gastroenterol. 1990 May;85(5): 487-96.

[9] Sabbagh C, Fuks D, Regimbeau JM. Non-hepatic gastrointestinal surgery in patients with cirrhosis. J Visc Surg. 2014 Jun;151(3):203-11. doi: 10.1016/j.jviscsurg.2014.04.004. Epub 2014 May 5.

[10] Im GY, Lubezky N, Facciuto ME, Schiano TD. Surgery in patients with portal hypertension: a preoperative checklist and strategies for attenuating risk. Clin Liver Dis. 2014 May;18(2):477-505. doi: 10.1016/j.cld.2014.01.006. Epub 2014 Feb 25.

[11] Lin TY, Liao JC, Chen WJ, Chen LH, Niu CC, Fu TS, Lai PL, Tsai TT. Surgical risks and perioperative complications of instrumented lumbar surgery in patients with liver cirrhosis. Biomed J. 2014 Jan-Feb;37(1):18-23. doi: 10.4103/2319-4170.113376.

[12] Jafarian A, Kasraianfard A, Najafi A, Salimi J, Moini M, Azmoudeh-Ardalan F, Ahmadinejad Z, Davoudi S, Sattarzadeh R, Seifi S, Moharari RS, Nejatisafa A, Saberi H, Aminian A, Kazemeini AR, Fakhar N, Makarem J, Yazdi NA, Sohrabpour AA, Dashti H, Nassiri-Toosi M. Patient outcomes in a liver transplant program in Iran. Exp Clin Transplant. 2014 Mar;12 Suppl 1:86-91.

[13] Ponziani FR, Zocco MA, Senzolo M, Pompili M, Gasbarrini A, Avolio AW. Portal vein thrombosis and liver transplantation: implications for waiting list period, surgical approach, early and late follow-up. Transplant Rev (Orlando). 2014 Apr;28(2): 92-101. doi: 10.1016/j.trre.2014.01.003. Epub 2014 Jan 27.

[14] Paolino J, Steinhagen RM. Colorectal surgery in cirrhotic patients. ScientificWorldJournal. 2014 Jan 15;2014:239293. doi: 10.1155/2014/239293. eCollection 2014.

[15] Wang WL, Zhu Y, Cheng JW, Li MX, Xia JM, Hao J, Yu L, Lv Y, Wu Z, Wang B,. Major hepatectomy is safe for hepatocellular carcinoma in elderly patients with cirrhosis. Eur J Gastroenterol Hepatol. 2014 Apr;26(4):444-51. doi: 10.1097/MEG. 0000000000000046.

[16] Kiamanesh D, Rumley J, Moitra VK. Monitoring and managing hepatic disease in anaesthesia. Br J Anaesth. 2013 Dec;111 Suppl 1:i50-61. doi: 10.1093/bja/aet378.

[17] Gopaldas RR, Chu D, Cornwell LD, Dao TK, Lemaire SA, Coselli JS, Bakaeen FG. Cirrhosis as a moderator of outcomes in coronary artery bypass grafting and off-pump coronary artery bypass operations: a 12-year population-based study. Ann Thorac Surg. 2013 Oct;96(4):1310-5. doi: 10.1016/j.athoracsur.2013.04.103. Epub 2013 Jul 25.

[18] Valentine E, Gregorits M, Gutsche JT, Al-Ghofaily L, Augoustides JG. Clinical update in liver transplantation. J Cardiothorac Vasc Anesth. 2013 Aug;27(4):809-15. doi: 10.1053/j.jvca.2013.03.031.

[19] , Liao JC, Chen WJ, Chen LH, Niu CC, Fu TS, Lai PL, Tsai TT. Complications associated with instrumented lumbar surgery in patients with liver cirrhosis: a matched co-

hort analysis. Spine J. 2013 Aug;13(8):908-13. doi: 10.1016/j.spinee.2013.02.028. Epub 2013 Mar 27.

[20] Pandey CK, Karna ST, Pandey VK, Tandon M, Singhal A, Mangla V. Perioperative risk factors in patients with liver disease undergoing non-hepatic surgery. World J Gastrointest Surg. 2012 Dec 27;4(12):267-74. doi: 10.4240/wjgs.v4.i12.267.

[21] Magoulas PL, El-Hattab AW. Glycogen storage disease type IV. In: Pagon RA, Adam MP, Ardinger HH, Bird TD, Dolan CR, Fong CT, Smith RJH, Stephens K, editors. GeneReviews® [Internet]. Seattle (WA): University of Washington, Seattle; 1993-2014. 2013 Jan 03.

[22] Khan N, Siddiq G. Outcome of laparoscopic cholecystectomy for gallstones disease in patients with liver cirrhosis. J Ayub Med Coll Abbottabad. 2013 Jan-Jun;25(1-2): 36-9.

[23] Kim MS, Lee JR. Assessment of liver stiffness measurement: novel intraoperative blood loss predictor?, World J Surg. 2013 Jan;37(1):185-91. doi: 10.1007/s00268-012-1774-y.

[24] Sugimura Y, Toyama M, Katoh M, Kato Y, Hisamoto K. Analysis of open heart surgery in patients with liver cirrhosis. Asian Cardiovasc Thorac Ann. 2012 Jun;20(3): 263-8. doi: 10.1177/0218492311435339.

[25] Nicoll A. Surgical risk in patients with cirrhosis. J Gastroenterol Hepatol. 2012 Oct; 27(10):1569-75. doi: 10.1111/j.1440-1746.2012.07205.x.

[26] Sirivatanauksorn Y, Taweerutchana V, Limsrichamrern S, Kositamongkol P, Mahawithitwong P, Asavakarn S, Tovikkai C. Recipient and perioperative risk factors associated with liver transplant graft outcomes. Transplant Proc. 2012 Mar;44(2):505-8. doi: 10.1016/j.transproceed.2012.01.065.

[27] Macaron C, Hanouneh IA, Suman A, Lopez R, Johnston D, Carey WW. Safety of cardiac surgery for patients with cirrhosis and Child-Pugh scores less than 8. Clin Gastroenterol Hepatol. 2012 May;10(5):535-9. doi: 10.1016/j.cgh.2011.12.030. Epub 2011 Dec 28.

[28] Raval Z, Harinstein ME, Skaro AI, Erdogan A, DeWolf AM, Shah SJ, Fix OK, Kay N, Abecassis MI, Gheorghiade M, Flaherty JD. Cardiovascular risk assessment of the liver transplant candidate. J Am Coll Cardiol. 2011 Jul 12;58(3):223-31. doi: 10.1016/j.jacc.2011.03.026.

[29] Bispo M, Marcelino P, Marques HP, Martins A, Perdigoto R, Aguiar MJ, Mourão L, Barroso E. Domino versus deceased donor liver transplantation: association with early graft function and perioperative bleeding. Liver Transpl. 2011 Mar;17(3):270-8. doi: 10.1002/lt.22210.

[30] Marrocco-Trischitta MM, Kahlberg A, Astore D, Tshiombo G, Mascia D, Chiesa R. Outcome in cirrhotic patients after elective surgical repair of infrarenal aortic aneur-

ysm. J Vasc Surg. 2011 Apr;53(4):906-11. doi: 10.1016/j.jvs.2010.10.095. Epub 2011 Jan 7.

[31] Tinti F, Umbro I, Meçule A, Rossi M, Merli M, Nofroni I, Corradini SG, Poli L, Pugliese F, Ruberto F, Berloco PB, Mitterhofer AP. RIFLE criteria and hepatic function in the assessment of acute renal failure in liver transplantation. Transplant Proc. 2010 May;42(4):1233-6. doi: 10.1016/j.transproceed.2010.03.128.

[32] Manousou P, Samonakis D, Cholongitas E, Patch D, O'Beirne J, Dhillon AP, Rolles K, McCormick A, Hayes P, Burroughs AK. Outcome of recurrent hepatitis C virus after liver transplantation in a randomized trial of tacrolimus monotherapy versus triple therapy. Liver Transpl. 2009 Dec;15(12):1783-91. doi: 10.1002/lt.21907.

[33] O'Leary JG, Yachimski PS, Friedman LS. Surgery in the patient with liver disease. Clin Liver Dis. 2009 May;13(2):211-31. doi: 10.1016/j.cld.2009.02.002.

[34] Dalmau A, Sabaté A, Aparicio I. Hemostasis and coagulation monitoring and management during liver transplantation. Curr Opin Organ Transplant. 2009 Jun;14(3): 286-90. doi: 10.1097/MOT.0b013e32832a6b7c.

[35] Frye JW, Perri RE. Perioperative risk assessment for patients with cirrhosis and liver disease. Expert Rev Gastroenterol Hepatol. 2009 Feb;3(1):65-75. doi: 10.1586/17474124.3.1.65.

[36] McAvoy NC, Kochar N, McKillop G, Newby DE, Hayes PC. Prevalence of coronary artery calcification in patients undergoing assessment for orthotopic liver transplantation. Liver Transpl. 2008 Dec;14(12):1725-31. doi: 10.1002/lt.21540.

[37] Dharancy S, Lemyze M, Boleslawski E, Neviere R, Declerck N, Canva V, Wallaert B, Mathurin P, Pruvot FR. Impact of impaired aerobic capacity on liver transplant candidates. Transplantation. 2008 Oct 27;86(8):1077-83. doi: 10.1097/TP.0b013e318187758b.

[38] Nanashima A, Sumida Y, Abo T, Tanaka K, Takeshita H, Hidaka S, Yano H, Sawai T, Obatake M, Yasutake T, Nagayasu T. Clinicopathological and intraoperative parameters associated with postoperative hepatic complications. Hepatogastroenterology. 2007 Apr-May;54(75):839-43.

[39] Moon YW, Kim YS, Kwon SY, Kim SY, Lim SJ, Park YS. Perioperative risk of hip arthroplasty in patients with cirrhotic liver disease. J Korean Med Sci. 2007 Apr;22(2): 223-6.

[40] Pulitanò C, Arru M, Bellio L, Rossini S, Ferla G, Aldrighetti L. A risk score for predicting perioperative blood transfusion in liver surgery. Br J Surg. 2007 Jul;94(7): 860-5.

[41] Santambrogio R, Opocher E, Ceretti AP, Barabino M, Costa M, Leone S, Montorsi M. Impact of intraoperative ultrasonography in laparoscopic liver surgery. Surg Endosc. 2007 Feb;21(2):181-8. Epub 2006 Nov 21.

[42] Harte B. What is the appropriate means of perioperative risk assessment for patients with cirrhosis? IMPACT consults. Proceedings of the 2nd Annual Cleveland Clinic Perioperative Medicine Summit. Cleve Clin J Med. 2006 Sep;73 Electronic Suppl 1:S10-1.

[43] Poon RT. Recent advances in techniques of liver resection. Surg Technol Int. 2004;13:71-7.

[44] Chang YC. Low mortality major hepatectomy. Hepatogastroenterology. 2004 Nov-Dec;51(60):1766-70.

[45] Suehiro T, Matsumata T, Shikada Y, Shimada M, Shirabe K, Sugimachi K. Change in alpha glutathione s-transferase levels during liver resection. Hepatogastroenterology. 2004 Nov-Dec;51(60):1747-50.

[46] Song TJ, Ip EW, Fong Y. Hepatocellular carcinoma: current surgical management. Gastroenterology. 2004 Nov;127(5 Suppl 1):S248-60.

[47] del Olmo JA, Flor-Lorente B, Flor-Civera B, Rodriguez F, Serra MA, Escudero A, Lledó S, Rodrigo JM. Risk factors for nonhepatic surgery in patients with cirrhosis. World J Surg. 2003 Jun;27(6):647-52. Epub 2003 May 13.

[48] Lentschener C, Ozier Y. Anaesthesia for elective liver resection: some points should be revisited. Eur J Anaesthesiol. 2002 Nov;19(11):780-8.

Chapter 2

New Perspective in HCV Clinical and Economical Management of the Current and Future Therapies

P. Pierimarchi, G. Nicotera, G. Sferrazza, F. Andreola, A. Serafino and P.D. Siviero

Additional information is available at the end of the chapter

http://dx.doi.org/10.5772/61187

Abstract

Hepatitis C virus (HCV) is a progressive disease that infects more than 185 million individuals worldwide and is associated with persistence of viral replication and ongoing necroinflammation and fibrosis. To date 20% of patients chronically infected with HCV progress to cirrhosis. Epidemiological studies demonstrate that the incidence of HCV is not well known, because acute infection is generally asymptomatic. The global prevalence is about 2.2% and there is a large degree of geographic variability. Before the 2011, the gold standard of therapy for the treatment of chronic hepatitis C (CHC) was based on the combination of pegylated Interferon (peg-IFN) and Ribavirin (RBV). However, several aspects related to safety profile limited their use in clinical practice. In the recent years, thanks to basic research on HCV structure and replicative cycle, it has been possible to develop direct acting antiviral drugs that have dramatically increased the viral clearance rate. Specifically, the advent of the triple therapy employing direct acting antivirals has dramatically increased the viral clearance rate, from less than 10%, with the initial regimen of IFN monotherapy, to more than 95% with the current therapy. Even though new medications for hepatitis C are effective disease modifiers and have the potential, in a long term perspective, to eradicate the pathology, the cost of new treatments are unlikely to be sustainable for the NHSs. The evidence documenting the effectiveness and tolerability of the new therapies for HCV and several pharmacoeconomic analysis, shows that despite the cost, the new treatments can be considered cost-effective in the long period. However, the health care systems are unable to compensate the height financial resources immediately needed for treating patients with the long terms savings that will be obtained from the eradication of HCV. Indeed, new pharmaceutical policy and a global commitment is required to improve strategies of treatment and price negotiation with pharmaceutical companies to move from a theoretical cost-effectiveness approach to a practical cost-sustainable reality.

Keywords: HCV, Hepatitis, DAAs

1. Introduction

Hepatitis C virus (HCV) is a progressive disease that infects more than 185 million individuals worldwide and is associated with persistence of viral replication and ongoing necroinflammation and fibrosis. To date, 20% of patients chronically infected with HCV progress to cirrhosis.

Epidemiological studies demonstrate that the incidence of HCV is not well known since acute infection is generally asymptomatic. The global prevalence is about 2.2%, and there is a large degree of geographic variability. Before the 2011, the gold standard of therapy for the treatment of chronic hepatitis C (CHC) was based on the combination of pegylated interferon (peg-IFN) and ribavirin (RBV). However, several aspects related to safety profile limited their use in clinical practice. In the recent years, thanks to basic research on HCV structure and replicative cycle, it has been possible to develop direct acting antiviral drugs that have dramatically increased the viral clearance rate. This new therapeutic strategy contemplates the use of interferon-free treatment protocols that are shorter and well tolerated, and this might improve the management of patients. These new medications for hepatitis C are effective disease modifiers and could potentially eradicate the infection in a long-term perspective. However, their costs are even high and unlikely sustainable for the National Health Systems (NHSs), and new pharmaceutical policy and a global commitment are required for achieving the universal access to new treatment strategies.

2. Structure and replicative cycle of HCV

The structure of the HCV virion remains poorly characterized despite several substantial progress in biochemical and morphological studies, and most of the HCV proteins are now actively being pursued as antiviral targets. HCV, discovered in 1989, is a positive-sense, single-stranded RNA virus, approximately 9600 nt in length, which belongs to the Flaviviridae family (*Flavivirus* genus), also including many arthropod-borne human pathogens such as yellow fever virus, West Nile virus, and dengue virus. HCV has been classified by the World Health Organization (WHO) as an oncogenic virus [1]. HCV-RNA encodes a polyprotein that is cleaved by cellular and viral proteases into structural and nonstructural proteins, each with a specific function. The structural proteins include two envelope glycoproteins E1 and E2, which are targets of the host antibody response and are crucial for viral entry and fusion, and a core protein (C), which interacts with the viral genome to form the nucleocapsid. The nonstructural proteins P7, NS2, NS3, NS4A, NS4B, NS5A, and NS5B form a complex with the RNA of the virus to initiate viral replication, which occurs by budding through intracellular membranes. Mature virions are released into the extracellular milieu by exocytosis, and nascent virions incorporate cellular lipoproteins and apolipoproteins (e.g., apoE and apoB) as lipoviral particles [2]. HCV specifically infects hepatocytes, entering the cells by receptor-mediated endocytosis. During primary infection, HCV particles are transported by the blood stream and come in contact with hepatocytes after spanning the fenestrated endothelium of the liver sinusoids. In the Disse space, virions are in direct contact with the basolateral surface of hepatocytes that interact with multiple cell surface molecules, including attachment factors

http://dx.doi.org/10.5772/61187

and receptors. Upon cell surface attachment, the subsequent steps of HCV entry are only partially known, but a putative mechanism has been described in analogy with other Flaviviridae [3]. The virus/receptor complex is internalized, and the nucleocapsid is released into the cytoplasm, decapsidated, and the free viral RNA is used for both polyprotein translation and replication in the cytoplasm. Replication and posttranslational processing seem to take place in a membranous site constituted by viral nonstructural proteins and host cell proteins, the *replication complex*, located in close contact with the perinuclear membranes. Genome encapsidation presumably takes place in the endoplasmic reticulum, and nucleocapsids are enveloped and matured into the Golgi apparatus before the release of new virions in the extracellular space by exocytosis [4]. There are seven main known genotypes (GT) of HCV (from GT-1 to GT-7) that have been classified into 67 subtypes with distinct geographic distributions, modality of transmission, and sensitivity to interferon-based treatments [5]. Estimates of genotype distribution within 98 countries show that the most widespread genotype is the GT-1 (46%), with the subtypes 1a and 1b that are the most common in the United States and in Europe, respectively. Afterward, there are the GT-3 (22%), frequent among drug users; the GT-2 (13%), mainly present in the Mediterranean area; and the GT-4 (13%), mainly present in Egypt and other Arabic countries. GT-7 is extremely rare, and the incidence and prevalence are not yet known [5]. These seven genotypes are responsible for 97% of all infections present worldwide [6]. Although there are no differences in the risk of cirrhosis among all genotypes, GT-3 and GT-1b are associated with increased rate of hepatic steatosis and of hepatocellular carcinoma, respectively [7]. In addition, all these genotypes show different frequencies of polymorphisms associated with resistance to several classes of virus-targeting drugs [8].

3. The role of immune response in HCV infection

HCV has a very high replicative capacity, and a viral titer of $>10^6$ IU/mL can be measured in the serum within days after infection (averages 1–2 weeks) [9]. Innate immune response is the first line of host defense during infection, and interferons (IFNs) are the family of cytokines specialized in coordinating immunity against viruses and for the induction of an antiviral state in cells, by activation and regulation of cellular components of innate immunity, such as natural killer (NK) cells [10]. Furthermore, the induction of the endogenous IFN system in the liver can be ineffective in clearing the infection and in preventing response to therapies with peg-IFN and RBV [11,12]. Types I and II IFNs are in general the major elements of the innate immune response against viruses [10]. Type III IFN family (also known as IFNs-λ) is composed of interleukins (IL)-29, IL-28A, and IL-28B and is induced in response to several viral pathogens. In the liver, type III IFN receptors are expressed at significant levels as a functional full-length form, suggesting intact type III IFN signaling as part of the intrahepatic innate immune response [13,14]. Genetic variants of the IFN-λ3 and IFN-λ4 locus are strongly associated with spontaneous clearance of HCV and with response to therapy with peg-IFN and RBV. The molecular mechanisms that link genetic variants near the IFN-λ4 gene with constitutive activation of the endogenous IFN system in the liver are not entirely known, but it might involve an ongoing stimulation of the JAK–STAT pathway by IFN-λ4 through the IFN-λ receptors on hepatocytes. In contrast to the innate immune response, which is induced within hours to days after infection, the adaptive immune response against HCV is not detectable before 6–8 weeks and involves all components of the adaptive immune system, i.e., humoral antibodies, $CD4^+$ T cells, and $CD8^+$ T cells [10]. All these three components were shown to be associated with viral clearance. A well-coordinated interaction of the different immune cells might be essential for a successful immune response against HCV; however, little is known about the precise dynamic of this cross-talk [15]. HCV-specific T cells are recruited to the liver, and the viral replication is inhibited by both noncytolytic and cytolytic mechanisms. In about 20% of patients, the immune reaction during acute hepatitis C is strong enough to eliminate the infection. Immunocompetent HCV-infected individuals produce antibodies against epitopes within the structural as well as nonstructural proteins. Most of them, however, have no relevant antiviral activity, and only a small fraction of antibodies is able to inhibit virus binding, entry, or uncoating. These "neutralizing antibodies" target linear as well as conformational discontinuous epitopes mainly located within the envelope glycoproteins E1 and E2. While strong data indicate the neutralizing activity of these antibodies *in vitro*, their efficiency *in vivo* is less understood [10,15]. HCV elimination is associated with strong and sustained $CD4^+$ and $CD8^+$ cell responses that target multiple epitopes within the different HCV proteins and that remain detectable long after resolution of infection [10,16,17]. They act noncytolytically, by secreting antiviral cytokines such as IFN-γ, as well as cytolytically, through perforin secretion and by engaging the FAS/FAS-L pathway [15]. Despite the intervention of both innate and adaptive immune response in CHC, the virus is able to escape from these barriers through yet unknown mechanisms.

4. Epidemiology and world impact of HCV

HCV infection is one of the main causes of chronic liver disease worldwide, and according to recent estimates, until now more than 185 million people around the world have been infected. In addition, annually there are three million of new infected people, and among them 350,000 die every year due to HCV-related disorders [18–21]. The prevalence of HCV varies greatly, depending on the geographical area and the population considered: in Western Europe, it ranges from 0.4% to 3%; in Eastern Europe and the Middle East, it is higher but not precisely known [22]. The majority of the infected people reside in Asian countries (Taiwan, Mongolia, and Pakistan), sub-Saharan Africa (Cameroon, Burundi, and Gabon), and the Eastern Mediterranean (Egypt), which holds the highest frequency, with more than 20% [18]. HCV is a major global public health issue due to its high prevalence, long-term unpredictable disease progression, and low diagnosis and treatment response rates. Despite the fact that HCV infection rates are decreasing, the clinical and economic impact of chronic HCV infection is expected to considerably grow in the next decade since a large population of individuals that acquired the virus in the 1960s developed disease-associated health issues through to the 1980s [23]. The dual therapy, based on the administration of peg-IFN and RBV, is successful only in 40–50% of patients infected with the GT-1, while untreated individuals or who failed treatment are at risk of developing severe liver injuries such as cirrhosis, liver transplantation, and hepatocellular carcinoma (HCC) [24]. In Europe, there are 30,000 people on the transplant waiting list but only 12,000 procedures per year, and the average cost of liver transplant in the United States varies between $139,000 and $400,000 [25]. Although HCV can be successfully treated by now using antiviral therapy based on the administration of new direct acting antivirals (DAAs), the economic burden of the disease, including complex regimens and the cost of treatment, remains high since health care costs continue to rise [26]. For this reason, many HCV-diagnosed patients around the world are left untreated or undertreated. A 2010 study performed on U.S. employments found that the cost of sick days and lower productivity per HCV-infected workers was US$8,352 per year [25]. A U.S. survey by the American Gastroenterological Association (AGA) indicated that the cost for 30,000 outpatient visits for HCV infection amounted to US$24 million in the 1998 [27]. The median cost for treating one patient with dual therapy (peg-IFN and RBV) ranges from €7,517 to €21,229, depending on the virus genotype, plus the costs of the new DAAs are about US$70,100 per quality-adjusted life years (QALY) for mild fibrosis and US$36,300 per QALY for advanced fibrosis [28].

5. Natural history of HCV infection

HCV transmission primarily occurs via parenteral routes. Before the 1990s, the main routes of transmission were unsafe blood transfusion procedures and injecting drug use. Currently, new infections are mainly due to the use of drugs and, to a lesser extent, to unsafe medical and surgical procedures, tattoos, and piercings. Distinctive HCV genotype distribution and prevalence worldwide are due primarily to differences in transmission routes and clinical care (Table 1) [29,30].

Patients
People who have received blood transfusions and solid organ transplant before 1992, or coagulation factor before 1987, or in countries where serological testing of blood donations for HCV is not routinely performed
Patients exposed to nosocomial infections such as employees in hemodialysis centers
Recipients of previously unscreened blood, blood products, and organs
Hemophiliacs
People with HIV infection
People exposed to unsterile medical or dental equipment in health care settings where infection control practices are substandard
Workers and other categories
Health care workers with occupational exposure to blood
Infants born from HCV-infected mothers
Injecting drug users and people using intranasal drugs
People receiving tattooing, body piercing, scarification procedures, and/or acupuncture with unsterile material
Prisoners
Sexual and household transmission are possible
10–40% with no identifiable risk factor

Table 1. Populations with high HCV prevalence or who have a history of HCV risk exposure/behavior

Acute HCV infections are often oligo- or asymptomatic. The long incubation period makes difficult to link related cases to the source of infection, and despite the high prevalence of disease, most infected people are unaware of their infection. The long-term impact of HCV infection is highly variable, ranging from minimal histological changes to extensive fibrosis and cirrhosis with or without HCC [31]. Spontaneous clearance in the chronic phase of the infection is rare and occurs only in 15–25% of cases. In 70–80% of infected patients, the virus persists and the infection becomes chronic. In most patients, CHC leads to different degrees of liver fibrosis, and one third (15–25%) of them could develop liver cirrhosis and HCC at a rate of 2–4% after 10 to 40 years (Figure 1) [10,18]. The progression of liver disease occurs over decades and is accelerated by alcohol consumption, diabetes/obesity, coinfections (human immunodeficiency virus [HIV] and hepatitis B virus), old age at the time of infection, cumulative exposure to hepatotropic viruses, and environmental hepatotoxins [32,33]. The extrahepatic manifestations of HCV infection include cryoglobulinemia, membranous glomerulonephritis, and some non-Hodgkin lymphomas [34]. In Europe, about 1/4 of HIV-infected patients have an HCV coinfection. Patients coinfected with HIV/HCV have a higher risk of cirrhosis and AIDS and a higher overall mortality [35]. Thanks to the growing knowledge on the pathophysiology of the disease, the development of diagnostic procedures, and the improvements in therapy and prevention, the clinical care for patients with HCV-related liver disease has considerably advanced during the last years.

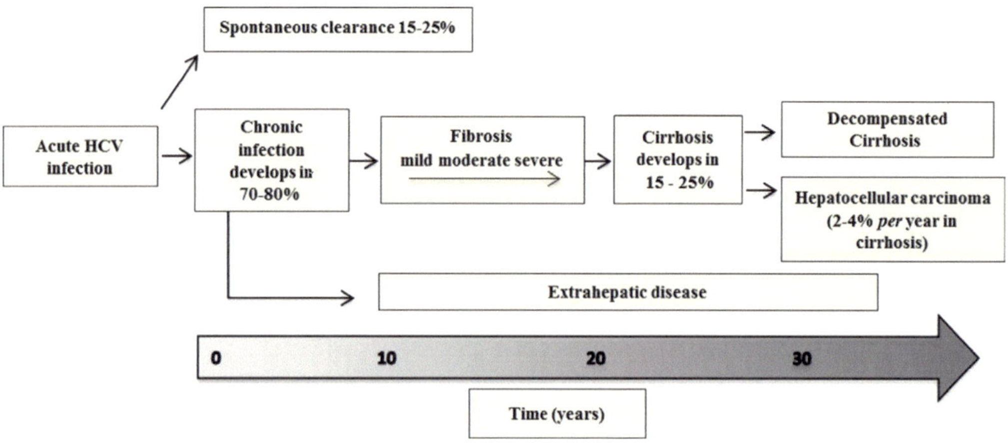

Figure 1. Natural history of HCV infection. In patients with HCV infection, the spontaneous clearance after the acute phase occurs only in 15–25% of cases; during the chronic phase, extrahepatic manifestations might occur. For patients who progress to decompensated cirrhosis, the survival rate at 5 years is about 50%, and among them, 2–4% per year develop hepatocellular carcinoma

6. Screening and diagnosis

Since many infected people are unknown to health care systems due to the asymptomatic nature of the disease, the management of HCV infection should focus not only on therapy but also on the screening of carrier individuals in order to prevent transmission [36]. In the case of a newly acquired infection, the diagnosis of CHC can be made 4–6 months after viral infection [30]. The HCV serologic testing should be offered to individuals who are part of a population with high HCV seroprevalence or who have a history of HCV risk exposure/behavior. It is also important to consider the possibility of infection with other blood-borne viruses in subjects with HCV, and to offer screening for tuberculosis, hepatitis B virus, and HIV, especially in some groups at risk, such as prisoners and people who inject drugs [18,26]. The current diagnostic techniques for HCV infection are based on a range of tests, including the detection of anti-HCV by enzyme immunoassay in the majority of patients. The test for HCV-RNA by real time polymerase chain reaction is considered the best technique to confirm the presence of viremia and represent the gold standard in HCV diagnosis [lower limit of detection <15 international units (IU)/mL] playing a crucial role in patient management and for choosing the best therapeutic regimen [30,31].

Following spontaneous or treatment-induced viral clearance, anti-HCV antibodies persist in the absence of HCV RNA but might decline and finally disappear in some individuals [37,38]. Additional tests include HCV genotype and subtype determination and host genetics. The improved safety and efficacy of the new DAAs across genotypes could allow a simplified approach to pretreatment screening, without requiring further baseline tests [39].

7. Assessment of liver disease severity

Due to the particularly high cost of the new DAAs, in the last 3 years, the access to treatment has been restricted and strictly regulated. For this reason, the decision regarding treatment initiation with DAAs mainly focus on the assessment of liver disease severity. In particular, individuals at more advanced stages and with compensated cirrhosis benefit more than people with less advanced cirrhosis since they are at higher dying risk.

Well-established panels of direct and indirect biomarkers have been studied for the assessment of fibrosis progression and for the diagnosis of cirrhosis. Indirect biomarkers reflect liver function while direct biomarkers reflect extracellular matrix turnover and include many molecules involved in hepatic fibrogenesis. The most commonly used indirect serum biomarkers comprise the following: (i) the AST platelet ratio index [APRI = (AST/upper limit of normal)× 100/platelet count] that was extensively validated in chronic HCV; (ii) Fibrotest, a patented biomarker panel using five biochemical markers and two clinical parameters, which was validated in several etiologies of cirrhosis and in the monitoring of fibrosis progression; and (iii) FIB4, a biomarker panel using age, AST, platelet count, and ALT [FIB4 = (age× AST) / (platelets × √ALT)], originally developed and validated in a cohort of HIV/HCV-coinfected patients [40]. The blood tests needed for calculating APRI and FIB4 scores are inexpensive and are available at the health facilities that provide treatment for HCV infection since they are also used to monitor patients before and after the commencement of treatment [18,26]. Liver biopsy remains the reference method for grading the activity and histological progression (staging) of the disease [30,31,41]. However, because of its invasiveness, patient discomfort, risk of complications, as well as the need for expert histological interpretation, transient ultrasound elastography (Fibroscan) is now used to assess liver disease severity prior to therapy at a safe level of predictability [42,43]. Fibroscan is a noninvasive method of measuring the mean stiffness of hepatic tissue, with hepatic rigidity considered a marker of progressive fibrosis. There are different scoring systems for assessing the severity of chronic liver disease. The major approach to classify CHC involves three separate considerations: (1) the etiology, which is determined on the basis of histological appearance and laboratory tests; (2) the severity and distribution of necroinflammatory activity; and (3) the degree of fibrosis [44]. The most common scoring methods to interpret a liver biopsy include the Metavir, the histologic activity index (HAI), also known as Knodell score, and the modified hepatic activity index (Ishak-modified Knodell score) [45].

Metavir is a scoring system used to assess inflammation and fibrosis by histopathological evaluation of a liver biopsy of patients with HCV. The scoring from A0 to A3 represents a grading system that gives an indication on the activity and degree of inflammation. The amount of inflammation is relevant since it is considered a precursor of fibrosis (Table 2). Metavir also includes a staging system that indicates the amount of fibrosis or scarring [46].

The Knodell score is a semiquantitative and reproducible histological scoring of liver biopsies, also commonly used for staging liver disease, that includes three categories of necroinflammatory activity: periportal injury with or without bridging necrosis, lobular injury, and portal inflammation. Lesions are assigned weighted numeric values that resulted in a combined score, the hepatic activity index (HAI) [47].

In the last years, the Knodell score has been partially replaced by the Ishak score, in which the major changes concern the modification of the HAI and the further division of necroinflammatory assessment in four categories [45].

Activity grade	A0	A1	A2	A3	
Definition	No activity	Mild activity	Moderate activity	Severe activity	
Fibrosis stage	F0	F1	F2	F3	F4
Definition	No fibrosis	Portal fibrosis without septa	Portal fibrosis with few septa	Numerous septa without cirrhosis	Cirrhosis

Table 2. Metavir liver biopsy scoring system

8. Predictors of treatment response to HCV

Several patient and viral-related factors that can affect the severity of the disease, its progression, and treatment outcome have been identified. The chronicity rate in HCV infection appears to be lower in young individuals, and several studies highlight that young age (age <40 years) is associated with more sustained virological response (SVR) [33,48]. The female sex is associated with a higher SVR rate than that of males, using the standard peg-IFN and RBV dual therapy [49]. Obesity is also a relevant predictor of disease progression, and prospective studies report that a body mass index of 25 kg/m^2 was associated with significant progression in the extent of fibrosis [50]. Furthermore, insulin resistance is extremely common in patients with chronic HCV infection and has been associated with increased disease severity, extrahepatic manifestations, and decreased response to antiviral therapy [51]. Many epidemiological studies showed an association between chronic HCV infection and the risk of developing type 1 and type 2 diabetes mellitus [52]. Taking into account the viral factors, HCV genotype is the strongest baseline predictor since there is a close correlation between the different genotypes and sensitivity to IFN-based therapies. GT-1 and GT-4 are intrinsically more resistant to IFN-α than GT-2 and GT-3, and for this reason, the viral clearance in patients who are IFN responders occurs much slower in GT-1 and 4, as compared to 2 and 3 [53]. Although viral load does not correlate with the severity of liver injury or the progression of the disease, a low baseline viral load (<600,000 IU/mL) is related with the SVR and the treatment outcome [54].

Genetic variations have long been sought to explain the differences in host antiviral response, and it is now well established that host genetics plays a role in the response to IFN-based therapy in HCV infection [55]. A number of polymorphisms related to the IFN gene (IL28B) have been involved in the immune response to HCV and appear to be strongly associated with SVR in all groups of patients [56]. There are three IL28B distinct genotypes known as CC, CT, and TT, which are strongly associated with race/ethnicity. People with the CC genotype have a stronger immune response to HCV infection than people with the CT or TT genotypes (called non-CC genotypes), and this polymorphism is strongly associated with a greater likelihood of spontaneous viral clearance [57]. In the context of peg-IFN/RBV therapy, the IL28B genotype could assist clinical decision making for the treatment of HCV infection. The first generation of DAAs, including nonstructural NS3/4A protease inhibitors, has shown promising outcomes when used in combination with peg-IFN/RBV in several clinical trials on GT-1-infected patients, with an SVR higher than the dual therapy [58,59]. The SVR rates in the SPRINT-2 and ADVANCE trials were higher in patients with CC (80% and 90%, in the two trials, respectively) compared with CT (71% and 71%) or TT (59% and 73%) [60–62]. It is not yet clear if IL28B polymorphism could still affect the treatment outcome with the interferon-free regimen since larger cohort sizes will be required to confirm its influence.

9. Current standard of care and future therapies for HCV infection

In the past few years, HCV therapy has quickly changed the natural history of this disease. Before 2011, the gold standard of therapy was based on the combination of peg-IFN and RBV that, however, acts by unspecific and not completely known mechanisms and exhibited low efficacy in some subgroup of population. The improvement of the knowledge on HCV life cycle allowed to identify innovative therapeutic targets and to develop new drugs known as direct acting antivirals (DAAs). These drugs target three of the main proteins involved in viral replication: the NS3/4A protease, the NS5B polymerase, and the NS5A. The addition of DAAs to peg-IFN and RBV and the development of new interferon-free regimen have dramatically increased clinical outcome leading SVR rates from 90 to 100% (Figure 2).

	Therapeutic target	Drugs	Mechanism	Activity
Indirect Drugs		Interferons	Trigger intracellular signaling that enhance the host-specific and non-specific antiviral immune responses	All HCV genotypes
		Ribavirin	Not fully understood; likely has both direct and indirect effects on HCV virus replication	All HCV genotypes
	Non-structural proteins			
Direct-Acting Antiviral Drugs	NS5B (RNA dependent RNA polymerase)	Sofosbuvir (NI) Dasabuvir (NNI)	Inhibit the RNA-dependent RNA polymerase by binding to the catalytic site of HCV polymerase (NIs) or near the active site of the enzyme (NNIs)	All HCV genotypes
	NS5A (Viral Replication or assembly)	Daclatasvir, Ledipasvir, ABT-267, MK8742, GS-5816, ABT-530	Not yet completely known; seem to inhibit viral RNA replication and assembly	All HCV genotypes
	NS4B (Membranous web formation)	n.a.	n.a.	n.a.
	NS4A, NS3 (Serine Protease)	Simperevir, Boceprevir, Telaprevir ABT-450, MK5172 ABT 493	Inhibit the HCV NS3/NS4 serine protease responsible for processing of HCV polyprotein and production of new infectious virions	Genotypes 1a and 1b
	NS2 (Protease)	n.a.	n.a.	n.a.
	P7 (Viral assembly)	n.a.	n.a.	n.a.
	Structural proteins Core E1 E2	n.a.	n.a	n.a

Figure 2. HCV protein products, mechanism of action, and activity of anti-HCV drugs. NIs: nucleoside inhibitors; NNIs: nonnucleoside inhibitors; n.a.: not available.

9.1. Endpoints of treatment

The goal of HCV therapy is to eradicate infection, thus limiting or preventing the development of disease complications. The most important endpoint, accepted by regulatory agencies for assessing the efficacy of the therapy, is the sustained virological response (SVR) (Table 3). SVR is defined as undetectable HCV RNA 12 weeks (SVR12) or 24 weeks (SVR24) after treatment completion. Achieving this result is associated with a reduced risk of disease progression in patients without cirrhosis, while those with cirrhosis remain at risk of life-threatening complications [30,31].

Responses to therapy	Features
Rapid virological response	Undetectable HCV RNA levels at week 4 of therapy, maintained until the end of treatment
Extended rapid virological response	Undetectable HCV RNA levels at weeks 4 and 12
Early virological response	HCV RNA detectable at week 4 but undetectable at week 12, maintained until the end of treatment
Delayed virological response	More than 2 log10 drop but still detectable HCV RNA at week 12, and undetectable at week 24, maintained until the end of treatment
Sustained virological response	Undetectable HCV RNA levels (<50 IU/mL), 24 weeks after completion of treatment
Partial response	More than 2 log10 IU/mL decrease in HCV RNA level from baseline at week 12 of therapy but still detectable at weeks 12 and 24
Null response	Less than 2 log10 IU/mL decrease in HCV RNA level from baseline at week 12 of therapy
Relapse	Undetectable HCV RNA levels at the end of treatment but detectable at any time within 24 weeks of follow-up
Breakthrough	Reappearance of HCV RNA at any time in the course of treatment

Table 3. Definition of responses to therapy according to the European Association for the Study of the Liver (EASL) (extracted from Conteduca et al. [75]).

9.2. Dual therapy: Pegylated-interferon and ribavirin

Until recently, the combination of peg-IFN and RBV was the "historical" standard of care for patients with HCV, and many regimens still contain one or both of these agents [8]. The IFNs are a family of proteins, naturally produced by cells of the immune system with antiviral, antiproliferative, and immunomodulatory activities. After administration, IFNs bind specifically to high-affinity receptors that are present on the surface of most cells, triggering a cascade of intracellular signaling responsible for the antiviral functions and immunomodulatory effects that enhance the host-specific antiviral immune responses [63]. However, in clinical practice, the efficacy of IFN is limited by short half-life and frequent administration (at least three times weekly, even better daily). These limitations have been resolved by developing a modified IFN conjugated with the polymer polyethylene glycol (peg). The introduction of pegylated forms of IFN-α has substantially improved SVR rates and pharmacokinetic profile, allowing once-weekly dosing without changing the safety profile [64]. RBV is an oral guanosine analog with broad antiviral activity against several RNA and DNA viruses. The exact mechanism of action has not yet been totally elucidated, although several hypotheses suggest that its biological action occurs through modest inhibition of viral replication, depletion of cellular guanosine triphosphate, immunomodulatory effects, and possible induction of viral mutagenesis [65]. The duration of combined therapy depends on genotype, viral load, and stage disease, with variable regimens from 24 to 48 weeks. Results from clinical practice showed that 45% of patients with GT-1 and GT-4 infection, 70–80% of those infected with GT-2 or GT-3, and 45–70% of patients with other genotypes achieved the SVR [66–72]. However, there were several limitations in treating patients with peg-IFN and RBV due to drug toxicities, low tolerability, or low efficacy (many patients do not respond or became intolerant) [69,70]. The safety profile is one of the limitations leading to dose reduction or treatment discontinuation. Adverse events caused by peg-IFN are fatigue, flu-like symptoms, depression, anemia, neutropenia, and thrombocytopenia, while those caused by RBV are blood and lymphatic disorder, nausea and vomiting, headache, anorexia, rash, and skin irritation [24,69].

9.3. NS3/4A inhibitors class

Protease inhibitors (PIs) act through reversible and covalent inhibition of the serine protease NS3/4A responsible for processing of HCV polyprotein and production of new infectious virions (Figure 2). These drugs can be structurally divided into two groups: linear tetrapeptide α-ketoamide derivatives and macrocyclic inhibitors. Generally, PIs have a remarkable antiviral activity and a low barrier to resistance and are selective against GT-1 infection. Furthermore, the most NS3/4A inhibitors interact with the cytochrome CYP3A4, one of the main enzymes responsible for drug metabolism, and this results in increased drug–drug interactions that can limit treatment regimen [8,73]. These limitations have been partially overcome by the advent of a new generation of PIs, which are also effective against genotypes other than the GT-1, and possess a higher barrier to viral resistance as well as lower propensity for toxicity and drug–drug interactions [8,74].

9.3.1. Telaprevir and Boceprevir

Telaprevir and boceprevir are the first generation of PIs approved by the Food and Drug Administration (FDA) and the European Medicines Agency (EMA). Telaprevir and boceprevir have been licensed in combination with peg-IFN and RBV, for the treatment of GT-1 infection in naive and experienced patients with compensated liver disease. Telaprevir and boceprevir improved SVR from 49% to 75% in naive patients as compared to the dual therapy [7,75]. Although these therapies have increased clinical outcome, their use is limited by increased rate of adverse effects, including hemolymphopoietic disorders and other reactions related to gastrointestinal system (nausea, diarrhea, vomiting, hemorrhoids, proctalgia, and pruritus). Furthermore, the drugs have a low genetic barrier to resistance [68] and extensive drug–drug interactions that limit their use in transplanted or coinfected patients [76–78].

9.3.2. Simeprevir

Simeprevir is a once-daily, second-wave protease inhibitor, licensed recently by the FDA and the EMA. This agent is indicated in association with peg-IFN and RBV for the treatment of GT-1 and GT-4 infection. This drug can be associated with sofosbuvir regardless of prior patient treatment history [79]. Simeprevir has a broad spectrum of activity against multiple HCV genotypes except for GT-3 [80]. Data from different trials show that it is highly effective and well tolerated. The most common adverse events are nausea, rash, pruritus, dyspnea, increment in bilirubin blood levels, and photosensitivity [8,74,79]. The NS3 Q80K polymorphism is commonly found in GT-1a viruses and is associated with resistance *in vitro* and impaired response to simeprevir. It is therefore recommended that patients infected with GT-1a must be screened for the presence of Q80K to evaluate the use of another agent in case of positive result [81]. The activity of simeprevir has been validated in several phase II/III studies: QUEST I, QUEST II, PROMISE, ASPIRE, and RESTORE.

In the QUEST I and QUEST II studies, 785 naive patients with GT-1 infection were randomized to placebo or simeprevir plus peg-IFN and RBV for 12 weeks. Eighty percent of patients treated with simeprevir achieved SVR12 compared with 50% in the placebo arm [81,82]. The PROMISE study randomized 393 relapsers with GT-1 infection to simeprevir or placebo for 12 weeks with peg-IFN plus RBV or RBV alone for additional 12–36 weeks, on a response-guided therapy basis. In this trial, 79% of simeprevir treated patients achieved an SVR at 12 weeks compared with 37% of patients in the placebo arm [83]. The efficacy of simeprevir in patients with GT-1 infection was evaluated also in the ASPIRE study that confirmed these results [84]. Finally, in the RESTORE trial, the efficacy of simeprevir in GT-4 infection was established [85].

9.3.3. Paritaprevir

Paritaprevir is an NS3/NS4A protease inhibitor that has been licensed by the FDA and the EMA in combination with ritonavir, ombitasvir, and dasabuvir with or without RBV. Paritaprevir is metabolized primarily by cytochrome CYP3A4 and is used in combination with ritonavir, a potent CYP3A4 inhibitor, in order to improve the exposures at acceptable dosing frequency [86,87].

9.4. NS5A inhibitors class

The nonstructural NS5A protein is critical for the virus functions, having a role in viral replication and assembly, and performing complex interactions with cellular functions. Because of this crucial role, NS5A has been identified as a suitable target for viral inhibition (Figure 2). NS5A inhibitors have a high antiviral potency, a pan-genotypic activity, and a genetic barrier to resistance from medium to high. They also possess a good pharmacokinetic and a safety profile that allow once-daily dosing [8,75,88]. Although several NS5A inhibitors are in clinical development or already approved, the exact mechanism is not yet completely known [89]. Recent evidence reported that some of these drugs inhibit formation of the *membranous web* (Figure 2) that is thought to be the site of viral RNA replication [88,90]; other hypotheses suggest that NS5A inhibitors induce rearrangement of NS5A from endoplasmic reticulum-derived foci and limit hyperphosphorylation of this nonstructural protein [91–93].

9.4.1. Daclatasvir

Daclatasvir is the first NS5A inhibitor that is active at picomolar concentrations with broad coverage of HCV genotypes [89]. Daclatasvir has been recently approved in combination with sofosbuvir with or without RBV for the treatment of GT-1, GT-3, and GT-4 chronic hepatitis C in naive and experienced patients. Daclatasvir has a pharmacokinetic profile that allows once-daily dosing, and a low potential of causing drug–drug interactions with other medications

[94]. Daclatasvir was studied in various combinations with NS3 and NS5B inhibitors and with peg-IFN and RBV.

In a phase II study, 395 naive patients with GT-1 and GT-4 infection were randomized to receive two doses of daclatasvir (20 or 60 mg) in combination with peg-IFN and RBV compared with peg-IFN and RBV plus placebo. The SVR24 was achieved by 59.2% of patients receiving 20 mg, 59.6% in those who received 60 mg, and 37.5% in the placebo group. In patients with GT-4 infection, the SVR24 was achieved by 66.7% and 100% of those who received 20 mg or 60 mg daclatasvir, respectively, vs 50.0% in the placebo group [95].

In the COMMAND trial, 151 treatment-naive patients with GT-2 and GT-3 infection were randomly assigned to receive daclatasvir or placebo plus peg-IFN and RBV for 24 weeks. SVR24 was achieved by 83% in GT-2 infection and by 69% in GT-3 infection, vs 63% in control arm [96]. The treatment is well tolerated, and the main adverse events reported are diarrhea, fatigue, headache, and nausea. The most significant resistant associated variants are 31V and Y93H for GT-1b, and 31V, Y93H M28, and Q30 for GT-1a [97].

9.4.2. Ledipasvir

Ledipasvir is a potent NS5A inhibitor against GT-1, GT-4, and GT-5 infection but has lower activity against GT-2 and GT-3 infection [89]. Ledipasvir was recently approved in combination with sofosbuvir with or without RBV for the treatment of GT-1-, GT-3-, and GT-4-infected patients, naive or experienced, and for the advanced liver disease [98]. This combination is one of the most emerging interferon-free therapies that present a better safety profile than standard therapy and an elevated efficacy with SVR rates from 90% to 100%.

9.4.3. Ombitasvir

Ombitasvir is a novel potent NS5A inhibitor with a promising efficacy particularly in difficult-to-treat patients, in association with other DAAs [99]. This drug has been licensed by the FDA and the EMA in combination with paritaprevir/ritonavir and Dasabuvir with or without RBV. The efficacy of this drug was proved in several clinical trials both in association with peg-IFN/RBV and in interferon-free regimens. In a study of treatment-naive GT-1-infected patients, ombitasvir in combination with peg-IFN and RBV showed an early virological response in 25 out of 28 patients receiving the NS5A inhibitor compared with 6 out of 9 patients in the placebo group [89,99,100].

9.5. NS5B inhibitors class

NS5B protein is responsible for replication of HCV RNA and represents one of DAAs therapeutic target (Figure 2). NS5B RNA polymerase inhibitors can be divided into two distinct categories: the nucleoside inhibitors (NIs) and the nonnucleoside inhibitors (NNIs). NIs act by binding to the active site of the enzyme and are integrated into the growing RNA chain, causing chain interruption. Nonnucleoside inhibitors (NNIs) bind outside the active site, leading to the allosteric inhibition of RNA polymerase activity [8,75]. NIs have pan-genotypic activity and a medium–high barrier to resistance; NNIs have a low–medium activity against different

HCV genotypes as well as a low barrier to resistance. These differences are explicated on the basis of different mechanisms of action because NIs act in a highly conserved region of the HCV genome while NNIs bind only one of the four binding sites, and this results in a lower efficacy against the different HCV genotypes [7,75].

9.5.1. Sofosbuvir

Sofosbuvir is the first NI approved by the FDA and the EMA in combination with other antiviral drugs for the treatment of all HCV genotypes in adults [101]. Recently, sofosbuvir was approved as a fixed-dose combination in a single tablet with ledipasvir [98]. Sofosbuvir has a potent activity against all HCV genotypes, a high barrier to resistance, an excellent tolerability, and a very favorable pharmacokinetic profile. The addition of sofosbuvir to peg-IFN and RBV did not increase the frequency or severity of side effects [101,102]. The main adverse events reported in clinical trials are fatigue, headache, and nausea. *In vitro* resistance is linked to the development of an S282T mutation in the NS5B gene, although this should be confirmed in higher numbers of patients [7,8]. The efficacy of sofosbuvir was evaluated in patients infected with GT-1 to GT-6 chronic hepatitis C and was licensed on the basis of the following three studies: NEUTRINO, PROTON, and ATOMIC.

The NEUTRINO was a phase III, single-arm study that investigated the efficacy and safety of sofosbuvir with peg-IFN and RBV in 327 naive patients with GT-1, GT-4, GT-5, or GT-6 infection. SVR rates at 12 weeks were 90% for GT-1 infection, 97% for GT-4/GT-5/GT-6 infections, and 80% in patients with cirrhosis [103]. In the PROTON study, 147 GT-1-infected patients were treated with sofosbuvir or placebo in combination with peg-IFN and RBV for 12 weeks. SVR12 rates were achieved by 91% in sofosbuvir arm and 58% in the placebo group [8,104]. Finally, results from ATOMIC study confirmed the high efficacy of sofosbuvir in these populations [105]. The introduction of this drug in clinical practice has changed the clinical outcome achieving SVR over 90% especially in difficult to treat population as the GT-1-infected one.

9.5.2. Dasabuvir

Dasabuvir is a nonnucleoside inhibitor and will be used as a part of the all-oral interferon-free HCV therapy in combination with ombitasvir and paritaprevir/ritonavir. This combined therapy has been recently approved by the FDA and the EMA. This combination has shown high efficacy in several clinical trials and is one of the most promising interferon-free regimen. Dasabuvir was developed to treat GT-1-infected patients while is inactive toward GT-2, GT-3, and GT-4 infection. Dasabuvir is well tolerated, and the main adverse events recorded, when in combination with other DAAs, were mild such as headache and fatigue [106,107].

9.6. Future therapies for HCV infection: interferon-free regimen

During the last year, the advent of interferon-free regimen has dramatically changed the standard of care of anti-HCV therapy. These therapies include molecules with different mechanisms of action, pan-genotypic activity that improve their safety, and efficacy profile, simplifying treatment duration. Several interferon-free combinations have been recently approved, and other trials are in ongoing with different DAAs. Results from recent clinical studies established that a permanent cure from infection could be achieved with interferon-free combinations [20].

9.6.1. Sofosbuvir plus ribavirin

Sofosbuvir was the first drug licensed by the FDA and the EMA as part of interferon-free regimen. Currently, sofosbuvir is indicated in combination with RBV for the treatment of patients with GT-2 and GT-3 infection, even at advanced stages of the disease, while for all the other genotypes, it is recommended only in patients ineligible or intolerant to peg-IFN. Sofosbuvir-based treatment has been evaluated in several clinical trials [101]: FISSION, POSITRON, VALENCE, and FUSION.

FISSION was a randomized study that evaluated 12 weeks of treatment with sofosbuvir and RBV compared with 24 weeks of treatment with peg-IFN and RBV in 499 treatment-naive patients with GT-2 or GT-3 infection. The SVR rates were 95% and 56% in GT-2- and GT-3-infected patients, respectively, for the treatment with sofosbuvir/RBV, vs 78% and 63% in the peg-IFN/RBV arm [103]. POSITRON study confirmed the clinical results obtained in FISSION study [108].

In the FUSION trial, the combination of sofosbuvir/RBV was evaluated in GT-2- or GT-3-infected patients, nonresponders to prior interferon-based treatment. SVR rates were 86–94% in patients with GT-2 infection and 30–62% in GT-3 infection, for 12 or 24 weeks of treatment, respectively [108]. The results obtained in the FISSION study for patients with GT-2 or GT-3 infection have been confirmed by the VALENCE trial [109].

Based on these studies, the combination of sofosbuvir and RBV showed high efficacy with SVR >90% in patients with GT-2 infection, while lower SVR rates were recorded in patients with GT-3 infection. This last population remains the most challenging group of patients to treat with interferon-free regimen.

9.6.2. Sofosbuvir/ledipasvir ± ribavirin

Recently, the FDA and the EMA approved the fixed combination of sofosbuvir/ledipasvir with or without RBV for 12 or 24 weeks for the treatment of GT-1, GT-3, and GT-4 chronic hepatitis C in naive and experienced patients and in patients who had liver peritransplant [98]. The efficacy of sofosbuvir/ledipasvir was evaluated in three phase III studies: ION-3, ION-2, and ION-1.

The phase III ION-3 study evaluated 8 weeks of treatment with ledipasvir/sofosbuvir with or without RBV and 12 weeks of treatment with ledipasvir/sofosbuvir, in 647 treatment-naive noncirrhotic patients with GT-1 infection. The SVR12 was 94% in ledipasvir/sofosbuvir, 93% ledipasvir/sofosbuvir plus RBV in patients who received 8 weeks, and 95% in patients who received 12 weeks of ledipasvir/sofosbuvir. These results showed no benefits with the addition of RBV in the regimen or with extension of the treatment duration to 12 weeks [110]. A similar rate of SVR was achieved in experienced patients with GT-1 infection in ION-2 and ION-1 studies, with clinical outcome ranging from 94% to 99% for subjects treated with ledipasvir/sofosbuvir ± ribavirin [111,112]. The treatment is well tolerated, and the most common side effects are fatigue and headache [98].

9.6.3. Sofosbuvir plus daclatasvir ± ribavirin

The combination of sofosbuvir plus daclatasvir with or without RBV for 12 or 24 weeks was evaluated in the AI444040 study in 211 patients infected with GT-1, GT-2, or GT-3, including treatment-naive individuals and who had failed prior therapy with boceprevir or telaprevir. SVR12 was achieved in 98% naive and experienced patients with GT-1 infection, 96% of those with GT-2 infection and 89% of those with GT-3 infection. The treatment was well tolerated, and the most common adverse events reported are fatigue, nausea, and headache. This results indicated that sofosbuvir plus daclatasvir is efficacious in GT-1-, GT-2-, or GT-3-infected patients and in nonresponders with GT-1 infection [94,113]. This therapeutic approach is now being tested in a phase III study, in subjects with GT-3 infection [114].

9.6.4. Sofosbuvir plus simeprevir ± ribavirin

The safety and efficacy of combined oral sofosbuvir plus simeprevir was evaluated in the COSMOS study. In this trial, 168 patients (treatment-naive patients and previous nonresponders) were randomized in two cohorts on the base of METAVIR scores (F0–F2 in cohort 1, F3–F4 in cohort 2) to receive 12 or 24 weeks of simeprevir and sofosbuvir with or without RBV. SVR was achieved by 92% in cohort 1 and 94% in cohort 2. This study suggested that the addition of RBV and treatment duration for 24 weeks did not clearly improve SVR rates. This combination therapy was well tolerated, and the most common adverse events were fatigue, headache, and nausea [115].

9.6.5. 3D regimen: paritaprevir/ritonavir, ombitasvir, dasabuvir ± ribavirin

The multitarget therapy, which includes all-oral combination of paritaprevir/ritonavir, ombitasvir, and dasabuvir, is one of the most promising interferon-free therapies. Paritaprevir/ritonavir and ombitasvir are coformulated as fixed combination in a single tablet. The therapeutic regimen "all in one" is completely oral, without interferon, and is the unique that provides three antiviral agents with direct action, each characterized by a different mechanism of action. The 3D regimen ± RBV is indicated for 12 or 24 weeks for the treatment of patients with GT-1 infection, while only paritaprevir/ritonavir and ombitasvir are indicated in GT-4 infection. The 3D regimen is also indicated in combination with RBV for 24 weeks in liver transplant recipients with GT-1 infection, in patients coinfected with HIV-1, and in patients receiving replacement therapy with opioids [116,117]. The safety and the efficacy of this regimen were based on the results of six clinical trials: SAPPHIRE I, SAPPHIRE II, PEARL II, PEARL III, PEARL IV, and TORQUOISE II.

In the phase III SAPPHIRE I study, 631 treatment-naive adults with GT-1 infection were treated for 12 weeks with 3D regimen in combination with RBV. The overall SVR12 was 96% [118].

The SAPPHIRE-II trial was conducted in 394 experienced patients with GT-1 infection without cirrhosis. The SVR rates were 95.3% among patients with a prior relapse, 100% among patients with a prior partial response, and 95.2% among patients with a prior null response [119].

The PEARL-III and PEARL-IV studies assessed the needing to include RBV in the 3D regimen in treatment-naive adults with GT-1 infection. Clinical results showed that SVRs are similar in GT-1a infection (99.5% *vs* 99% with or without RBV, respectively), while patients with GT-1b infection achieved higher SVR12 in RBV group (97.0% vs 90.2%, with or without RBV, respectively) [120]. Similar results were obtained in the PEARL-II, in experienced patients with GT-1b infection [121]. The efficacy of paritaprevir/ritonavir and ombitasvir in treatment-naive or experienced patients with GT-4 infection was proved in the PEARL-I. In this trial, 90.9% of naive patients treated with 3D regimen without RBV and 100% of naive and experienced patients treated with 3D regimen plus RBV achieved SVR12 [122].

In the TURQUOISE-II study, the efficacy and the safety of 12 or 24 weeks with 3D regimen with RBV were assessed in patients with advanced disease and GT-1 infection. Ninety-two percent of patients achieved SVR rates at 12 weeks, vs 96% at 24 weeks. Experienced patients with GT-1a infection had a better response from 24 weeks of treatment [123]. The resistance profile observed in these clinical trials seems to have little impact on the likelihood of achieving SVR, given the low virological failure rates recorded. The 3D regimen has shown high efficacy in patients with GT-1 infection (90–100%) and is well tolerated. The main adverse events reported are moderate, mainly pruritus, fatigue, and headache [117,118]. This interferon-free regimen is now being tested in different clinical trials in association with other DAAs.

New interferon-free combinations are under investigation in phase II/III clinical trials. New compounds seem to have a more potent activity vs different genotypes than the DAAs of second generation. The aim of these new therapies is to treat HCV infection through shorter regimen. Grazoprevir and elbasvir ± sofosbuvir and sofosbuvir and ledipasvir plus GS-9451 are the most promising combination in clinical development. A six-week interferon-free oral treatment regimen for HCV GT-1 infection will be likely available in the near future [124–127].

9.7. Special population

9.7.1. Liver transplanted patients

HCV infection is one of the risk factors of liver transplantation and an important cause of morbidity and mortality in these patients [128]. HCV infection recurrence occurs in 50% of subjects with detectable HCV RNA at the time of liver transplantation [31,129]. Dual therapy based on peg-IFN/RBV was the standard of care and is associated with low SVR rates at 24 weeks (20–25%). Telaprevir and boceprevir improved SVR until 67%, but drug–drug interaction with immunosuppressive agents and serious adverse events can limit their use [8,130,131]. The introduction of DAAs has improved the efficacy of HCV therapy in patients before and after liver transplantation.

The first interferon-free regimen evaluated in pretransplant setting was 48 weeks of sofosbuvir and RBV for all HCV genotypes. The posttransplant follow-up showed that sofosbuvir and RBV prevented recurrence of HCV infection in 70% of patients [132]. Similar SVRs were obtained in patients that had received liver transplant and then relapsed. The safety profile is better than standard therapy on the base of adverse events reported [133,134].

The SOLAR-1 Phase II study analyzed the combination of sofosbuvir and ledipasvir for 12 or 24 weeks, in naive and experienced patients with a relapse of GT-1/GT-4 infection after liver transplantation. The results showed that 96–98% of patients with F0-F3 fibrosis, 96% with Child–Pugh–Turcotte A cirrhosis, 85–83% with Child–Pugh–Turcotte B cirrhosis, and 60–67% with Child–Pugh–Turcotte C achieved the SVR12. The treatment was generally safe and well tolerated [135]. Finally, in the CORAL-I study, the safety and the efficacy of 24 weeks of 3D regimen with RBV were studied in 34 GT-1-infected liver transplant recipients with none or mild fibrosis. The SVR was achieved in 97.1% of patients [136].

9.7.2. HIV-coinfected patients

Due to shared modalities of transmission, the infection with HCV is often widespread among HIV-infected people. In the last decade, the rate of HCV coinfection was increased, and it has been estimated that about 15–30% of HIV-infected patients are also infected with HCV. HIV/HCV-infected patients are more difficult to treat since the coinfection decrease HCV clearance. The standard of care of these patients was the combination of peg-IFN and RBV, but the coadministration of several agents leads to increased drug–drug interaction and adverse events and requires dose adjustment [137,138]. Similarly to that reported for HCV monoinfected patients, the development of DAAs and interferon-free regimens has substantially increased the treatment outcome. The combination of sofosbuvir and RBV was explored in two studies. PHOTON-1 showed that 76%, 88%, and 67% of treatment-naive patients with GT-1, GT-2, or GT-3 infection, respectively, achieved the SVR12. Sofosbuvir has minimal or none interactions with a wide range of antiretroviral drugs, and treatment was well tolerated [139,140]. Similar results have been obtained from PHOTON-2 [141]. The combination of sofosbuvir and ledipasvir was evaluated in the ERADICATE study. In this trial, 100% of untreated and antiretroviral-treated patients achieved the SVR12 [142]. Finally, the results from TURQUOISE-I study showed that 93.5% of patients achieved SVR12 with 3D regimen plus RBV [143].

10. Conclusions and challenges for the future

The advent of DAAs and interferon-free strategies has substantially improved the clinical outcome in HCV therapy. Some interferon-free regimens have recently been licensed, and some other are in clinical development. These new combinations have shown high SVR, ranging from 90% to 100% even with shorter courses (8–12 weeks) of treatment, especially in low responsive population with dual and triple therapies. Current studies focus on the clinical development of a new generation of DAAs, such as the combination of ABT 493 and ABT 530, sofosbuvir, and GS-5816, gazoprevir, and elbasvir, which will be available in the near future as therapeutic strategies with high efficacy and short regimen (4–8 weeks). However, both scientific and economic unresolved issues are still present.

For the scientific perspectives, new and larger clinical studies are required in subjects infected with GT-3, in treatment-experienced patients and at advanced stages of the disease, which remain the most difficult subpopulations to be treated [144,145].

From the economic point of view, even though the new medications for hepatitis C are effective disease modifiers and have the potential, in a long-term perspective, to eradicate the pathology, the costs of new treatments are unlikely to be sustainable for the NHSs. Indeed, new pharmaceutical policy and a global commitment are required to improve strategies of treatment and price negotiation with pharmaceutical companies to move from a theoretical cost-effectiveness approach to a practical cost-sustainable reality. Even if curing hepatitis C saves lives and prevents a lot of downstream health care costs related to the progression of the disease, including liver cancer or requirement of transplant, payers and politicians are in an uproar for a variety of reasons, not least the fact that the drug is priced much higher in the United States than in the rest of the world. For example, in Europe, where the government negotiates the price, the cost of sofosbuvir is on the order of $55,000/patient. The ongoing discussion about the sustainability of the new treatments demonstrates the limit of the current health technology assessment classical approach. Indeed, the new products can be cost-effective in a long-term perspective, considering the avoidance of further hospitalization and medicalization costs related with transplantation. Until it will not be possible to reorganize the complete process of therapy, to be able to capitalize the expected savings, the cost-effectiveness evaluation will remain just a theory, posing concrete challenge to the sustainability of NHS systems. On the other hand, the proposed cost of treatment is still considered too high in relation to the prevalence of the pathology. This situation has opened the discussion on the necessity to find new reimbursement approaches and new level of cooperation between different States. In Europe, for example, bracket list price (min–max) for sofosbuvir has been proposed, to be adjusted for instance by GDP/Pro-capita income (e.g., differential price), prevalence (price/volume), and/or adaptive reimbursement considering genotyping, subclusters, and time to event. None of the possible solutions have been implemented in a coordinated manner, but the access to HCV new treatments stimulated, among health care decision makers, the consciousness of the need of a new global synergistic approach.

Author details

P. Pierimarchi*, G. Nicotera, G. Sferrazza, F. Andreola, A. Serafino and P.D. Siviero

*Address all correspondence to: pasquale.pierimarchi@ift.cnr.it

Institute of Translational Pharmacology, National Research Council of Italy, Rome, Italy

References

[1] Marinho RT, Barreira DP. Hepatitis C, stigma and cure. World J Gastroenterol. 2013 Oct 28;19(40):6703–9. doi: 10.3748/wjg.v19.i40.6703.

[2] Paul D, Madan V, Bartenschlager R. Hepatitis C virus RNA replication and assembly: living on the fat of the land. Cell Host Microbe. 2014 Nov 12;16(5):569–79. doi: 10.1016/j.chom.2014.10.008.

[3] Dubuisson J, Cosset FL. Virology and cell biology of the hepatitis C virus life cycle—an update. J Hepatol. 2014 Nov;61(Suppl 1):S3–13. doi: 10.1016/j.jhep.2014.06.031.

[4] Penin F, Dubuisson J, Rey FA, Moradpour D, Pawlotsky JM. Structural biology of hepatitis C virus. Hepatology. 2004; 39: 5–19.

[5] Smith DB, Bukh J, Kuiken C, Muerhoff AS, Rice CM, Stapleton JT, et al. Expanded classification of hepatitis C virus into 7 genotypes and 67 subtypes: updated criteria and assignment web resource. Hepatology. 2014 Jan;59(1):318–27. doi: 10.1002/hep.26744.

[6] Gower E, Estes C, Blach S, Razavi-Shearer K, Razavi H. Global epidemiology and genotype distribution of the hepatitis C virus infection. J Hepatol. 2014 Nov;61(Suppl 1):S45–57. doi: 10.1016/j.jhep.2014.07.027.

[7] Kohli A, Shaffer A, Sherman A, Kottilil S. Treatment of hepatitis C: a systematic review. JAMA. 2014 Aug 13;312(6):631–40. doi: 10.1001/jama.2014.7085.

[8] Feeney ER, Chung RT. Antiviral treatment of hepatitis C. BMJ. 2014;349:g3308. doi: 10.1136/bmj.g3308

[9] Ozaras R, Tahan, V, Acute hepatitis C: prevention and treatment. Expert Rev Anti Infect Ther. 2009 Apr;7(3):351–61. doi: 10.1586/eri.09.8.

[10] Heim MH, Thimme R, Innate and adaptive immune responses in HCV infections. J Hepatol. 2014 Nov;61(Suppl 1):S14–25. doi: 10.1016/j.jhep.2014.06.035.

[11] Sarasin-Filipowicz M, Oakeley EJ, Duong FH, Christen V, Terracciano L, Filipowicz W, et al. Interferon signaling and treatment outcome in chronic hepatitis C. Proc Natl Acad Sci U S A. 2008 May 13;105(19):7034–9. doi: 10.1073/pnas.0707882105.

[12] Heim MH. Innate immunity and HCV. J Hepatol. 2013 Mar;58(3):564–74. doi: 10.1016/j.jhep.2012.10.005.

[13] Park H, Serti E, Eke O, Muchmore B, Prokunina-Olsson L, Capone S, et al. IL-29 is the dominant type III interferon produced by hepatocytes during acute hepatitis C virus infection. Hepatology. 2012 Dec;56(6):2060–70. doi: 10.1002/hep.25897.

[14] Gao B, Radaeva S, Park O. Liver natural killer and natural killer T cells: immunobiology and emerging roles in liver diseases. J Leukoc Biol. 2009 Sep;86(3):513–28. doi: 10.1189/JLB.0309135.

[15] Neumann-Haefelin C, Thimme R. Adaptive immune responses in hepatitis C virus infection. Curr Top Microbiol Immunol. 2013;369:243–62. doi: 10.1007/978-3-642-27340-7_10.

[16] Thimme R, Oldach D, Chang KM, Steiger C, Ray SC, Chisari FV. Determinants of viral clearance and persistence during acute hepatitis C virus infection. J Exp Med 2001;194:1395–1406.

[17] Takaki A, Wiese M, Maertens G, Depla E, Seifert U, Liebetrau A, et al. Cellular immune responses persist and humoral responses decrease two decades after recovery from a single-source outbreak of hepatitis C. Nat Med 2000; 6:578–582.

[18] WHO: Guidelines for the screening, care and treatment of persons with hepatitis C infection. April 2014. http://www.who.int/mediacentre/news/releases/2014/hepatitis-guidelines/en/ (accessed 17 February 2015).

[19] Negro F. Epidemiology of hepatitis C in Europe. Dig Liver Dis. 2014 Dec 15;46(Suppl 5):S158–64. doi: 10.1016/j.dld.2014.09.023.

[20] Lavanchy D. The global burden of hepatitis C. Liver Int. 2009 Jan;29(Suppl 1):74–81. doi: 10.1111/j.1478-3231.2008.01934.x.

[21] Alter MJ. Epidemiology of hepatitis C virus infection. World J Gastroenterol. 2007 May 7;13(17):2436–41.

[22] Hahné SJ, Veldhuijzen IK, Wiessing L, Lim TA, Salminen M, Laar Mv. Infection with hepatitis B and C virus in Europe: a systematic review of prevalence and cost-effectiveness of screening. BMC Infect Dis. 2013 Apr 18;13:181. doi: 10.1186/1471-2334-13-181.

[23] McHutchison JG, Bacon BR. Chronic hepatitis C: an age wave of disease burden. Am J Manag Care. 2005 Oct;11(Suppl 10):S286–95; quiz S307-11.

[24] McHutchison JG, Lawitz EJ, Shiffman ML, Muir AJ, Galler GW, McCone J, et al. Peginterferon Alfa-2b or Alfa-2a with ribavirin for treatment of hepatitis C infection. N Engl J Med. 2009 Aug 6;361(6):580–93. doi: 10.1056/NEJMoa0808010.

[25] Economist Intelligence Unit. The silent pandemic: tackling hepatitis C with policy innovation. http://www.janssen-emea.com/The-silent-pandemic (accessed 17 February 2015).

[26] World Health Organization. Media Centre: Hepatitis C. Fact sheet no. 164. April 2014.http://www.who.int/mediacentre/factsheets/fs164/en/ (accessed 17 February 2015).

[27] McHutchison JG, Bacon BR, Owens GS. Making it happen: managed care considerations in vanquishing hepatitis C. Am J Manag Care. 2007 Dec;13(Suppl 12):S327–36; quiz S337-40.

[28] Blachier M, Leleu H, Peck-Radosavljevic M, Valla DC, Roudot-Thoraval F. The burden of liver disease in Europe: a review of available epidemiological data. J Hepatol. 2013 Mar;58(3):593–608. doi: 10.1016/j.jhep.2012.12.005.

[29] Preciado MV, Valva P, Escobar-Gutierrez A, Rahal P, Ruiz-Tovar K, Yamasaki L, et al. Hepatitis C virus molecular evolution: transmission, disease progression and antiviral therapy. World J Gastroenterol. 2014 Nov 21;20(43):15992–6013. doi:10.3748/wjg.v20.i43.15992.

[30] Mutimer D, Aghemo A, Diepolder H, Negro F, Robaeys G, Ryder S, et al. EASL Clinical Practice Guidelines: management of hepatitis C virus infection. J Hepatol. 2014 Feb;60(2):392–420. doi: 10.1016/j.jhep.2013.11.003.

[31] European Association for the Study of the Liver. EASL recommendations on treatment of hepatitis C 2014. J Hepatol. 2014 Aug;61(2):373–95. doi: 10.1016/j.jhep.2014.05.001.

[32] Carrion AF, Martin P. Viral hepatitis in the elderly. Am J Gastroenterol. 2012 May;107(5):691–7. doi: 10.1038/ajg.2012.7. Epub 2012 Jan 31.

[33] Chen SL, Morgan TR. The natural history of hepatitis C virus (HCV) infection. Int J Med Sci 2006; 3(2):47–52. doi:10.7150/ijms.3.47

[34] Ko HM, Hernandez-Prera JC, Zhu H, Dikman SH, Sidhu HK, Ward SC, et al. Morphologic features of extrahepatic manifestations of hepatitis C virus infection. Clin Dev Immunol. 2012;2012:740138. doi: 10.1155/2012/740138.

[35] Andreoni M, Giacometti A, Maida I, Meraviglia P, Ripamonti D, Sarmati L. HIV-HCV co-infection: epidemiology, pathogenesis and therapeutic implications. Eur Rev Med Pharmacol Sci. 2012 Oct;16(11):1473–83.

[36] Zaghloul H, El-Shahat M. Recombinase polymerase amplification as a promising tool in hepatitis C virus diagnosis. World J Hepatol. 2014 Dec 27;6(12):916–22. doi: 10.4254/wjh.v6.i12.916.

[37] Chevaliez S, Pawlotsky JM. Diagnosis and management of chronic viral hepatitis: antigens, antibodies and viral genomes. Best Pract Res Clin Gastroenterol 2008;22:1031–1048.

[38] Kamili S, Drobeniuc J, Araujo AC, Hayden TM. Laboratory diagnostics for hepatitis C virus infection. Clin Infect Dis 2012;55:S43–S48

[39] Ford N, Swan T, Beyer P, Hirnschall G, Easterbrook P, Wiktor S. Simplification of antiviral hepatitis C virus therapy to support expanded access in resource-limited settings. J Hepatol. 2014 Nov;61(Suppl 1):S132–8. doi: 10.1016/j.jhep.2014.09.019.

[40] Sharma S, Khalili K, Nguyen GC. Non-invasive diagnosis of advanced fibrosis and cirrhosis. World J Gastroenterol. 2014 Dec 7;20(45):16820–30. doi: 10.3748/wjg.v20.i45.16820.

[41] Papastergiou V, Tsochatzis E, Burroughs AK. Non-invasive assessment of liver fibrosis. Ann Gastroenterol. 2012;25(3):218–231.

[42] Castera L, Sebastiani G, Le Bail B, de Ledinghen V, Couzigou P, Alberti A. Prospective comparison of two algorithms combining non-invasive methods for staging liver fibrosis in chronic hepatitis C. J Hepatol. 2010 Feb;52(2):191–8. doi: 10.1016/j.jhep.2009.11.008.

[43] Wilder J, Patel K. The clinical utility of FibroScan(®) as a noninvasive diagnostic test for liver disease. Med Devices (Auckl). 2014 May 3;7:107–14. doi: 10.2147/MDER.S46943.

[44] Shiha G., Zalata K. Ishak versus METAVIR: terminology, convertibility and correlation with laboratory changes in chronic hepatitis C. InTech; 2011. P155–171.

[45] Theise ND. Liver biopsy assessment in chronic viral hepatitis: a personal, practical approach. Mod Pathol. 2007 Feb;20(Suppl 1):S3–14. doi:10.1038/modpathol.3800693

[46] Mannan R, Misra V, Misra SP, Singh PA, Dwivedi M. A comparative evaluation of scoring systems for assessing necro-inflammatory activity and fibrosis in liver biopsies of patients with chronic viral hepatitis. J Clin Diagn Res. 2014 Aug;8(8):FC08–12. doi: 10.7860/JCDR/2014/8704.4718.

[47] Brunt EM. Grading and staging the histopathological lesions of chronic hepatitis: the Knodell histology activity index and beyond. Hepatology. 2000 Jan;31(1):241–6.

[48] Antonucci G, Angeletti C, Vairo F, Longo MA, Girardi E. Age and prediction of sustained virological response to hepatitis C virus (HCV) infection treatment based on 28-day decrease in HCV RNA levels. J Infect Dis. 2009 Nov 1;200(9):1484–5; author reply 1485. doi: 10.1086/644507.

[49] Yu JW, Sun LJ, Zhao YH, Kang P, Yan BZ. Impact of sex on virologic response rates in genotype 1 chronic hepatitis C patients with peginterferon alpha-2a and ribavirin treatment. Int J Infect Dis. 2011 Nov;15(11):e740–6. doi: 10.1016/j.ijid.2011.05.018.

[50] Navaneethan U, Kemmer N, Neff GW. Predicting the probable outcome of treatment in HCV patients. Therap Adv Gastroenterol. 2009 Sep;2(5):287–302. doi: 10.1177/1756283X09339079.

[51] El-Zayadi AR, Anis M. Hepatitis C virus induced insulin resistance impairs response to anti viral therapy. World J Gastroenterol. 2012 Jan 21;18(3):212–24. doi: 10.3748/wjg.v18.i3.212.

[52] Antonelli A, Ferrari SM, Giuggioli D, Di Domenicantonio A, Ruffilli I, Corrado A, Fabiani S, Marchi S, Ferri C, Ferrannini E, Fallahi P. Hepatitis C virus infection and type 1 and type 2 diabetes mellitus. World J Diabetes. 2014 Oct 15;5(5):586–600. doi: 10.4239/wjd.v5.i5.586.

[53] Strahotin CS, Babich M. Review article: hepatitis C variability, patterns of resistance, and impact on therapy. Adv Virol. 2012;2012:267483. doi: 10.1155/2012/267483.

[54] Zhu Y, Chen S. Antiviral treatment of hepatitis C virus infection and factors affecting efficacy. World J Gastroenterol. 2013 Dec 21;19(47):8963–73. doi: 10.3748/wjg.v19.i47.8963.

[55] Jensen DM, Pol S. IL28B genetic polymorphism testing in the era of direct acting antivirals therapy for chronic hepatitis C: ten years too late? Liver Int. 2012 Feb;32(Suppl 1):74–8. doi: 10.1111/j.1478–3231.2011.02712.x.

[56] Balagopal A, Thomas DL, Thio CL. IL28B and the control of hepatitis C virus infection. Gastroenterology. 2010 Dec;139(6):1865–76. doi: 10.1053/j.gastro.2010.10.004.

[57] Ge D, Fellay J, Thompson AJ, Simon JS, Shianna KV, Urban TJ, et al. Genetic variation in IL28B predicts hepatitis C treatment-induced viral clearance. Nature. 2009 Sep 17;461(7262):399–401. doi: 10.1038/nature08309.

[58] Zeuzem S, Andreone P, Pol S, Lawitz E, Diago M, Roberts S, et al. Telaprevir for retreatment of HCV infection. N Engl J Med. 2011 Jun 23;364(25):2417–28. doi: 10.1056/NEJMoa1013086.

[59] Jacobson IM, McHutchison JG, Dusheiko G, Di Bisceglie AM, Reddy KR, Bzowej NH, et al. Telaprevir for previously untreated chronic hepatitis C virus infection. N Engl J Med. 2011 Jun 23;364(25):2405–16. doi: 10.1056/NEJMoa1012912.

[60] Poordad F, McCone J Jr, Bacon BR, Bruno S, Manns MP, Sulkowski MS, et al. Boceprevir for untreated chronic HCV genotype 1 infection. N Engl J Med. 2011 Mar 31;364(13):1195–206. doi: 10.1056/NEJMoa1010494.

[61] Jacobson IM, Catlett I, Marcellin P, Bzowej H, Muir AJ, Adda N, et al. Telaprevir substantially improved SVR rates across all IL28B genotypes in the ADVANCE trial. J Hepatol. 2011;54(Suppl 1): S542

[62] Poordad F, Bronowicki JP, Gordon SC, Zeuzem S, Jacobson IM, Sulkowski MS, et al. Factors that predict response of patients with hepatitis C virus infection to boceprevir. Gastroenterology. 2012 Sep;143(3):608–18.e1-5. doi: 10.1053/j.gastro.2012.05.011.

[63] Chung R.T, Gale M. Jr, Polyak S.J, Lemon S.M, Liang T.J, Hoofnagle J.H. Mechanisms of action of interferon and ribavirin in chronic hepatitis C: summary of a workshop. Hepatology. 2008 January; 47(1): 306–320. doi:10.1002/hep.22070.

[64] Wedemeyer H, Wiegand J, Cornberg M, Manns MP. Polyethylene glycol–interferon: current status in hepatitis C virus therapy. J Gastroenterol Hepatol. 2002 Dec; 17(Suppl 3):S344–50. doi: 10.1046/j.1440-1746.17.s3.26.x

[65] Feld JJ, Hoofnagle JH. Mechanism of action of interferon and ribavirin in treatment of hepatitis C. Nature. 2005 Aug 18;436(7053):967–72.

[66] Di Bisceglie AM, Hoofnagle JH. Optimal therapy of hepatitis C. Hepatology. 2002 Nov;36(5 Suppl 1):S121–7. doi: 10.1053/jhep.2002.36228

[67] Ghany MG, Strader DB, Thomas DL, Seeff LB. Diagnosis, management, and treatment of hepatitis C: an update. Hepatology. 2009 Apr;49(4):1335–74. doi: 10.1002/hep.22759.

[68] Liang TJ, Ghany MG. Current and future therapies for hepatitis C virus infection. N Engl J Med. 2013 May 16;368(20):1907–17. doi: 10.1056/NEJMra1213651.

[69] Manns MP, McHutchison JG, Gordon SC, Rustgi VK, Shiffman M, Reindollar R, et al. Peginterferon alfa-2b plus ribavirin compared with interferon alfa-2b plus ribavirin for initial treatment of chronic hepatitis C: a randomized trial. Lancet. 2001 Sep 22;358(9286):958–65. doi:10.1016/S0140-6736(01)06102-5

[70] Fried MW, Shiffman ML, Reddy KR, Smith C, Marinos G, Gonçales FL Jr, et al. Peginterferon alfa-2a plus ribavirin for chronic hepatitis C virus infection. N Engl J Med. 2002 Sep 26;347(13):975–82. doi: 10.1056/NEJMoa020047

[71] Mangia A, Santoro R, Minerva N, Ricci GL, Carretta V, Persico M, et al. Peginterferon alfa-2b and ribavirin for 12 vs 24 weeks in HCV genotype 2 or 3. N Engl J Med. 2005 Jun 23;352(25):2609–17.

[72] McHutchison JG, Lawitz EJ, Shiffman ML, Muir AJ, Galler GW, McCone J, et al. Peginterferon alfa-2b or alfa-2a with ribavirin for treatment of hepatitis C infection. N Engl J Med. 2009 Aug 6;361(6):580–93. doi: 10.1056/NEJMoa0808010.

[73] Lange CM, Zeuzem S. Perspectives and challenges of interferon-free therapy for chronic hepatitis C. J Hepatol. 2013 Mar;58(3):583–92. doi: 10.1016/j.jhep.2012.10.019.

[74] Clark VC, Peter JA, Nelson DR. New therapeutic strategies in HCV: second-generation protease inhibitors. Liver Int. 2013 Feb;33(Suppl 1):80–4. doi: 10.1111/liv.12061

[75] Conteduca V, Sansonno D, Russi S, Pavone F, Dammacco F. Therapy of chronic hepatitis C virus infection in the era of direct-acting and host targeting antiviral agents. J Infect. 2014 Jan;68(1):1–20. doi: 10.1016/j.jinf.2013.08.019.

[76] Garg V, van Heeswijk R, Lee JE, Alves K, Nadkarni P, Luo X. Effect of telaprevir on the pharmacokinetics of cyclosporine and tacrolimus. Hepatology. 2011 Jul;54(1):20–7. doi: 10.1002/hep.24443.

[77] Thomas DL, Bartlett JG, Peters MG, Sherman KE, Sulkowski MS, Pham PA. Provisional guidance on the use of hepatitis C virus protease inhibitors for treatment of hepatitis C in HIV-infected persons. Clin Infect Dis. 2012 Apr;54(7):979–83. doi: 10.1093/cid/cir882.

[78] Kiser JJ, Burton JR, Anderson PL, Everson GT. Review and management of drug interactions with boceprevir and telaprevir. Hepatology. 2012 May;55(5):1620–8. doi: 10.1002/hep.25653.

[79] European Medicines Agency. Olysio: EPAR—Product Informationhttp. http://www.ema.europa.eu/ema/index.jsp?curl=pages/medicines/human/medicines/002777/human_med_001766.jsp&mid=WC0b01ac058001d124 (accessed 17 February 2015).

[80] Moreno C, Berg T, Tanwandee T, Thongsawat S, Van Vlierberghe H, Zeuzem S, et al. Antiviral activity of TMC435 monotherapy in patients infected with HCV genotypes 2–6: TMC435-C202, a phase IIa, open-label study. J Hepatol. 2012 Jun;56(6):1247–53. doi: 10.1016/j.jhep.2011.12.033.

[81] Jacobson IM, Dore GJ, Foster GR, Fried MW, Radu M, Rafalsky VV, et al. Simeprevir (TMC435) with pegylated interferon alfa 2a plus ribavirin in treatment-naive patients with chronic hepatitis C virus genotype 1 infection (QUEST-1): a phase 3, randomised, doubleblind, placebo-controlled trial. Lancet. 2014 Aug 2;384(9941):403–13. doi: 10.1016/S0140-6736(14)60494-3.

[82] Manns M, Marcellin P, Poordad F, de Araujo ES, Buti M, Horsmans Y, et al. Simeprevir with pegylated interferon alfa 2a or 2b plus ribavirin in treatment-naive patients with chronic hepatitis C virus genotype 1 infection (QUEST-2): a randomised, double-blind, placebo-controlled, phase 3 trial. Lancet. 2014 Aug 2;384(9941):414–26. doi: 10.1016/S0140-6736(14)60538-9.

[83] Forns X, Lawitz E, Zeuzem S, Gane E, Bronowicki JP, Andreone P, et al. Simeprevir with peginterferon and ribavirin leads to high rates of SVR in patients with HCV genotype 1 who relapsed after previous therapy: a phase 3 trial. Gastroenterology. 2014 Jun;146(7):1669–79.e3. doi: 10.1053/j.gastro.2014.02.051.

[84] Zeuzem S, Berg T, Gane E, Ferenci P, Foster GR, Fried MW, et al. Simeprevir increases rate of sustained virologic response among treatment-experienced patients with HCV genotype-1 infection: a phase IIb trial. Gastroenterology. 2014 Feb;146(2):430–41.e6. doi: 10.1053/j.gastro.2013.10.058

[85] Moreno C, Hezode C, Marcellin P, Bourgeois S, Francque S, Samuel D, et al. Efficacy and safety of simeprevir with PegIFN/ribavirin in naive or experienced patients infected with chronic HCV genotype 4. J Hepatol. 2015 Jan 14. pii: S0168–8278(15)00002-1. doi: 10.1016/j.jhep.2014.12.031.

[86] Gentile I, Borgia F, Buonomo AR, Zappulo E, Castaldo G, Borgia G. ABT-450: a novel protease inhibitor for the treatment of hepatitis C virus infection. Curr Med Chem. 2014;21(28):3261–70. doi:10.2174/0929867321666140706125950.

[87] Poordad F, Hezode C, Trinh R, Kowdley KV, Zeuzem S, Agarwal K, et al. ABT-450/r–ombitasvir and dasabuvir with ribavirin for hepatitis C with cirrhosis. N Engl J Med. 2014 May 22;370(21):1973–82. doi: 10.1056/NEJMoa1402869

[88] Eyre NS, Beard MR. HCV NS5A inhibitors disrupt replication factory formation: a novel mechanism of antiviral action. Gastroenterology. 2014 Nov;147(5):959–62. doi: 10.1053/j.gastro.2014.09.024.

[89] Pawlotsky JM. NS5A inhibitors in the treatment of hepatitis C. J Hepatol. 2013 Aug; 59(2):375–82. doi: 10.1016/j.jhep.2013.03.030.

[90] Berger C, Romero-Brey I, Radujkovic D, Terreux R, Zayas M, Paul D, et al. Daclatasvir-like inhibitors of NS5A block early biogenesis of hepatitis C virus-induced membranous replication factories, independent of RNA replication. Gastroenterology. 2014 Nov;147(5):1094–105.e25. doi: 10.1053/j.gastro.2014.07.019

[91] Targett-Adams P, Graham EJ, Middleton J, Palmer A, Shaw SM, Lavender H, et al. Small molecules targeting hepatitis C virus-encoded NS5A cause subcellular redistribution of their target: insights into compound modes of action. J Virol. 2011 Jul; 85(13):6353–68. doi: 10.1128/JVI.00215-11.

[92] Qiu D1, Lemm JA, O'Boyle DR 2nd, Sun JH, Nower PT, Nguyen V, et al. The effects of NS5A inhibitors on NS5A phosphorylation, polyprotein processing and localization. J Gen Virol. 2011 Nov;92(Pt 11):2502–11. doi: 10.1099/vir.0.034801-0

[93] Fridell RA, Qiu D, Valera L, Wang C, Rose RE, Gao M., et al. Distinct functions of NS5A in hepatitis C virus RNA replication uncovered by studies with the NS5A inhibitor BMS-790052. J Virol. 2011 Jul;85(14):7312–20. doi: 10.1128/JVI.00253-11.

[94] European Medicines Agency. Daklinza: EPAR—Product Information. http://www.ema.europa.eu/ema/index.jsp?curl=pages/medicines/human/medicines/003768/human_med_001792.jsp&mid=WC0b01ac058001d124 (accessed 17 February 2015)

[95] Hézode C, Hirschfield GM, Ghesquiere W, Sievert W, Rodriguez-Torres M, Shafran SD, et al. Daclatasvir plus peginterferon alfa and ribavirin for treatment-naive chronic hepatitis C genotype 1 or 4 infection: a randomised study. Gut. 2014 Jul 30. pii: gutjnl-2014-307498. doi: 10.1136/gutjnl-2014-307498.

[96] Dore GJ, Lawitz E, Hézode C, Shafran SD, Ramji A, Tatum HA, et al. Daclatasvir plus peginterferon and ribavirin is noninferior to peginterferon and ribavirin alone, and reduces the duration of treatment for HCV genotype 2 or 3 infection. Gastroenterology. 2015 Feb;148(2):355–366.e1. doi: 10.1053/j.gastro.2014.10.007.

[97] Gao M, Nettles RE, Belema M, Snyder LB, Nguyen VN, Fridell RA, et al. Chemical genetics strategy identifies an HCV NS5A inhibitor with a potent clinical effect. Nature. 2010 May 6;465(7294):96–100. doi: 10.1038/nature08960.

[98] European Medicines Agency. Harvoni: EPAR—Product Information. http://www.ema.europa.eu/ema/index.jsp?curl=pages/medicines/human/medicines/003850/human_med_001813.jsp&mid=WC0b01ac058001d124 (accessed 17 February 2015)

[99] Krishnan P, Beyer J, Mistry N, Koev G, Reisch T, DeGoey D. In vitro and in vivo antiviral activity and resistance profile of ombitasvir, an inhibitor of hepatitis C virus

NS5A. Antimicrob Agents Chemother. 2015 Feb;59(2):979–87. doi: 10.1128/AAC.04226-14

[100] Kowdley KV, Lawitz E, Poordad F, Cohen DE, Nelson DR, Zeuzem S, et al. Phase 2b trial of interferon-free therapy for hepatitis C virus genotype 1. N Engl J Med. 2014 Jan 16;370(3):222–32. doi: 10.1056/NEJMoa1306227.

[101] European Medicines Agency. Sovaldi: EPAR - Product Information http://www.ema.europa.eu/ema/index.jsp?curl=pages/medicines/human/medicines/002798/human_med_001723.jsp&mid=WC0b01ac058001d124 (accessed 17 February 2015)

[102] Cholongitas E, Papatheodoridis GV. Sofosbuvir: a novel oral agent for chronic hepatitis C. Ann Gastroenterol. 2014;27(4):331–337.

[103] Lawitz E, Mangia A, Wyles D, Rodriguez-Torres M, Hassanein Tarek, Gordon SC, et al. Sofosbuvir for previously untreated chronic hepatitis C infection. N Engl J Med 2013; 368:1878–1887

[104] Lawitz E, Lalezari JP, Hassanein T, Kowdley KV, Poordad FF, Sheikh AM, et al. Sofosbuvir in combination with peginterferon alfa-2a and ribavirin for non-cirrhotic, treatment-naive patients with genotypes 1, 2, and 3 hepatitis C infection: a randomised, double-blind, phase 2 trial. Lancet Infect Dis 2013;13:401–8.

[105] Kowdley KV, Lawitz E, Crespo I, Hassanein T, Davis MN, DeMicco M, et al. Sofosbuvir with pegylated interferon alfa-2a and ribavirin for treatment-naive patients with hepatitis C genotype-1 infection (ATOMIC): an open-label, randomised, multicentre phase 2 trial. Lancet. 2013 Jun 15;381(9883):2100–7. doi: 10.1016/S0140-6736(13)60247-0

[106] Kati W, Koev G, Irvin M, Beyer J, Liu Y, Krishnan P, et al. In vitro activity and resistance profile of dasabuvir, a non-nucleoside HCV polymerase inhibitor. Antimicrob Agents Chemother. 2015 Mar;59(3):1505–11. doi: 10.1128/AAC.04619-14.

[107] Trivella JP, Gutierrez J, Martin P. Dasabuvir: a new direct antiviral agent for the treatment of hepatitis C. Expert Opin Pharmacother. 2015 Mar;16(4):617–24. doi: 10.1517/14656566.2015.1012493.

[108] Jacobson IM, Gordon SC, Kowdley KV, Yoshida EM, Rodriguez-Torres M, Sulkowski MS, et al. Sofosbuvir for hepatitis C genotype 2 or 3 in patients without treatment options. N Engl J Med. 2013 May 16;368(20):1867–77. doi: 10.1056/NEJMoa1214854

[109] Zeuzem S, Dusheiko GM, Salupere R, Mangia A, Flisiak R, Hyland RH, et al. Sofosbuvir and ribavirin in HCV genotypes 2 and 3. N Engl J Med. 2014 May 22;370(21):1993–2001. doi: 10.1056/NEJMoa1316145

[110] Kowdley KV, Gordon SC, Reddy KR, Rossaro L, Bernstein DE, Lawitz E, et al. Ledipasvir and sofosbuvir for 8 or 12 weeks for chronic HCV without cirrhosis. N Engl J Med. 2014 May 15;370(20):1879–88. doi: 10.1056/NEJMoa1402355.

[111] Afdhal N, Reddy KR, Nelson DR, Lawitz E, Gordon SC, Schiff E, et al. Ledipasvir and sofosbuvir for previously treated HCV genotype 1 infection. N Engl J Med. 2014 Apr 17;370(16):1483–93. doi: 10.1056/NEJMoa1316366.

[112] Afdhal N, Zeuzem S, Kwo P, Chojkier M, Gitlin N, Puoti M, et al. Ledipasvir and sofosbuvir for untreated HCV genotype 1 infection. N Engl J Med. 2014 May 15;370(20): 1889–98. doi: 10.1056/NEJMoa1402454

[113] Sulkowski MS, Gardiner DF, Rodriguez-Torres M, Reddy KR, Hassanein T, Jacobson I, et al. Daclatasvir plus sofosbuvir for previously treated or untreated chronic HCV infection. N Engl J Med. 2014 Jan 16;370(3):211–21. doi: 10.1056/NEJMoa1306218.

[114] Nelson DR, Cooper JN, Lalezari JP, Lawitz E, Pockros PJ, Gitlin N, et al. All-oral 12-week treatment with daclatasvir plus sofosbuvir in patients with hepatitis C virus genotype 3 infection: ALLY-3 phase 3 study. Hepatology. 2015 Jan 23. doi: 10.1002/hep.27726.

[115] Lawitz E, Sulkowski MS, Ghalib R, Rodriguez-Torres M, Younossi ZM, Corregidor A, et al. Simeprevir plus sofosbuvir, with or without ribavirin, to treat chronic infection with hepatitis C virus genotype 1 in non-responders to pegylated interferon and ribavirin and treatment-naive patients: the COSMOS randomised study. Lancet. 2014 Nov 15;384(9956):1756–65. doi: 10.1016/S0140-6736(14)61036-9.

[116] Electronic Medicines Compendium. Summary of Product Characteristics: Viekirax tablets. http://www.medicines.org.uk/emc/medicine/29784 (accessed 18 February 2015)

[117] Electronic Medicines Compendium. Summary of Product Characteristics: Exviera tablets http://www.medicines.org.uk/emc/medicine/29785 (accessed 18 February 2015)

[118] Feld JJ, Kowdley KV, Coakley E, Sigal S, Nelson DR, Crawford D, et al. Treatment of HCV with ABT-450/r-ombitasvir and dasabuvir with ribavirin. N Engl J Med. 2014 Apr 24;370(17):1594–603. doi: 10.1056/NEJMoa1315722.

[119] Zeuzem S, Jacobson IM, Baykal T, Marinho RT, Poordad F, Bourlière M, et al. Retreatment of HCV with ABT-450/r-ombitasvir and dasabuvir with ribavirin. N Engl J Med. 2014 Apr 24;370(17):1604–14. doi: 10.1056/NEJMoa1401561.

[120] Ferenci P, Bernstein D, Lalezari J, Cohen D, Luo Y, Cooper C, et al. ABT- 450/r-ombitasvir and dasabuvir with or without ribavirin for HCV. N Engl J Med. 2014 May 22;370(21):1983–92. doi: 10.1056/NEJMoa1402338

[121] Andreone P, Colombo MG, Enejosa JV, Koksal I, Ferenci P, Maieron A, et al. ABT-450, ritonavir, ombitasvir, and dasabuvir achieves 97% and 100% sustained virologic response with or without ribavirin in treatment-experienced patients with HCV genotype 1b infection. Gastroenterology. 2014 Aug;147(2):359–365.e1. doi: 10.1053/j.gastro.2014.04.045.

[122] Pol S, Reddy KR, Hezode C, Hassanein T, Marcellin P, Berenguer M, et al. Interferon-free regimens of ombitasvir and ABT-450/r with or without ribavirin in patients with HCV genotype 4 Infection: PEARL-I study results. Nov 7–11 2014 Boston, MA, 65th Annual Meeting of the American Association for the Study of Liver Diseases.

[123] Poordad F, Hezode C, Trinh R, Kowdley KV, Zeuzem S, Agarwal K, et al. ABT-450/r-ombitasvir and dasabuvir with ribavirin for hepatitis C with cirrhosis. N Engl J Med. 2014 May 22;370(21):1973–82. doi: 10.1056/NEJMoa1402869

[124] Lawitz E, Gane E, Pearlman B, Tam E, Ghesquiere W, Guyader D, et al. Efficacy and safety of 12 weeks versus 18 weeks of treatment with grazoprevir (MK-5172) and elbasvir (MK-8742) with or without rivavirin for hepatitis C virus genotype 1 infection in previously untreated patients with cirrhosis and patients with previous null response with or without cirrhosis (C-WORTHY): a randomised, open-label phase 2 trial. Lancet. 2014 Nov 11. pii: S0140–6736(14)61795–5. doi: 10.1016/S0140-6736(14)61795-5.

[125] Sulkowski M, Hezode C, Gerstoft J, Vierling JM, Mallolas J, Pol S, et al. Efficacy and safety of 8 weeks versus 12 weeks of treatment with grazoprevir (MK-5172) and elbasvir (MK-8742) with or without ribavirin in patients with hepatitis C virus genotype 1 mono-infection and HIV/hepatitis C virus co-infection (C-WORTHY): a randomised, open-label phase 2 trial. Lancet. 2014 Nov 11. pii: S0140–6736(14)61793–1. doi: 10.1016/S0140-6736(14)61793-1.

[126] Lawitz E, Poordad F, Gutierrez JA, Evans B, Hwang P, Howe A, et al. C-SWIFT: grazoprevir (MK-5172) + elbasvir (MK-8742) + sofosbuvir in treatment-naive patients with hepatitis C virus genotype 1 infection, with and without cirrhosis, for durations of 4, 6, or 8 weeks (interim results). Nov 7–11 2014 Boston, MA, 65th Annual Meeting of the American Association for the Study of Liver Diseases

[127] Kohli A, Sims Z, Marti M, Nelson A, Osinusi A, Bon D, et al. Combination oral, hepatitis C antiviral therapy for 6 or 12 weeks: final results of the SYNERGY trial. March 3–6, 2014. Boston, MA. 21st Conference on Retroviruses and Opportunistic Infections

[128] Carvalho-Filho RJ, Feldner AC, Silva AE, Ferraz ML. Management of hepatitis C in patients with chronic kidney disease. World J Gastroenterol. 2015 Jan 14;21(2):408–22. doi: 10.3748/wjg.v21.i2.408.

[129] Joshi D, Pinzani M, Carey I, Agarwal K. Recurrent HCV after liver transplantation-mechanisms, assessment and therapy. Nat Rev Gastroenterol Hepatol. 2014 Dec; 11(12):710–21. doi: 10.1038/nrgastro.2014.114.

[130] Wang CS, Ko HH, Yoshida EM, Marra CA, Richardson K. Interferon-based combination anti-viral therapy for hepatitis C virus after liver transplantation: a review and quantitative analysis. Am J Transplant. 2006 Jul;6(7):1586–99. doi: 10.1111/j.1600-6143.2006.01362.x

[131] Pungpapong S, Aqel BA, Koning L, Murphy JL, Henry TM, Ryland KL, et al. Multicenter experience using telaprevir or boceprevir with peginterferon and ribavirin to

treat hepatitis C genotype 1 after liver transplantation. Liver Transpl. 2013 Jul;19(7): 690–700. doi: 10.1002/lt.23669.

[132] Curry MP, Forns X, Chung RT, Terrault NA, Brown R Jr, Fenkel JM, et al. Sofosbuvir and ribavirin prevent recurrence of HCV infection after liver transplantation: an open-label study. Gastroenterology. 2015 Jan;148(1):100–107.e1. doi: 10.1053/j.gastro. 2014.09.023.

[133] Charlton M, Gane E, Manns MP, Brown RS Jr, Curry MP, Kwo PY, et al. Sofosbuvir and ribavirin for treatment of compensated recurrent hepatitis C virus infection after liver transplantation. gastroenterology. 2015 Jan;148(1):108–17. doi: 10.1053/j.gastro. 2014.10.001

[134] Mathias A, Cornpropst M, Clemons D, Denning J, Symonds WT. No clinically significant pharmacokinetic drug–drug interactions between sofosbuvir (GS-7977) and the immunosuppressants, cyclosporine A or tacrolimus in healthy volunteers. Nov 2012 Boston Annual Meeting of the American Association for the Study of Liver Diseases

[135] Rajender Reddy K, Everson GT, Flamm SL, Denning JM, Arterburn S, Brandt-Sarif T, et al. Ledipasvir/sofosbuvir with ribavirin for the treatment of HCV in patients with post-transplantrecurrence: preliminary results of a prospective, multicenter study. Nov 7–11 2014 Boston, MA, 65th Annual Meeting of the American Association for the Study of Liver Diseases

[136] Kwo PY, Mantry PS, Coakley E, Te HS, Vargas HE, Brown R Jr, et al. An interferon-free antiviral regimen for HCV after liver transplantation. N Engl J Med. 2014 Dec 18;371(25):2375–82. doi: 10.1056/NEJMoa1408921.

[137] Sulkowski MS. Management of acute and chronic HCV infection in persons with HIV coinfection. J Hepatol. 2014 Nov;61(Suppl 1):S108–19. doi: 10.1016/j.jhep. 2014.08.006.

[138] Naggie S, Sulkowski MS. Management of patients coinfected with HCV and HIV: a close look at the role for direct-acting antivirals. Gastroenterology. 2012 May;142(6): 1324–1334.e3. doi: 10.1053/j.gastro.2012.02.012

[139] Sulkowski MS, Naggie S, Lalezari J, Fessel WJ, Mounzer K, Shuhart M, et al. Sofosbuvir and ribavirin for hepatitis C in patients with HIV-1 coinfection. JAMA. 2014 Jul 23–30;312(4):353–61. doi: 10.1001/jama.2014.7734.

[140] Kirby B, Mathias A, Rossi S, Moyer C, Shen G, Kearney BP. No clinically significant pharmacokinetic drug interactions between sofosbuvir (GS-7977) and HIV antiretrovirals atripla, rilpivirine, darunavir/ritonavir, or raltegravir in healthy volunteers. Nov 9–12 2012 Boston, MA, 63rd Annual Meeting of the American Association for the Study of Liver Diseases

[141] Molina JM, Orkin C, Iser DM, Zamora FX, Nelson M, Stephan C, et al. Sofosbuvir plus ribavirin for treatment of hepatitis C virus in patients co-infected with HIV

(PHOTON-2): a multicentre, open-label, non-randomised, phase 3 study. Lancet. 2015 Feb 3. pii: S0140–6736(14)62483–1. doi: 10.1016/S0140-6736(14)62483-1.

[142] Osinusi A, Townsend K, Nelson N, Kohli A, Meissner E, Gross C, et al. Use of sofosbuvir/ledipasvir fixed dose combination for treatment of hcv genotype-1 infection in patients coinfected with HIV (interim results). April 9–13 London, United Kingdom EASL—The International Liver Congress 2014 49th Annual Meeting of the European Association for the Study of the Liver.

[143] Eron JJ, Wyles D, Sulkowski MS, Trinh R, Lalezari J, Slimet J, et al. Turquoise-I: safety and efficacy of abt-450/r/ombitasvir, dasabuvir, and ribavirinin patients co-infected with hepatitis C and HIV-1. September 5–9, 2014 Washington, DC ICAAC 2014 54th Interscience Conference on Antimicrobial Agents and Chemotherapy

[144] Petta S, Craxì A. Current and future HCV therapy: do we still need other anti-HCV drugs? Liver Int. 2015 Jan;35(Suppl 1):4–10. doi: 10.1111/liv.12714.

[145] Pawlotsky JM. Reviews in basic and clinical gastroenterology and hepatology. Gastroenterology. 2014 May;146(5):1176–92. doi: 10.1053/j.gastro.2014.03.003

Chapter 3

Advances in HCV Therapy

Eric Hilgenfeldt and Roberto J. Firpi

Additional information is available at the end of the chapter

http://dx.doi.org/10.5772/60986

Abstract

Hepatitis C is a devastating illness which has the potential in the majority of cases to lead to significant morbidity and mortality. Worldwide, the number living with chronic hepatitis C approaches 185 million. Up until recently, the regimen of peg-IFN and ribavirin stood as the standard of care and is still commonly used as first line therapy. This is rapidly changing. Direct acting antivirals have altered the landscape drastically. By understanding the genome of the hepatitis C virus, scientists and researchers have been able to exploit its mechanism of transmission by creating inhibitors against several of the nonstructural proteins that are integral to HCV replication and function [NS3/4 protease, NS5A polymerase, and NS5B polymerases (nucleoside and non-nucleoside)]. The previously reported 50%-70% SVR rates achieved with peg-IFN and RBV are no longer the standard of care. Thanks to direct acting antivirals, IFN free as well as "all oral" regimens are being used to treat HCV. In addition to this, ribavirin-free regimens are also available. These highly effective therapies also provide far less side effects and accomplish better results in less time, thus shortening treatment duration significantly. Additionally, even in the notoriously difficult -to-treat populations, results have been promising.

Keywords: Hepatitis C Virus, Direct Acting Antiviral, Treatment, Sustained Virologic Response

1. Introduction

Hepatitis C virus (HCV) infection is a devastating illness, which has the potential in the majority of cases to lead to significant morbidity and mortality. Worldwide, the number living with chronic HCV approaches 185 million. Until recently, the regimen of pegylated interferon (peg-IFN) and ribavirin (RBV) stood as the standard of care and is still commonly used as first-line therapy in some countries. This is rapidly changing. Direct acting antivirals (DAA) have altered the landscape dramatically. By understanding the genome of the HCV, scientists and researchers have been able to exploit its mechanism of transmission by creating inhibitors against several of the nonstructural proteins that are integral to HCV replication and function. Sustained virological response (SVR), which is commonly defined as a lack of HCV viral detection 12-24 weeks following treatment, with ribavirin and pegylated interferon alone, was marginal but has continued to improve. Despite the improvement, the introduction of DAAs has made the previously reported 50-70% SVR rates fall far short of rates achieved with DAAs.

NS3/4 Protease Inhibitors	NS5A Inhibitors	Nucleos(t)ide NS5B Polymerase Inhibitors	Nonnucleos(t)ide NS5B Polymerase Inhibitors
Boceprevir	Daclatasvir	Mericitabine	*Dasabuvir*
Telaprevir	Elbasvir	*Sofosbuvir*	Deleobuvir
Simeprevir	*Ledipasvir*	VX-135	Lomibuvir
Parotaprevir	*Ombitasvir*		Tegobuvir
Asunaprevir	Samatasvir		ABT-072
Faldaprevir	ACH-2928		BMS-791325
Danoprevir	BMS824393		GS-9669
Grazoprevir	PPI-461		
Sovaprevir	PPI-668		
Vedroprevir	GS-5816		
Vaniprevir			
IDX320			

Legend: Drugs in italics have received FDA approval as of January 2015

Adapted from www.hepatitis.va.gov

Table 1. FDA approved and investigated drugs by mechanism of action

As it currently stands, four classes of DAA exist, which can be categorized according to the protein they inhibit. These four include inhibitors of the NS3/4 protease, NS5A polymerase, and NS5B polymerases (nucleoside and nonnucleoside). The approval of two NS3/4 protease inhibitors, telaprevir (TEL) and boceprevir (BOC), occurred in 2011 and marked the beginning of the age of DAAs. This was followed 2 years later by the approval of sofosbuvir (SOF), a nucleoside NS5B inhibitor, and simeprevir (SIM), an NS3/4 protease inhibitor, further expanded the available treatment options. In 2014, a combination of IFN-free regimen utilizing SOF and an NS5A inhibitor, ledipasvir (LED), was approved. Closely following this, the four-drug combination pack of an NS5A inhibitor, NS3/4A inhibitor, and a nonnucleoside NS5B inhibitor of ombitasvir (OMB), paritaprevir (PARr), and dasabuvir (DAS), respectively, gained Food and Drug Administration (FDA) approval in the United States. In addition to the DAAs in the four-drug combination pack, ritonavir has been added due to its potent inhibition of

CYP3A4, increasing the effect of paritaprevir. Several other agents are currently undergoing late stage clinical trials and are expected to be approved in the near future (Table 1).

2. Epidemiology

In the most recent National Health and Nutrition Examination Survey (NHANES), the estimated prevalence of HCV infection is approximately 3.6 million in the United States alone, with an estimated 2.7 of these having chronic infection. Worldwide, the World Health Organization (WHO) estimates that nearly 150 million people have chronic HCV infection. In both the United States and worldwide, estimates likely fall significantly short given that nearly half of all infected patients have never been tested for HCV. Additionally, the incidence among prisoners and the homeless are not known and in less developed nations are often not recorded [1]. HCV is thought to be the causal factor of up to one-third of cases of cirrhosis worldwide [2, 3].

In a study done by Shepherd *et al.* [4], analysis of positive HCV seroprevalence throughout some of the most populous nations of the world revealed an overall worldly prevalence rate of 2%, or roughly 123 million people. Given the limitations that widespread detection and recording pose, one would expect the actual prevalence to be larger. Individual analysis of many nations including China, Pakistan, and Egypt revealed estimated HCV seroprevalence well above this range. Disease transmission patterns again reveal that the majority of transmission of HCV is thought to be from unscreened blood donation, injection drug use, unsafe therapeutic injection, or other health care-related procedures. As medical practices become safer and blood screening continues to occur, the rates of HCV transmission from injection drug use will become the predominant mode of transmission as it has in developed countries like Australia, England, and the United States. Despite its success in the United States, several barriers to improving the safety of blood transfusions have remained throughout nations across the world [4-6]. As it stands, the WHO's global database estimates that among the 97 of 164 countries that provided data, 89% of donated blood is being screened following basic quality procedures [7].

HCV cirrhosis remains the primary indication for liver transplant (LT) in the United States with over 15,000 patients currently listed on the United Network for Organ Sharing (UNOS) list [8]. In year 2013 alone, over 6,400 patients underwent LT in the United States, increasing steadily from 1,700 in 1988 [9]. The United States leads in amount of deceased donor liver transplantations followed by China, with roughly 2,000 in 2010 [10].

3. Economic impact

As is the case with most newly discovered pharmaceuticals, recently approved DAAs carry with them a financial cost so high that it is a barrier to treatment. At around $1,000 U.S. dollars per pill, a 12-week regimen would run the patient and their insurance provider approximately

$84,000 with other DAA sharing similar price tags. The endeavor of validating coverage depends upon the tangible and the intangible, the objective and subjective, the cold hard science, and the cold hard dollars. Like prior novel pharmaceuticals before them, DAAs will need full support from the respective government in which the regimen is being distributed, as it does in the United States. Governing medical councils such as the FDA, the Health Products and Food Branch (HPFB) of Health Canada, the State Food and Drug Administration (SFDA) in China, and so on, will need to first approve drug regimens and define which population is to receive them.

It is difficult to estimate the exact savings per patient due to the multitude of confounding variables. All things considered, if a patient with HCV progresses naturally without treatment to the point of being considered to have end-stage liver disease. The equivalent of hundreds of thousands of medical dollars will have been spent in order to treat and care for these patients. In addition to the cost savings achieved by no longer needing to treat the manifestations of chronic hepatitis C, the cure of hepatitis C has been also been shown to provide benefits. Beside the improvement in psychological and social well-being, which accompanies cure of HCV, treatment has been shown to decrease and potentially reverse cirrhosis, esophageal varices, and the risk for the development of hepatocellular carcinoma [11-13].

Notably, incomplete treatment, unsuccessful treatment, and reinfection are always possible, particularly in patients with comorbid psychiatric illness, concomitant drug addiction, and poor social support, all known risks factors for contracting HCV [3]. In the long run, this issue should continue to fade in its controversy given that the minimum manufacturing costs for producing direct acting antivirals have been estimated at $100-250 for a 12-week course of treatment once patent expires and production of generic versions are widely available [14]. Additionally, immediate treatment upon detection as opposed to delay in therapy has shown cost-effectiveness [15].

4. Past therapy

Over the past several years, more so recently, treatment options for HCV have exponentially grown. Treatment for HCV began with the FDA approval of interferon (IFN) in 1991, followed by combined IFN and RBV in 1998, and later with peg-IFN in 2001. The regimen of peg-IFN and RBV once stood as the standard of care, and still does in many nations, until recently. DAAs, which target nonstructural proteins involved in replication and infection of HCV, were first approved in 2011.

Peg-IFN and RBV historically have been shown to result in SVR rates of 75% in patients with genotypes 2 or 3, but only of 40% in patients with genotype 1 [16]. The duration of therapy often depended on both patient's genotype and their response to therapy as measured by HCV RNA viral load following initiation of treatment [17]. In one-third of all patients being treated with peg-IFN and RBV, adverse side effects were noted. These ranged from an influenza-like illness, characterized by fatigue, headache, fever, and rigors as well as complaints of depression, irritability, or insomnia. In addition to the side effects, therapy with peg-IFN was a tedious experience. Treatment often included weekly subcutaneous injections of peg-IFN in addition to daily oral RBV for up to 48 weeks. In addition to this, patients required at least monthly appointments for the first 12 weeks for monitoring of side effects and blood work, including HCV viral load monitoring. The tedious schedule and weekly subcutaneous injections lead many to either not enroll for therapy or undergo incomplete treatment.

As it stands now, the time of weekly injections and unfavorable side effects are gone. In 2014, new IFN-free regimens became available. The previous peg-IFN and RBV therapy or even triple therapy involving TEL or BOC is quickly becoming extinct. In 2015 onward, IFN-containing regimens will be replaced by all-oral, IFN-free therapies. Additionally, RBV-free regimens are also becoming widely available, and RBV will likely go the way of peg-IFN due to its unfavorable side effect of anemia.

5. Direct acting antiviral therapy

As noted thus far, the groundbreaking development of DAAs has appeared to instantaneous change a bleak and dismal diagnosis to one filled with hope and promise. HCV seems to be paralleling HIV in that it was once considered a death sentence where treatment was harsh and limited but has now changed to something treatable with a pill. Additionally, one can now expect to live a near normal lifespan and be contributors to society.

The genome of HCV is now well understood, and because of this, scientists have been able create inhibitors against components of the genome integral to HCV replication and function. As it currently stands, four classes of DAAs exist and include the NS3/4 protease inhibitors, NS5A polymerase inhibitors, and the NS5B polymerases (nucleoside and nonnucleoside) inhibitors. Starting with protease inhibitors in 2011, BOC and TEL changed the game and raised SVR to impressive levels in treatment-naive patients. Shortly after, SOF, a nucleoside NS5B inhibitor, and SIM, another NS3/4 protease inhibitor, were approved and progress soared. It was not long before the old regimen of peg-IFN was being disposed of for more convenient and more tolerable agents. In the past months, additional agents have been approved and include LED, OMB, PARr, and DAS. Many more are under investigation and will likely be approved by the time of this publication.

The treatment of HCV centers on achieving SVR because if one can achieve this then life expectancy approaches near normal [18]. Without a detectable HCV viral load, cirrhosis is not expected to be occurring, and therefore neither are the complications thereof. Historically, achieving SVR in unique patient populations has proven difficult. Additionally, patients with certain factors often did not tolerate treatment well. In these populations, treatment was not approved, i.e., post liver transplant HCV patients. Genotypic analysis has also helped to identify unique populations. It has been established that some strains of HCV appear to possess an innate resistance to peg-IFN and RBV. Further exploration into genotypic and polymorphic variation and its effect on treatment response is needed, particularly now that these new agents with different mechanisms of action than peg-IFN and RBV are being utilized.

5.1. Genotype specific

HCV is classified into 11 genotypes with the first 6 of these garnering the majority of attention. Interestingly, various genotypes possess a geographic predominance [19] (Table 2).

Genotype	Geographic distribution
1	United States, Europe, Japan
2	Mediterranean, Europe, Japan, North America
3	Southeast Asia, Europe, United States
4	Egypt, North Africa, sub-Saharan Africa, Middle East
5	South Africa
6-11	China, Korea, Taiwan, Southeast Asia

Table 2. HCV genotype geographic distribution

Genotype 1 is the most prevalent genotype in the world and until recently had been the most difficult genotype to treat due to its poor SVR rates in response to peg-IFN and RBV. Treatment over the years has evolved significantly and the newest available guidelines support the use of the SOF/LED combination or the OMB/PARr/DAS/RBV combination [20-27]. Alternatively, data also indicate that use of SOF, SIM with or without RBV, achieved acceptable rates of SVR and can also be considered for use [28]. In patients with genotype 1 HCV infection, new SVR targets are now at greater than 90%. Newer therapies will need to measure up to these results. New agents remain under study, but preliminary results have been as impressive as the above regimens, and thus the market for treatment of genotype 1 infection will be saturated before we know it [29, 30] (Table 3).

Genotype 2 is found in clusters in the Mediterranean region and has historically responded well to the previous standard of peg-IFN and RBV. Genotype 3, now becoming the most difficult genotype to treat, has the unique characteristic of being associated with intravenous drug use. Recent studies using the newer DAAs show increased rates of SVR. Current recommendations for treatment suggest ample success is possible by utilizing a SOF and RBV regimen [31-36]. Building on excellent results of a phase II trial, an ongoing phase III trial is pending and expected to show widespread success with the use of daclatasvir (DAC) in combination with SOF [37, 38]. DAC, an NS5A inhibitor, has shown similar promising results throughout all genotypes as expected given its pan-genotypic treatment effect. Other promising regimens include SOF/LED combination, as well as GS-5816, a pan-genotypic NS5A inhibitor in combination with RBV [39, 40] (Table 4).

Genotype 4 is found mostly in Egypt, the Middle East, and northern Africa. Although rare in the United States, in Egypt, the prevalence of HCV is upwards of 15% and thus remains an important research focus. Similarly, genotypes 5 and 6 are rare in the United States and are more frequently found in southern Africa, Southeast Asia, China, and Korea. Given the geographic distribution, few genotype 4-6 patients have been enrolled in clinical trials. More

http://dx.doi.org/10.5772/60986

research is needed, but SOF-based regimens are likely to be significantly effective in the meantime [31, 41-46] (Table 5).

Trial	Phase	*n*	Regimen	SVR	Comments
ION-1 [20]	III	865	SOF/LED ± RBV for 12 or 24 wks	>97%	Included patients with compensated cirrhosis
ION-2 [20]	III	440	SOF/LED ± RBV for 12 or 24 wks	>94%	Previously treated patients with and without cirrhosis. Lower SVR was observed in the 12-week group without RBV.
ION-3 [21]	III	647	SOF/LED ± RBV for 8 or 12 wks	>93%	Included patients with compensated cirrhosis in 12 week arm
SAPPHIRE-I [22]	III	631	OMB/PARr/DAS + RBV for 12 wks	>95%	Absence of cirrhosis required
SAPPHIRE-II [25]	III	297	OMB/PARr/DAS + RBV for 12 wks	>96%	Previously treated patients without cirrhosis. SVR similar regardless of previously treatment failure.
PEARL-III [23]	III	305	OMB/PARr/DAS ± RBV for 12 wks	>90%	G-1a patients
PEARL-IV [23]	III	419	OMB/PARr/DAS ± RBV for 12 wks	>99%	G-1b patients
TURQUOISE-II [24]	III	380	OMB/PARr/DAS + RBV for 12 or 24 wks	>92%	Patients with compensated cirrhosis
COSMOS [28]	II	167	SOF/SIM ± RBV for 12 or 24 wks	>90%	Extending treatment and RBV did not significantly improve SVR, phase III trial ongoing(OPTIMIST)
SIRIUS [27]	II	155	SOF/LED for 24 wks or SOF/LED + RBV for 12 wks	>96%	Previously treated patients with and without cirrhosis. 12 week course proved as effective.
C-WORHTY [26]	II	253	GRZ/ELB ± RBV for 12 or 18 wks	>90%	Previously treated and untreated with and without cirrhosis

Legend: Wks: week; GRZ: grazoprevir; ELB: elbasvir

Table 3. Results of DAA treatment in genotype 1 patients

Trial	Phase	*n*	Regimen	SVR	Comments
FISSION [31]	III	499	SOF + RBV for 12 wks	97%	Compared to previous standard, SOF greatly improved SVR rates from 78% to 97%
POSITRON [32]	III	278	SOF + RBV for 12 wks vs placebo	78%	SVR was higher for G-2(93%) vs G3(61%)

Trial	Phase	*n*	Regimen	SVR	Comments
VALENCE [33]	III	419	SOF + RBV for 12 or 24 wks	>78%	G-2 was treated for 12 wk and G-3 was treated for 24 wks in patients with and without cirrhosis who were and were not previously treated. Lowest SVR(78%) was noted in the previously treated, cirrhotic genotype 3 patients.
FUSION [32]	III	201	SOF + RBV for 12 or 16 wks	>86%	Previously treated patients with and without cirrhosis.
LONESTAR II [34]	II	47	SOF + RBV + peg-IFN for 12 wks	>96%	Previously treated patients with and without cirrhosis
A144040 [37]	II	44	DAC + SOF ± RBV for 24 wks	>88%	
PROTON [35]	II	25	SOF + RBV + peg-IFN for 12 wks	92%	
ELECTRON [36]	II	50	SOF + RBV ± peg-IFN for 12 wks	100%	Among the SOF + RBV arms of the study SVR was high, the SOF only group reported an SVR of 60%

Legend: Wks: week; DAC: daclatasvir

Table 4. Results of DAA treatment in genotypes 2 and 3 patients

Trial	Phase	*n*	Regimen	SVR	Comments
NEUTRINO [31]	III	327*	SOF + RBV + peg-IFN for 12 wks	96%	Patients with genotypes 1, 4, 5, and 6. Of these 27/28 genotype 4 patients and 7/7 genotype 5 and 6 achieved SVR.
Egypt Ancestry Trial [41]	II	60	SOF + RBV for 12 or 24 wks	>79%	SVR was lowest in the 12-wk, treatment naïve group.
RESTORE [42]	III	107	SIM + RBV + peg-IFN for 12 wks	>65%	SVR of 83% in the treatment naïve group, 40% in the prior null responders
PEARL I [43, 44]	II	86	OMB/PARr ± RBV for 12 wks	>91%	Preliminary data, patients in the RBV group achieved 100% SVR

Trial	Phase	*n*	Regimen	SVR	Comments
SYNERGY [45]	II	21	LED/SOF for 12 wks	95%	Preliminary data, included previously treated patients
ATOMIC [46]	II	316	SOF + RBV + peg-IFN for 12 or 24 wks	>82%	Patients with genotypes 1, 4, 5 and 6; 9/11 genotype 4 and 5/5 genotype 6 achieved SVR
Legend:*Of the 327, only 28 patients were genotype 4; Wks: week					

Table 5. Results of DAA treatment in genotype 4, 5 and 6 patients

6. Unique populations

Large phase III trials convincingly show favorable SVR in patients who are naive to treatment, noncirrhotic, and in non-HIV coinfected. However, what about patients who do not fit into these categories? Furthermore, concern for side effect profile, inadequate practitioner training, and concern for drug-drug interaction have led to avoidance in all but treatment-naive and otherwise healthy patients.

In addition to the unique groups of patients described below, other factors should also be taken into consideration as they can complicate the decision as to which treatment should be initiated. These include patients with renal failure, heart failure, and comorbid psychiatric illness to name a few. The medical comorbidities of each individual is a hornet's nest of potential failure, and as such, each case embarked upon should be done so with careful consideration of all coexisting medical and psychological conditions. To ensure of this, it is helpful to have a trained multidisciplinary team made up of physicians, pharmacists, nurses, psychologists, and social workers. Aside from making medication dose adjustments when required, current guidelines recommend that in the presence of complex comorbid medical conditions, treatment of HCV be initiated and managed by a hepatologist and potentially at a medical center affiliated with liver transplantation [47].

6.1. Treatment experienced

Patients who have been previously treated pose perhaps one of the most common dilemmas that practitioners face. Often times, patients get retreated due to initial therapeutic failure (typically to peg-IFN and RBV) or HCV relapse. Patients may be presenting for retreatment following previous partial treatment or after being lost to follow-up. Rarely, patients can become reinfected with HCV. In all scenarios, therapy with new HCV drug regimens should be offered.

Initial studies with TEL, BOC, and SIM showed encouraging results. In the REALIZE trial, nonresponders, partial responders, or those who have suffered a relapse were randomized into three treatment groups separated by treatment duration. An SVR rate of 66% was achieved in the 12-week treatment arm of TEL, peg-IFN, and RBV [48]. Similarly, BOC in combination peg-IFN and RBV was able to achieve rates of SVR of 63% overall, however only 38% in prior nonresponders [49]. Larger trials and trials utilizing SIM showed similar results [50-53]. In general, all studies reported adverse side effects of severe anemia, requiring treatment discontinuation, dose reduction, or transfusion. Given the poor response of prior null responders, treatment utilizing TEL, BOC, or SIM in combination with peg-IFN and ribavirin is not recommended in the treatment experienced population.

Several promising trials evaluating the therapeutic benefit of newer DAAs have been reported with high overall SVRs, few side effects, and minimal drug interactions. (Tables 3-5). Based on these trials, recommendations regarding appropriate therapy as tailored to the genotype have been made. In general, genotype 1 patients have several options as convincing results as to effectiveness has been produced with either SOF/LED, SOF/SIM, or the four-drug combination of PARr/OMB/DAS/RBV. For those with genotype 2 or 3, reassuring data from the LONE-STAR-2 trial that achieved SVR rates of 83-96% in these patients confirmed that a 12-week regimen of SOF, RBV, and peg-IFN be used [34]. For those not eligible for peg-IFN, SVRs of 80-90% were still achievable with SOF and RBV alone [32, 33]. In genotype 4 patients, options include SOF/LED, SOF/RBV with or without peg-IFN, or the four-drug combination of PARr/OMB/DAS/RBV. As with the treatment-naive patients, genotype 5 or 6 has few reported data, but an SOF-based regimen will likely be efficacious.

6.2. Decompensated cirrhosis

Cirrhosis, regardless of its level of compensation, is known to result in a decreased SVR in patients being treated for HCV. On decompensation with the development of ascites, variceal hemorrhage, encephalopathy, or coagulopathy, the probability of survival is only 50% at 5 years, with a median survival of only 2 years [54, 55]. Thus, it remains imperative to provide rapid and effective treatment for HCV.

A meta-analysis done by Vierling *et al.* [56] examined several phase III clinical trials of patients undergoing HCV treatment with biopsy proven cirrhosis. In the trials of patients receiving the standard therapy of peg-IFN and RBV, an overall SVR of 20% was found. In 2011, riding the momentum of improved SVR in noncirrhotic patients receiving triple therapy, BOC, TEL, and SIM were given in combination with peg-IFN and RBV, and the rate of SVR increased significantly to 55% and 74%, respectively, in this previously dismal population [53, 56]. Improvement in SVR was not without its drawbacks. In the BOC- and TEL-treated groups, significant side effects of anemia and diarrhea were noted. Slightly less severe side effects of flulike illness and pruritus were noted in those treated with SIM; however, significant resistance was found in genotype 1A patients who possessed a specific genetic polymorphism known as the Q80K mutation. A screening test for detection of this mutation is available, and given that nearly 50% of United States and 20% of European patients had the mutation at baseline, testing should be conducted prior to treatment with SIM [57].

Following on the success of a trial conducted by Gane *et al.* [58], which showed an SVR in 9 out of 9 patients with decompensated cirrhosis treated with SOF, LED, and RBV, the SOLAR-1 trial was conducted. This trial was a multicenter, randomized trial of 108 patients with genotypes 1 and 4 HCV whom also had Child-Pugh class B or C cirrhosis. Excluding 6 patients who underwent eventual liver transplant, an SVR of 87% and 89% was attained in the 12- and 24-week treatment groups, respectively. Given the larger chance of adverse events observed in the 24-week group, consensus guidelines for treating genotypes 1 and 4 patients with decompensated cirrhosis support a 12-week course of SOF, LED, and RBV [47]. Most importantly, the patients with virologic response had significant improvement in liver function, including improvements in bilirubin, albumin, modified end-stage liver disease (MELD) scores, and Child-Pugh scores. These guidelines recommend that for genotypes 2 and 3, daily SOF and RBV should be utilized up to 48 weeks for treatment. These recommendations are based on sparse data showing an achieved SVR in 10 of 11 patients [59]. Further data is needed in this group and is expected to change guidelines further. Preliminary data reported on the use of SOF, LED, and RBV for 12 weeks in genotype 3 patients showed favorable results with an SVR being achieved in all 26 patients treated [60].

Further research is needed in this group, including studies evaluating larger groups of patients to delineate a specific regimen. As it stands, similar to other unique populations, it appears that second-generation agents such as SOF, LED, and the like provide a superior benefit to first-generation protease inhibitors like SIM, TEL, and BOC. In addition to the pan-genomic action, improved dosing regimens, less drug-drug interactions, and more tolerable side effect profiles make them a first choice in patients with decompensated cirrhosis regardless of liver transplant candidacy.

6.3. HIV coinfected

HIV-infected individuals with concomitant hepatitis C are known to have an increased morbidity and mortality [61]. Following the development of highly active antiretroviral therapy (HAART), there has been an ever-increasing percentage of HIV-infected patients who are dying from liver disease. In HIV-infected patients, death from liver disease remains far more prevalent than death attributable to HIV-related complications [62, 63].

Historically, having coinfection with HIV also leads to poor responses to peg-IFN and RBV therapy [64, 65]. Additionally, coinfection with HIV also lead to increased risk for progression to cirrhosis [66]. On a molecular level, it has been postulated that the higher viral load of HCV RNA noted in this population is secondary to both increased replication of HCV RNA by HIV proteins as well as a generalized state of immunodeficiency [67, 68].

Up until recently, treating patients with coinfection of HIV was felt to be difficult secondary to the historically poorer responses to peg-IFN and RBV. Recently, however, concern regarding potential drug-drug interactions has existed and has lead to practitioner trepidation [69, 70]. This has fortunately not panned out, and several large trials have shown excellent results in treatment of the HCV/HIV coinfected.

With protease inhibitors approved first, trials utilizing a triple therapy of either TEL or BOC in combination with peg-IFN and RBV were conducted. Sulkowski *et al.* [71] treated 62 coinfected genotype 1 patients with TEL, peg-IFN, and RBV achieved an SVR of 74%. In another study, using triple therapy with BOC in combination with peg-IFN and RBV, an SVR of 63% was attained; however, significant side effects leading to dropout in 12 of 65 patients occurred. This dropout continues to be a concern and is thought to be secondary to side effects, high pill burden, and pharmacokinetic interactions between HCV NS3/4A protease inhibitors and antiretroviral drugs [72, 73].

Following on the success of first-generation DAAs, trials utilizing SOF were later conducted. In a study of genotype 1 patients, Osinusi *et al.* [74] treated 50 HCV and HIV coinfected patients with 12 weeks of SOF and LED. Grouping based on HAART naive versus on HAART showed no difference in the 100% SVR rates achieved in both groups. No adverse events or discontinuations were noted during the treatment period. Sulkowski *et al.* [75] was able to achieve an SVR of 67-88% based on genotype following a 12- to 24-week course of SOF and RBV. Of note, this approach was void of significant drug-drug interactions. In an even larger trial conducted by Molina *et al.* [76], 275 patients with genotypes 1-4 HCV underwent treatment with a 12-week course of SOF and RBV. The overall SVR rate achieved was 85% in genotype 1, 88% in genotype 2, 89% in genotype 3, and 84% in patients with genotype 4. Given the results of these trials, an SOF-based regimen, free of peg-IFN, is recommended; however, with new drug regimens being approved, further studies and head-to-head trials will need to be conducted in order to truly determine the best choice for these select patients.

6.4. Recurrence after liver transplant

Graft failure and fibrosis remain a feared complications among patients transplanted for HCV. Invariably, HCV recurs in all patients following transplantation. Similar to the pretransplant state, patients with HCV progress to fibrosis and eventual decompensation of the transplanted liver. Patients who undergo liver transplantation as a whole have been shown to have higher rates of mortality for this reason [77-79]. Routine monitoring has gone far to anticipate these changes; however, treatment needs continued improvement. Until recently, treatment with peg-IFN and RBV was only marginally effective, and use in this population was off-label. With the newly discovered DAAs, great promise for treatment exists. In addition to the superb ability to achieve SVR, DAAs offer favorable side effect profiles with manageable drug interactions with common immunosuppressive regimens. Some of the DAAs have been shown to do this better than others.

Complicating factors that must be discussed in this patient population include donor and recipient variables. Independent of the treatment regimen, certain characteristics have been shown in large retrospective analysis to negatively impact progression to fibrosis and cirrhosis following LT. The presence of advanced donor age or steatosis as well as specific genetic polymorphisms in both the donor and the recipient can lead to advanced progression of fibrosis [80-83]. Factors such as living vs. deceased donor, human leukocyte antigen (HLA) matching, and HCV positive donor status have not been shown to reliably contribute to fibrosis progression [84, 85]. Within the context of HCV-related liver transplantation, several studies have also attempted to identify specific allelic variants that may contribute to either poor response to standard antiviral therapy or a more rapid progression of fibrosis [86, 87]. Further studies are needed to confirm these, however, and as it stands due to the limited supply, the

http://dx.doi.org/10.5772/60986

allocation of available livers for transplant based on the presence of nucleotide polymorphisms is not practiced (Table 6).

Donor Factors	Recipient Factors
Age >50 years	Genotype 1B
Liver steatosis >30%	IL28B Genotype CT and TT
IL28B Genotype CT and TT	
Lack of DDX58 polymorphism	

Table 6. Factors leading to worse outcomes following liver transplantation

Currently, three treatment strategies for management of HCV in the transplant setting are being used. The first strategy involves treatment of patients currently listed for transplantation. Until recently, the barrier with this strategy has been that with peg-IFN, RBV and the early DAAs patients often either do not tolerate therapy or do not achieve SVR [88]. The second strategy that is not being used thus far involves treating HCV recurrence immediately following liver transplantation. Whether or not this method of treatment increases in popularity will be determined by the tolerability and side effects of the new DAAs. The third and most commonly used strategy involves initiating treatment after several months following transplantation and noted progression of HCV.

Several trials have evaluated the effectiveness of using peg-IFN and RBV in order to treat HCV recurrence in patients following LT. The results have not been favorable, and side effects, particularly anemia, have posed barriers to treatment completion. Overall SVR, in patients with minimal fibrosis, following 48 weeks of therapy was only 48% [89]. Follow-up studies have had even less favorable results [90]. Therefore, peg-IFN and RBV alone is not recommended in this treatment group.

In the largest series evaluating the use of TEL and BOC for the treatment of HCV recurrence following liver transplantation, Burton et al. [91] successfully treated 81 patients with genotype 1 HCV and achieved an SVR at 12 weeks of 63%. Despite its success, TEL and BOC in combination with peg-IFN and RBV led to severe side effects of anemia requiring a transfusion in nearly 50% of patients. Additionally, close monitoring of immunosuppressant drug levels was required, and frequent dose adjustments were needed. Given these results, the use of BOC and TEL are not recommended unless newer, better-tolerated agents are unavailable.

Recent trials report favorable tolerability and highly effective results with the use of new DAAs. In a trial evaluating 40 patients treated with RBV and SOF, an SVR12 of 70% was achieved [92]. Slightly better results were achieved in the HCV-TARGET consortium, which evaluated 189 patients being treated with SOF-based regimens. Overall, SVR among the groups ranged from 69% to 88%. Additionally, SOF and SIM regimens achieved SVR12 of 80-88% depending if RBV was used [93]. The utilization of SOB in combination with LED is also being looked at and has shown that in patients with compensated disease and minimal cirrhosis, a highly favorable SVR12 of 96% could be attained. This regimen is also appealing as it only required 12 weeks of therapy [94]. Current guidelines put in place by the AASLD-ISDA recommend treatment of genotype 1 infection with combination SOF and SIM. For genotype 2 or 3, SOF or RBV alone is recommended [47]. These recommendations are likely subject to change given approval of LED as well as favorable results of a trial looking at ritonavir-boosted paritaprevir, coformulated with ombitasvir, plus dasabuvir [95]. The treatment of post-LT patients with more advanced cirrhosis (Child-Pugh B or C) continues to require further study; however, preliminary results reveal that even in this highly difficult-to-treat group, an SVR of 81% could be achieved [94]. Other regimens continue to be under investigation at this time.

It is anticipated that all-oral DAA regimens will be both highly effective as well as highly tolerated in the liver transplant setting. Continued research evaluating safety profiles of these medications should be done, but in the meantime, given the amount of evidence currently available and in accordance with current guidelines, the initiation of a sofosbuvir-based regimen in this patient population is highly recommended.

7. Future therapy

As alluded to in the sections above, DAA research is producing large quantities of favorable data, particularly in genotypes prevalent in Europe and the United States. Numerous clinical trials have been completed. More trials are ongoing or are recruiting. Naturally, head-to-head trials are needed to differentiate between many of the already known successful regimens, but few will agree to this in the short term. Future research should aim to improve the currently available classes of HCV drugs with the goal of limiting significant side effects. Specifically, we hope that all newly developed NS3-4A protease inhibitors, nucleoside/nucleotide analogues, nonnucleoside inhibitors of HCV NS5B, and NS5A inhibitors share a similar high-potency, pan-genotypic antiviral activity, and high barrier to resistance. In the distant future, perhaps DAAs will have lost their utility as research on vaccination continues [96].

8. Summary

Therapy for HCV has seemed to exponentially grow over the past 4 years. Because of DAAs, IFN-free as well as all-oral regimens are being used to treat HCV. In addition to this, ribavirin-free regimens are also available. Thus far, these highly effective therapies have proven to provide fewer side effects and achieve better results, all the while in less time. Hope for cure and eradication remains paramount and is now achievable. With appropriate allocation of resources, physician training, and available treatment, the cure of HCV is possible. Doing so will drastically decrease overall health care costs, improve quality of life, and decrease the number of liver transplants needed.

http://dx.doi.org/10.5772/60986

Author details

Eric Hilgenfeldt[1*] and Roberto J. Firpi[2]

*Address all correspondence to: eric.hilgenfeldt@medicine.ufl.edu

1 Department of Internal Medicine, University of Florida College of Medicine, Gainesville, FL, USA

2 Department of Gastroenterology, Hepatology and Nutrition, University of Florida College of Medicine, Gainesville, FL, USA

References

[1] WHO. *Hepatitis C*. WHO 2014 2014-07-28 11:19:38. Available from: http://www.who.int/mediacentre/factsheets/fs164/en/

[2] Denniston, M.M., et al., *Chronic hepatitis C virus infection in the United States, National Health and Nutrition Examination Survey 2003 to 2010*. Ann Intern Med, 2014. 160(5): 293-300.

[3] Alter, M.J., *Epidemiology of hepatitis C virus infection*. World J Gastroenterol, 2007. 13(17):2436-41.

[4] Shepard, C.W., L. Finelli, and M.J. Alter, *Global epidemiology of hepatitis C virus infection*. Lancet Infect Dis, 2005. 5(9):558-67.

[5] Dhingra, N., *Blood safety in the developing world and WHO initiatives*. Vox Sang, 2002. 83 Suppl 1:173-7.

[6] Shan, H., et al., *Blood banking in China*. Lancet, 2002. 360(9347):1770-5.

[7] WHO. *Global database on blood safety*. WHO 2014 2014-07-25 14:56:12. Available from: http://www.who.int/bloodsafety/global_database/en/

[8] O'Leary, J.G., R. Lepe, and G.L. Davis, *Indications for liver transplantation*. Gastroenterology, 2008. 134(6):1764-76.

[9] OPTN. *Organ Procurement and Transplantation Network*. 2014. Available from: http://optn.transplant.hrsa.gov/latestData/rptData.asp

[10] Services, U.S.D.o.H.a.H. *OPTN/SRTR 2011 Annual Data Report: international data*. 2011; 199-226]. Available from: http://srtr.transplant.hrsa.gov/annual_reports/2011/pdf/08_intl_12.pdf

[11] Morgan, R.L., et al., *Eradication of hepatitis C virus infection and the development of hepatocellular carcinoma: a meta-analysis of observational studies.* Ann Intern Med, 2013. 158(5 Pt 1):329-37.

[12] Bruno, S., et al., *Sustained virologic response prevents the development of esophageal varices in compensated, Child-Pugh class A hepatitis C virus-induced cirrhosis. A 12-year prospective follow-up study.* Hepatology, 2010. 51(6):2069-76.

[13] Poynard, T., et al., *Impact of pegylated interferon alfa-2b and ribavirin on liver fibrosis in patients with chronic hepatitis C.* Gastroenterology, 2002. 122(5):1303-13.

[14] Hill, A., et al., *Minimum costs for producing hepatitis C direct-acting antivirals for use in large-scale treatment access programs in developing countries.* Clin Infect Dis, 2014. 58(7): 928-36.

[15] Leidner, A.J., et al., *Cost-effectiveness of hepatitis C treatment for patients in early stages of liver disease.* Hepatology, 2015.

[16] Ghany, M.G., et al., *Diagnosis, management, and treatment of hepatitis C: an update.* Hepatology, 2009. 49(4):1335-74.

[17] Jacobson, I.M., *Treatment options for patients with chronic hepatitis C not responding to initial antiviral therapy.* Clin Gastroenterol Hepatol, 2009. 7(9):921-30.

[18] van der Meer, A.J., et al., *Life expectancy in patients with chronic HCV infection and cirrhosis compared with a general population.* JAMA, 2014. 312(18):1927-8.

[19] Hnatyszyn, H.J., *Chronic hepatitis C and genotyping: the clinical significance of determining HCV genotypes.* Antivir Ther, 2005. 10(1):1-11.

[20] Afdhal, N., et al., *Ledipasvir and sofosbuvir for previously treated HCV genotype 1 infection.* N Engl J Med, 2014. 370(16):1483-93.

[21] Kowdley, K.V., et al., *Ledipasvir and sofosbuvir for 8 or 12 weeks for chronic HCV without cirrhosis.* N Engl J Med, 2014. 370(20):1879-88.

[22] Feld, J.J., et al., *Treatment of HCV with ABT-450/r-ombitasvir and dasabuvir with ribavirin.* N Engl J Med, 2014. 370(17):1594-603.

[23] Ferenci, P., et al., *ABT-450/r-ombitasvir and dasabuvir with or without ribavirin for HCV.* N Engl J Med, 2014. 370(21):1983-92.

[24] Poordad, F., et al., *ABT-450/r-ombitasvir and dasabuvir with ribavirin for hepatitis C with cirrhosis.* N Engl J Med, 2014. 370(21):1973-82.

[25] Zeuzem, S., et al., *Retreatment of HCV with ABT-450/r-ombitasvir and dasabuvir with ribavirin.* N Engl J Med, 2014. 370(17):1604-14.

[26] Bourliere, M., J. Bronowicki, V. de Ledinghen, et al., *Ledipasvir/sofosbuvir fixed dose combination is safe and efficacious in cirrhotic patients who have previously failed protease-inhibitor based triple therapy.* Boston, Massachusetts Program and abstracts of the 65th

Annual Meeting of the American Association for the Study of Liver Diseases, November 7-11, 2014. Abstract LB-6.

[27] Lawitz, E., et al., *Efficacy and safety of 12 weeks versus 18 weeks of treatment with grazoprevir (MK-5172) and elbasvir (MK-8742) with or without ribavirin for hepatitis C virus genotype 1 infection in previously untreated patients with cirrhosis and patients with previous null response with or without cirrhosis (C-WORTHY): a randomised, open-label phase 2 trial.* Lancet, 2014.

[28] Lawitz, E., et al., *Simeprevir plus sofosbuvir, with or without ribavirin, to treat chronic infection with hepatitis C virus genotype 1 in non-responders to pegylated interferon and ribavirin and treatment-naive patients: the COSMOS randomised study.* Lancet, 2014. 384(9956):1756-65.

[29] *Phase III Hallmark DUAL: ASV+DCV (Nulls/Partials, Intolerants/Ineligibles. Naives)—Full Text View—ClinicalTrials.gov.* 2015. Available from: https://clinicaltrials.gov/ct2/show/NCT01581203

[30] *Study to Assess Efficacy, Safety, Tolerability and Pharmacokinetics of Simeprevir, Daclatasvir and Sofosbuvir in Treatment-naive Participants with Chronic Hepatitis C Virus Genotype 1 Infection—Full Text View—ClinicalTrials.gov.* 2015. Available from: https://clinicaltrials.gov/ct2/show/NCT02349048?term=Daclatasvir+plus+Sofosbuvir&rank=3

[31] Lawitz, E., et al., *Sofosbuvir for previously untreated chronic hepatitis C infection.* N Engl J Med, 2013. 368(20):1878-87.

[32] Jacobson, I.M., et al., *Sofosbuvir for hepatitis C genotype 2 or 3 in patients without treatment options.* N Engl J Med, 2013. 368(20):1867-77.

[33] Zeuzem, S., et al., *Sofosbuvir and ribavirin in HCV genotypes 2 and 3.* N Engl J Med, 2014. 370(21):1993-2001.

[34] Lawitz, E., et al., *Sofosbuvir with peginterferon-ribavirin for 12 weeks in previously treated patients with hepatitis C genotype 2 or 3 and cirrhosis.* Hepatology, 2014.

[35] Lawitz, E., et al., *Sofosbuvir in combination with peginterferon alfa-2a and ribavirin for non-cirrhotic, treatment-naive patients with genotypes 1, 2, and 3 hepatitis C infection: a randomised, double-blind, phase 2 trial.* Lancet Infect Dis, 2013. 13(5):401-8.

[36] Gane, E.J., et al., *Nucleotide polymerase inhibitor sofosbuvir plus ribavirin for hepatitis C.* N Engl J Med, 2013. 368(1):34-44.

[37] Sulkowski, M.S., et al., *Daclatasvir plus sofosbuvir for previously treated or untreated chronic HCV infection.* N Engl J Med, 2014. 370(3):211-21.

[38] Nelson, D.R., et al., *All-oral 12-week treatment with daclatasvir plus sofosbuvir in patients with hepatitis C virus genotype 3 infection: ALLY-3 phase 3 study.* Hepatology, 2015.

[39] Gane, J., R. Hyland, and D. An, *Sofosbuvir/ledipasvir fixed dose combination is safe and effective in difficult-to-treat populations including genotype-3 patients, decompensated geno-*

type-1 patients, and genotype-1 patients with prior sofosbuvir treatment experience. Abstract O6. 49th European Association for the Study of the Liver International Liver Congress; London, April 9-13, 2014.

[40] *Comparison of Sofosbuvir/GS-5816 Fixed Dose Combination for 12 Weeks with Sofosbuvir and Ribavirin for 24 Weeks in Adults with Chronic Genotype 3 HCV Infection—Full Text View—ClinicalTrials.gov.* 2015. Available from: https://clinicaltrials.gov/ct2/show/NCT02201953

[41] Ruane, P.J., et al., *Sofosbuvir plus ribavirin for the treatment of chronic genotype 4 hepatitis C virus infection in patients of Egyptian ancestry.* J Hepatol, 2014.

[42] Moreno, C., et al., *Simeprevir with peginterferon/ribavirin in treatment-naive or -experienced patients with chronic HCV genotype 4 infection: a phase III study. Abstract PS9/6.* 14th European AIDS Conference; Brussels, 2013.

[43] *A Study to Evaluate the Safety and Effect of Co-administration of ABT-450 with Ritonavir (ABT-450/r) and ABT-267 in Adults with Chronic Hepatitis C Virus Infection—Full Text View—ClinicalTrials.gov.* 2015. Available from: https://clinicaltrials.gov/ct2/show/NCT01685203

[44] *Results from Phase 2 PEARL-I Study in Genotype 4 Chronic Hepatitis C Patients at the Liver Meeting.* Nov 11, 2014. Available from: http://abbvie.mediaroom.com/2014-11-11-AbbVie-to-Present-Results-from-Phase-2-PEARL-I-Study-in-Genotype-4-Chronic-Hepatitis-C-Patients-at-The-Liver-Meeting-2014

[45] Kapoor, R., A. Kohli, and S. Sidharthan, *Treatment of hepatitis C genotype 4 with ledipasvir and sofosbuvir for 12 weeks: results of the SYNERGY trial. Abstract 240.* American Association for the Study of Liver Diseases (AASLD) Liver Meeting; Boston, November 7-12, 2014.

[46] Kowdley, K.V., et al., *Sofosbuvir with pegylated interferon alfa-2a and ribavirin for treatment-naive patients with hepatitis C genotype-1 infection (ATOMIC): an open-label, randomised, multicentre phase 2 trial.* Lancet, 2013. 381(9883):2100-7.

[47] AASLD-ISDA. *Full Report | Recommendations for Testing, Managing, and Treating Hepatitis C.* 2015. Available from: http://www.hcvguidelines.org/full-report-view

[48] Zeuzem, S., et al., *Telaprevir for retreatment of HCV infection.* N Engl J Med, 2011. 364(25):2417-28.

[49] Vierling, J.M., et al., *Boceprevir for chronic HCV genotype 1 infection in patients with prior treatment failure to peginterferon/ribavirin, including prior null response.* J Hepatol, 2014. 60(4):748-56.

[50] Bacon, B.R., et al., *Boceprevir for previously treated chronic HCV genotype 1 infection.* N Engl J Med, 2011. 364(13):1207-17.

[51] Hézode, C., et al., *Effectiveness of telaprevir or boceprevir in treatment-experienced patients with HCV genotype 1 infection and cirrhosis.* Gastroenterology, 2014. 147(1):132-142.e4.

[52] Zeuzem, S., et al., *Simeprevir increases rate of sustained virologic response among treatment-experienced patients with HCV genotype-1 infection: a phase IIb trial.* Gastroenterology, 2014. 146(2):430-41.e6.

[53] Forns, X., et al., *Simeprevir with peginterferon and ribavirin leads to high rates of SVR in patients with HCV genotype 1 who relapsed after previous therapy: a phase 3 trial.* Gastroenterology, 2014. 146(7):1669-79.e3.

[54] Fattovich, G., et al., *Morbidity and mortality in compensated cirrhosis type C: a retrospective follow-up study of 384 patients.* Gastroenterology, 1997. 112(2):463-72.

[55] D'Amico, G., G. Garcia-Tsao, and L. Pagliaro, *Natural history and prognostic indicators of survival in cirrhosis: a systematic review of 118 studies.* J Hepatol, 2006. 44(1):217-31.

[56] Vierling, J.M., et al., *Safety and efficacy of boceprevir/peginterferon/ribavirin for HCV G1 compensated cirrhotics: meta-analysis of 5 trials.* J Hepatol, 2014. 61(2):200-9.

[57] *The FDA & the Janssen Briefing Documents Oct 24 Hearing*. FDA antiviral drugs advisory committee meeting 2015 [cited 2013 October 24th]; Background package for NDA 205123 Simeprevir (TMC 435)]. Available from: http://www.natap.org/2013/HCV/102313_02.htm

[58] Gane, E.J., et al., *Efficacy of nucleotide polymerase inhibitor sofosbuvir plus the NS5A inhibitor ledipasvir or the NS5B non-nucleoside inhibitor GS-9669 against HCV genotype 1 infection.* Gastroenterology, 2014. 146(3):736-743.e1.

[59] Curry, M.P., et al., *Sofosbuvir and ribavirin prevent recurrence of HCV infection after liver transplantation: an open-label study.* Gastroenterology, 2015. 148(1):100-107.e1.

[60] Gane, E., R. Hyland, and D. An, *High efficacy of LDV/SOF regimens for 12 weeks for patients with HCV genotype 3 or 6 infection. [Abstract LB11.].* 65th Annual Meeting of the American Association for the Study of Liver Diseases (AASLD). November 7-11, 2014; Boston, MA.

[61] Zeremski, M., A.D. Martinez, and A.H. Talal, *Editorial commentary: management of hepatitis C virus in HIV-infected patients in the era of direct-acting antivirals.* Clin Infect Dis, 2014. 58(6):880-2.

[62] Weber, R., et al., *Liver-related deaths in persons infected with the human immunodeficiency virus: the D:A:D study.* Arch Intern Med, 2006. 166(15):1632-41.

[63] Sherman, K.E., *Treatment of hepatitis C virus and human immunodeficiency virus co-infection.* Clin Gastroenterol Hepatol, 2005. 3(10 Suppl 2):S118-21.

[64] Torriani, F.J., et al., *Peginterferon Alfa-2a plus ribavirin for chronic hepatitis C virus infection in HIV-infected patients.* N Engl J Med, 2004. 351(5):438-50.

[65] Opravil, M., et al., *The dose-response relationship of peginterferon alfa-2a and ribavirin in the treatment of patients coinfected with HIV-HCV.* HIV Clin Trials, 2012. 13(1):33-45.

[66] Benhamou, Y., et al., *Factors affecting liver fibrosis in human immunodeficiency virus-and hepatitis C virus-coinfected patients: impact of protease inhibitor therapy.* Hepatology, 2001. 34(2):283-7.

[67] Deng, A., et al., *Human immunodeficiency virus type 1 Vpr increases hepatitis C virus RNA replication in cell culture.* Virus Res, 2014. 184:93-102.

[68] Di Martino, V., et al., *The influence of human immunodeficiency virus coinfection on chronic hepatitis C in injection drug users: a long-term retrospective cohort study.* Hepatology, 2001. 34(6):1193-9.

[69] Chen, E.Y., et al., *Knowledge and attitudes about hepatitis C virus (HCV) infection and its treatment in HCV mono-infected and HCV/HIV co-infected adults.* J Viral Hepat, 2013. 20(10):708-14.

[70] Karageorgopoulos, D.E., et al., *Drug interactions between antiretrovirals and new or emerging direct-acting antivirals in HIV/hepatitis C virus coinfection.* Curr Opin Infect Dis, 2014. 27(1):36-45.

[71] Sulkowski, M.S., et al., *Combination therapy with telaprevir for chronic hepatitis C virus genotype 1 infection in patients with HIV: a randomized trial.* Ann Intern Med, 2013. 159(2):86-96.

[72] Beste, L.A., P.K. Green, and G.N. Ioannou, *Boceprevir and telaprevir-based regimens for the treatment of hepatitis C virus in HIV/HCV coinfected patients.* Eur J Gastroenterol Hepatol, 2015. 27(2):123-9.

[73] Montes, M., et al., *Telaprevir combination therapy in HCV/HIV co-infected patients (INSIGHT study): sustained virologic response at 12 weeks final analysis.* J Int AIDS Soc, 2014. 17(4 Suppl 3):19626.

[74] Osinusi, A., et al., *Re-treatment of chronic hepatitis C virus genotype 1 infection after relapse: an open-label pilot study.* Ann Intern Med, 2014. 161(9):634-8.

[75] Sulkowski, M.S., et al., *Sofosbuvir and ribavirin for hepatitis C in patients with HIV coinfection.* JAMA, 2014. 312(4):353-61.

[76] Molina, J.M., et al., *Sofosbuvir plus ribavirin for treatment of hepatitis C virus in patients co-infected with HIV (PHOTON-2): a multicentre, open-label, non-randomised, phase 3 study.* Lancet, 2015.

[77] Berenguer, M., *Natural history of recurrent hepatitis C.* Liver Transpl, 2002. 8(10 Suppl 1):S14-8.

[78] Busuttil, R.W., et al., *Analysis of long-term outcomes of 3200 liver transplantations over two decades: a single-center experience.* Ann Surg, 2005. 241(6):905-16; discussion 916-8.

[79] Forman, L.M., et al., *The association between hepatitis C infection and survival after orthotopic liver transplantation.* Gastroenterology, 2002. 122(4):889-96.

[80] Cameron, A.M., et al., *Effect of nonviral factors on hepatitis C recurrence after liver transplantation.* Ann Surg, 2006. 244(4):563-71.

[81] Briceño, J., et al., *Impact of donor graft steatosis on overall outcome and viral recurrence after liver transplantation for hepatitis C virus cirrhosis.* Liver Transpl, 2009. 15(1):37-48.

[82] Prieto, M., et al., *High incidence of allograft cirrhosis in hepatitis C virus genotype 1b infection following transplantation: relationship with rejection episodes.* Hepatology, 1999. 29(1):250-6.

[83] Firpi, R.J., et al., *CC genotype donors for the interleukin-28B single nucleotide polymorphism are associated with better outcomes in hepatitis C after liver transplant.* Liver Int, 2013. 33(1):72-8.

[84] Shiffman, M.L., et al., *Histologic recurrence of chronic hepatitis C virus in patients after living donor and deceased donor liver transplantation.* Liver Transpl, 2004. 10(10):1248-55.

[85] Akamatsu, N. and Y. Sugawara, *Liver transplantation and hepatitis C.* Int J Hepatol, 2012. 2012:686135.

[86] Biggins, S.W., et al., *Differential effects of donor and recipient IL28B and DDX58 SNPs on severity of HCV after liver transplantation.* J Hepatol, 2013. 58(5):969-76.

[87] Féray, C., et al., *Influence of the genotypes of hepatitis C virus on the severity of recurrent liver disease after liver transplantation.* Gastroenterology, 1995. 108(4):1088-96.

[88] Verna, E.C., et al., *High post-transplant virological response in hepatitis C virus infected patients treated with pretransplant protease inhibitor-based triple therapy.* Liver Int, 2014.

[89] Carrión, J.A., et al., *Efficacy of antiviral therapy on hepatitis C recurrence after liver transplantation: a randomized controlled study.* Gastroenterology, 2007. 132(5):1746-56.

[90] Bzowej, N., et al., *PHOENIX: a randomized controlled trial of peginterferon alfa-2a plus ribavirin as a prophylactic treatment after liver transplantation for hepatitis C virus.* Liver Transpl, 2011. 17(5):528-38.

[91] Burton, J.R., et al., *A US multicenter study of hepatitis C treatment of liver transplant recipients with protease-inhibitor triple therapy.* J Hepatol, 2014. 61(3):508-14.

[92] Charlton, M., et al., *Sofosbuvir and ribavirin for treatment of compensated recurrent hepatitis C virus infection after liver transplantation.* Gastroenterology, 2015. 148(1):108-17.

[93] Brown, R., et al., *Safety and efficacy of new DAA-based therapy for hepatitis C post-transplant: interval results from HCV-TARGET longitudinal, observational study.* Program and abstracts of the 65th Annual Meeting of the American Association for the Study of Liver Diseases, Nov 2014. 60 Supplement 1.

[94] Reddy, K.R., et al., *Ledipasvir/sofosbuvir with ribavirin for the treatment of HCV in patients with post transplant recurrence: pre- liminary results of a prospective, multicenter*

study. Program and abstracts of the 65th Annual Meeting of the American Association for the Study of Liver Diseases, Nov 2014. 60 Supplement 1.

[95] Kwo, P.Y., et al., *An interferon-free antiviral regimen for HCV after liver transplantation.* N Engl J Med, 2014. 371(25):2375-82.

[96] Swadling, L., et al., *A human vaccine strategy based on chimpanzee adenoviral and MVA vectors that primes, boosts, and sustains functional HCV-specific T cell memory*. 2014.

Chapter 4

Hepatitis C — Overview and Update in Treatment

Abdullah Saeed Gozai Al-Ghamdi

Additional information is available at the end of the chapter

http://dx.doi.org/10.5772/60949

Abstract

Hepatitis C virus (HCV) infection is one of the main causes of chronic liver disease worldwide, making it a major public health issue. The World Health Organization (WHO) estimates a worldwide prevalence of 3%. Each year, three to four million people are newly diagnosed with HCV, and it remains endemic in many countries of the world. According to the WHO, there are at least 21.3 million HCV carriers in Eastern Mediterranean countries, a figure close to the combined number of estimated carriers in the Americas and Europe. The purpose of this chapter is to give an overview and update in treatment of HCV patients by a broad search of published literature on aspect of epidemiology, natural history, risk factors, diagnosis and treatment of HCV, graded on the best available evidence. All that to improve HCV patient care, and to promote and improve the multidisciplinary care required in the treatment of these patients.

Keywords: HCV, hepatitis C treatment, sofosbuvir, Sovaldi, daclatasvir, ledipasvir/sofosbuvir, Harvoni, Viekira Pak, Viekirax, Exviera, simeprevir

1. Introduction

Hepatitis C virus (HCV) infection is one of the main causes of progressive liver disease worldwide, making it a major public health issue. World Health Organization (WHO) estimates indicate that more than 185 million people around the world have been infected with HCV, of whom 350,000 die each year [1].

HCV induces chronic infection in up to 80% of infected individuals. One third of those who become chronically infected are predicted to develop cirrhosis or hepatocellular carcinoma. Despite its high prevalence, most people infected with the virus are unaware of their infection.

The purpose of this chapter is to give an overview on HCV and existing treatments and to outline recent innovations in the treatment of HCV patients. To do this, a broad search of the published literature has been undertaken. The search included epidemiology of HCV, its natural history, the risk factors involved, as well as the diagnosis and treatment of HCV, all of which have been graded on the best available evidence. The ultimate purpose is to improve HCV patient care and to promote and encourage the multidisciplinary care required in the treatment of these patients.

2. Epidemiology

In most countries, surveys undertaken to establish the prevalence of HCV have focused on specific groups of individuals, for example, drug users, those indulging in high-risk sexual behavior, and blood donors who are not representative of the general population. Consequently, global estimates of HCV prevalence in the year 2008 are still not accurate [2].

Overall, the available data suggest that 130-170 million individuals are infected with HCV (approximately 2.2-3.0%) worldwide, with its highest prevalence occurring in Eastern Mediterranean and African regions [2,3].

Previously undertaken analyses on global, regional, and country levels have mostly failed to estimate the correct HCV disease burden with studies based on age distribution and active infection. Most country-level studies have been carried out on the adult population; however, when these estimates were applied to a country's entire population, the disease burden was probably overestimated. In addition, studies focused on anti-HCV (antibody positive) testing overestimated the disease burden because they often included those subjects who have been cured, either spontaneously or after treatment [4].

Globally, genotype 1 (G1) has been found to account for 46% of all anti-HCV infections among adults, making it the most common, followed by G3 (22%), G2 (13%), G4 (13%), G6 (2%), and G5 (1%). Undefined or combination genotypes accounted for 3% of total HCV infections [4]. Genotype 1b was the most common subtype, accounting for 22% of all infections. However, significant regional, country, and local variations were found to exist. Infections in North America, Latin America, and Europe were predominately G1 (62-71%), with G1b accounting for 26%, 39%, and 50% of all cases, respectively. North Africa and the Middle East had a large G4 population (71%), which was attributable to the high prevalence of G4 in Egypt. When Egypt was excluded, genotype 4 accounted for 34% of all infections, and the genotype distribution of this region was dominated by G1 (46%). Asia was predominately G3 (39%) followed by G1 (36%), largely driven by the HCV infections in India and Pakistan. G1b accounted for 25% of all infections in this region. In Australasia, G1 dominated (53%), followed by G3 (39%). G1b was present in 16% of cases [4].

3. Virology

The hepatitis C virus is a hepatotropic RNA virus of the genus *Hepacivirus* in the Flaviviridae family, originally cloned in 1989 as the causative agent of non-A, non-B hepatitis [5,6,7]. HCV is a positive-sense, single-stranded enveloped RNA virus approximately 9600 nucleotides in length. Approximately 10^{12} viral particles are generated daily in chronically HCV-infected patients [5,8]. The genome is organized to include nontranslated RNA segments (NTRs) at 5 and 3 ends and a single large open reading frame (ORF) encoding a giant 327 kDa polyprotein that is processed by cellular and virally encoded proteases into three structural proteins (core, E1, E2) and seven nonstructural proteins (p7, NS2, NS3, NS4A, NS4B, NS5A, and NS5B) [9].

The HCV 5 NTR contains 341 nucleotides located upstream of the coding region and is composed of four domains (numbered I to IV) with highly structured RNA elements, including numerous stem loops and a pseudoknot. The 5 NTR also contains the internal ribosome entry site (IRES), which initiates the cap-independent translation of HCV genome into a single polyprotein by recruiting both viral proteins and cellular proteins such as eukaryotic initiation factors (eIF) 2 and 3 [5].

The core protein is the viral capsid protein with a length of 191 amino acids (p21c). It can be further cleaved to generate a smaller 179-amino-acid core protein (p19c). The core protein has numerous functionalities involving RNA binding, immune modulation, cell signaling, oncogenic potential, and autophagy [5,9,10]. E1 and E2 are the two viral envelope proteins that surround the viral particles. p7 contains two transmembrane domains and is required for viral assembly and release. NS2 is the viral autoprotease that likely contains at least four transmembrane domains and plays a key role in viral assembly, mediating the cleavage between NS2 and NS3 [5,9,11,12]. NS3 protease plays a critical role in HCV processing by cleaving downstream of NS3 at four sites (between NS3/4A, NS4A/4B, NS4B/NS5A, and NS5A/NS5B) [5,9]. NS4A is a cofactor for the NS3 protease, and NS5B is the viral RNA polymerase. The functions of NS4B and NS5A are not totally clear, but they are probably involved in viral RNA replication and pathogenesis. All of these HCV proteins are believed to form replication complexes on intracellular membranes for either viral morphogenesis or RNA replication [5,9,13-15].

4. Natural history and clinical presentation

Hepatitis C is a heterogeneous disease with considerable morbidity and mortality rates. More than 80% of infected individuals develop chronic infection; the remaining 10-20% develop spontaneous clearance with natural immunity. The acute infection has an incubation period of 7 weeks (range, 4-20 weeks) and is symptomatic in only 20% of patients and rarely severely icteric. Serum aminotransferase levels generally increase to more than 10 times the normal range and go back to normal once the disease symptoms resolve themselves. HCV antibodies usually develop at the time of onset of symptoms. HCV RNA appears even earlier, during the incubation period, with an increase in titer at the time of the manifestation of symptoms, and then disappears once the disease disappears. Once acute HCV infection has established itself, around 85% of patients develop chronic infection, which is generally asymptomatic. In these patients, HCV RNA remains present and in approximately 75% of patients, alanine aminotransferases (ALT), and aspartate aminotransferases (AST) remain elevated at more than 1.5 times the upper normal limit. The course of chronic hepatitis C is variable, with vague, intermittent, and nonspecific symptoms of chronic fatigue and malaise, which usually present in less than 20% of patients. Extrahepatic manifestations of HCV, including glomerulonephritis and cryoglobulinemia, can develop in a small percentage of patients. The development of progressive liver injury, fibrosis, and cirrhosis can occur in 20% to 30% of chronically infected patients over a period of 20-30 years. In patients presenting with chronic hepatitis C, fibrosis progression is extremely variable over time and can be partially predicted based on the age of the patient at infection, disease duration, liver histologic activity and stage of fibrosis, and ALT profile. However, it is often difficult to predict clinical outcomes in individual cases. In patients who have developed cirrhosis, the 5-year risk of decompensation is between 15% and 20% and that of hepatocellular carcinoma around 10%. The relationship between virus load, HCV genotype, quasi-species variability, and progression of liver disease is controversial. Acquired infection after age 40 years, being male, excessive alcohol consumption, hepatitis B virus (HBV) or HIV coinfection, steatosis, and immunosuppressed state have all been identified as cofactors associated with progression of fibrosis and development of cirrhosis. Once cirrhosis develops, symptoms are more common, and the signs of end-stage liver disease can appear, manifesting themselves as jaundice, weakness, wasting, and gastrointestinal bleeding. The incidence of developing hepatocellular carcinoma is 2-5% per year in patients with hepatitis C-related cirrhosis. Thus, this important liver disease has protean manifestations but is often insidious and can often lead to end-stage liver disease that needs liver transplantation, despite the presence of few overt symptoms and signs of illness [16-20].

5. Risk factors

The risk factors for the transmission of HCV infection vary substantially between countries and geographic regions. HCV is spread primarily by contact with blood and blood products. With the introduction in 1991 of routine blood screening for HCV antibodies and improvements in the test in mid-1992, transfusion-related hepatitis C has virtually disappeared. Illicit use of injectable drugs is currently the main source of HCV infections in most developed countries (e.g., Western Europe, US) and is becoming a major source of infection in transitional economy and developing countries, accounting for 40% or more of those infected. Of the estimated 16 million people in 148 countries who actively inject drugs, 10 million are infected with HCV [2,21,22]. In developing and transitional economy countries, the nosocomial transmission of new HCV infections is a major problem because of the reuse of contaminated or inadequately sterilized syringes and needles used in medical, paramedical, and dental procedures, with an estimated 2.3-4.7 million new infections occurring each year [2,23-25]. In patients on chronic hemodialysis, overall, the current prevalence of HCV is below 5% in most of Northern Europe, around 10% in most of Southern Europe and the US, but between 10%

and 50% and up to 70% in many parts of the developing world, including many Asian, Latin American, and North African countries. It is important to emphasize that the prevalence of HCV is highly variable from unit to unit within the same country, with recent reports from some dialysis units in the US reporting a prevalence above 20% [26]. The risk of transmission of HCV from a mother to her child occurs in 4-8% of births to women with HCV infection and in 17-25% of births to women with HIV and HCV coinfection. The risk posed to the infant from breastfeeding is negligible, and nonsexual intrafamilial transmission is very rare [27,28]. The risk of heterosexual transmission is low, while recent data indicate that promiscuous male homosexual activity is related to HCV infection [29]. Folk medicine practices, including acupuncture and ritual scarification, as well as body piercing, tattooing, and commercial barbering are potential modes for transmission of HCV infection when performed without appropriate infection control measures [30,31].

6. Laboratory testing

6.1. Serologic and molecular assays

The test for anti-HCV is usually performed in the presence of an elevated ALT level and a positive history of risk factors for HCV infection, or physical findings suggest the presence of chronic liver disease. WHO recommends that HCV serology testing be performed on individuals who are part of a population with high HCV seroprevalence or who have a history of HCV risk exposure and/or behavior rather than at the time of presentation with symptomatic disease. The application of this recommendation will require taking into consideration which populations meet these criteria. In some countries with a high seroprevalence of HCV or a low level of infection control, HCV testing might be recommended for the general population. Clearly, this would have significant resource implications [1]. Diagnosis of HCV infection is based on the detection of anti-HCV antibodies by enzyme immunoassay and the detection of HCV RNA by a sensitive molecular method, ideally a real-time PCR assay. These assays have no role in the assessment of disease severity or its prognosis [32,33]. Genotyping is useful in epidemiological studies, and also in clinical management, for predicting the likelihood of response and determining the optimal duration of therapy. Several commercial assays are available to determine HCV genotypes using direct sequence analysis of the 5 noncoding region, which includes Trugene 5 NC HCV genotyping kit, reverse hybridization analysis using genotype-specific oligonucleotide probes located in the 5 noncoding region, INNO-LiPa HCV II, and Versant HCV Genotyping Assay 2.0 [34,35].

6.2. Defining disease severity

Laboratory tests that are commonly obtained following the initial diagnosis of chronic hepatitis C include liver enzymes and function tests, a complete blood cell count, tests for coinfection with HBV or HIV, tests for immunoglobulin G antibody to hepatitis A virus (anti-HAV) to determine if immunity is present or if vaccination is recommended, and antinuclear antibody to exclude coexistent autoimmune hepatitis.

Elevated blood levels of liver enzymes ALT and AST occur when the membrane of the liver cells is damaged and liver enzymes leak into the blood stream, thus indicating ongoing liver injury. The degree of elevation of liver enzymes present in the blood correlates with the severity of liver cell injury. However, blood levels of liver enzymes do not correlate with the degree or severity of hepatic fibrosis. The important tests that reflect liver synthetic function are serum bilirubin, albumin, and international normalized ratio (INR). Abnormal serum albumin, bilirubin, or prothrombin time may be seen in the setting of impaired hepatic synthetic function. Some models used to evaluate liver disease severity are helpful for the assessment of liver function, for example, the model for end-stage liver disease (MELD). The MELD score was adopted by UNOS in 2002 for use in deceased donor liver allocation for adults with cirrhosis. MELD is a prospectively developed and validated chronic liver disease severity scoring system that uses a patient's laboratory values for serum bilirubin, serum creatinine, and INR to predict a 3-month survival [36]. The MELD equation that is currently used by UNOS for prioritizing allocation of deceased donor livers for transplantation is as follows: MELD = 3.8*$\log_e$(serum bilirubin [mg/dL]) + 11.2*$\log_e$(INR) + 9.6*$\log_e$(serum creatinine [mg/dL]) + 6.4. Patients with the combination of serum creatinine ≤1 mg/dl, serum bilirubin ≤1 mg/dl, and INR ≤1 will receive the minimum score of 6 MELD points. In addition, UNOS has set an upper limit for the MELD score at 40 points. However, there is no need to go through the above time-consuming equation because several online tools are available for calculating the MELD score [37-39].

7. Tests of fibrosis

7.1. Noninvasive laboratory tests

Noninvasive tests of hepatic fibrosis are used for the staging of fibrosis in patients with chronic liver disease. The tests are often used to differentiate patients with significant fibrosis (F2 to F4) from those with minimal or no fibrosis (F0 to F1). There are four commercial serum marker systems that have been validated: FibroTest/FibroSure (marketed in the United States by LabCorp), Hepascore (Quest Diagnostics), FibroSpect (Prometheus Corp), and the European Liver Fibrosis Study Group panel (not available in the United States). In addition, the aspartate aminotransferase-to-platelet ratio (APRI) has also been studied. The APRI has the advantage of being easily calculated using data available from routine laboratory tests.

All the serum tests have limitations: (a) they typically reflect the rate of matrix turnover, not deposition, and thus tend to be more elevated when there is high inflammatory activity. By contrast, extensive matrix deposition can go undetected if there is minimal inflammation. (b) None of the markers are liver specific, and concurrent sites of inflammation may contribute to serum levels. (c) Serum levels are affected by clearance rates, which may be impaired due to either sinusoidal endothelial cell dysfunction or impaired biliary excretion. (d) They are surrogates, not biomarkers [40].

7.2. Elastogram (Fibroscan)

Fibroscan can quantify fibrosis in the liver by means of elastography. Tissue elasticity is acquired through pulse-echo ultrasound, measuring shear wave velocity, the S-wave. The wave travels faster in less elastic and stiff livers. Results of liver elasticity are expressed in kilopascals (kPa). The scan can be performed easily; it is inexpensive and produces no side effects. The position of the patient is similar to when performing a liver biopsy, that is, on the back, with the right hand under the head. Patients only feel the probe pressure in the intercostal space without anticipated pain. It is possible to measure liver elasticity from different angles in the right as well as the left lobe. A liver stiffness measurement using Fibroscan is reproducible and independent of the operator, and explores a volume of liver parenchyma, which can be approximated to a cylinder of 1 cm in diameter and 4 cm in length. This volume is 100 times larger than the biopsy specimen volume and is thus much more representative of the entire hepatic parenchyma. Some extensive studies have demonstrated that the measurement of liver stiffness with Fibroscan is a good alternative for liver biopsy. The amount of fibrosis can be quantified very easily and reliably and is feasible in more than 95% of the patients. Obesity, ascites, and narrow intercostal spaces are physiological boundaries that can hamper the accuracy of the test. Acute hepatitis and liver congestion as in cardiac failure can cause false high scores, and they need to be ruled out before carrying out Fibroscan. Sometimes it may be virtually impossible to take measurements in such patients [41, 42]. Fibroscan value ranged from 2.4 to 75.5 kPa with a cutoff value of 7.1 kPa for $F \geq 2$, 9.5 kPa for $F \geq 3$, and 12.5 kPa for $F = 4$ (according to Metavir histological classification system) [41, 43]. One of the studies comparing elastography to histological examination on 327 patients concluded that liver stiffness measurements and fibrosis grades correlated well, with increasing reliability in more extensive fibrosis ($F \geq 3$) or cirrhosis. It was impossible to determine a cutoff value to differentiate between F0 and F1 by Fibroscan [41,44].

7.3. Liver biopsy

Percutaneous liver biopsy is the gold standard for grading and staging of liver disease, which can help to determine the extent of progress of hepatic fibrosis and inflammation. It is important in clinical practice, where it may reflect the severity of liver disease and predict response to treatment. Liver biopsy is an invasive procedure associated with discomfort and, in rare cases, with serious complications. The accuracy of liver biopsy is limited and prone to sampling error and interpretational variability. Although this procedure continues to be recommended, current practice is changing for two main reasons: first, treatment is being shown to be more effective, and second, biochemical tests, serological tests, and elastograms can all provide a great deal of information on disease progression. Pathologists can increase the importance and utility of liver biopsy in chronic hepatitis C, providing information not only on the stage of fibrosis and necro-inflammatory activity but also on the grade of steatosis and iron accumulation, which are implicated in disease progression. Moreover, other diseases, such as steatohepatitis and hereditary hemochromatosis can be identified by liver biopsy. Nevertheless, the use of serological and radiological tests will reduce the indications for liver biopsy [45].

8. Hepatitis C treatments

The ultimate goal of treatment in patients with chronic HCV is to eradicate HCV RNA, which is associated with decreases in all-cause mortality, liver-related death, need for liver transplantation, hepatocellular carcinoma rates, and liver-related complications.

Since interferon-alpha (IFN-α) was first introduced for treatment of non-A, non-B hepatitis 1990, therapy for patients with chronic HCV has improved dramatically. Sustained virological response rates (SVRs) have increased from 5% to 10% with standard interferon therapy, to over 40% when standard interferon is combined with ribavirin. The modification of interferon (pegylation) to improve its pharmacokinetics has further increased rates of SVR. Two types of pegylated interferon, pegylated interferon α2a and pegylated interferon α2b,which differ in their pharmacokinetics and chemical properties, were approved by the FDA in 2001. Treatment with combined pegylated interferon and ribavirin may result in SVR in 42% to 52% of genotype 1 infected patients, 70% to 80% of genotype 2 or 3 infected patients, and 54-68% of genotype 4 infected patients [46,47].

The landscape of treatment for HCV infection has evolved substantially since the introduction of highly effective HCV protease inhibitor therapies, namely, boceprevir and telaprevir, in 2011. Both drugs were approved as directly acting antiviral treatments for use in HCV genotype 1 infection, in combination with pegylated interferon and ribavirin. These NS3/4A protease inhibitors have been shown to substantially increase rates of SVR to 59-75% in both treatment-naive and previously treated patients, compared with dual therapy [48-52]. Although their development was a major advance, both agents are associated with significant toxicity, numerous drug-drug interactions, and low response rates in those patients with cirrhosis and nonresponders to previous treatment. In addition, boceprevir and telaprevir required the addition of pegylated interferon and ribavirin for 24 to 48 weeks, which markedly increased the overall cost of therapy, and are associated with the emergence of resistance-associated variants in the majority of patients who fail treatment [53].

In 2013 and 2014, the FDA approved new direct acting antiviral treatments, including second generation protease inhibitors, NS5A inhibitors, and NS5B RNA-dependent RNA polymerase inhibitors with HCV eradication rates of >95%.

The eradication of HCV RNA is predicted by the achievement of SVR and defined by the absence of HCV RNA by polymerase chain reaction three to 6 months after stopping treatment. An SVR is associated with a 99% chance of being HCV RNA negative during long-term follow-up and can therefore be considered an indication of a cure of the HCV infection. With the growing availability of highly effective interferon-free regimens for HCV infection, a curative all-oral treatment is becoming a possibility for the vast majority of patients. The second-generation protease inhibitors that have been approved for treatment of HCV and are available in the market are simeprevir, sofosbuvir, ledipasvir/sofosbuvir, daclatasvir, and the combination of ombitasvir-paritaprevir-ritonavir and dasabuvir. Trials are still ongoing on other new products, many of which are expected to appear in the near future.

8.1. Simeprevir (Olysio®, Janssen Therapeutics)

This is the first available second-generation protease inhibitor (NS3/4A protease inhibitor) indicated for the treatment of chronic hepatitis C infection as a component of a combination antiviral treatment regimen [54]. Simeprevir is available in 150 mg capsules to be taken orally once daily with food. The elimination of simeprevir is by the liver, and no dose adjustment is required in the setting of renal impairment [55]. Simeprevir is not recommended in patients with hepatic impairment Child-Pugh Class B and C because of two- to five-fold increases in exposure. In general, simeprevir is well tolerated. Its most common adverse effects are rash (including a potentially serious photosensitivity reaction), pruritus, and nausea. The photosensitivity reaction that related to simeprevir usually occurs during the first 4 weeks of therapy but can develop at any time on treatment. Patients taking simeprevir may experience transient increases in serum bilirubin levels that peak at week 2 of treatment, but these are typically mild in severity and not associated with elevated hepatic aminotransferase levels [56,57]. The coadministration of simeprevir with substances that are moderate or strong inducers or inhibitors of cytochrome P450 3A (CYP3A) is not recommended, as this may lead to significantly lower or higher exposure of simeprevir, respectively, which may result in reduced therapeutic effect or adverse reactions. A number of compounds are contraindicated in patients receiving simeprevir, including the following:

1. Antibiotics (erythromycin, clarithromycin, telithromycin, rifampin, rifabutin, rifapentine)
2. Systemically administered antifungals (itroconazole, ketoconazole, voriconazole, posaconazole, fluconazole)
3. Anticonvulsants (carbamazepine, oxcarbazepine, phenobarbital, phenytoin)
4. Systemically administered dexamethasone
5. Herbal products (milk thistle, St. John's wort)
6. A number of antiretroviral drugs, including cobicistat-based regimens, efavirenz, delavirdine, etravirine, nevirapine, ritonavir, and any HIV protease inhibitor, boosted or not by ritonavir.

Simeprevir is safe in patients using immunosuppressants, such as cyclosporine and tacrolimus, with no dose adjustment, and safe in those using lamivudine, emtricitabine, tenofovir, abacavir, raltegravir, maraviroc, and rilpivirine. The dose of simeprevir needs adjustment with some antiarrhythmics, warfarin, HMG Co-A reductase inhibitors, sedative/anxiolytics, and calcium channel blockers [58-64].

8.2. Sofosbuvir (Sovaldi®, Gilead Sciences)

This is an HCV nucleotide analog NS5B polymerase inhibitor indicated for the treatment of chronic hepatitis C infection as a component of a combination antiviral treatment regimen. Sofosbuvir is available as a 400-mg tablet. The recommended dose of sofosbuvir is 400 mg taken orally once daily, with or without food, regardless of the patient's genotype or prior hepatitis C treatment experience. No dose adjustment is needed for mild-to-moderate renal impairment or with mild, moderate, or severe hepatic impairment. Currently, no dose recommendation can be given for patients with severe renal impairment (estimated glomerular filtration rate <30 ml/min) or with end-stage renal disease due to higher exposures (up to 20-fold) of the predominant sofosbuvir metabolite. Sofosbuvir has pan-genotypic HCV activity and is effective in treatment-naive, treatment-experienced, and HIV-coinfected patients with compensated cirrhosis, and in patients with hepatocellular carcinoma meeting Milan criteria awaiting liver transplantation. Sofosbuvir has been very well tolerated in clinical trials. The most common adverse effects (≥20%) observed with sofosbuvir, when used in combination with ribavirin, have been fatigue and headaches. The most common adverse events (≥20%) observed in combination with pegylated IFN-α and ribavirin were fatigue, headaches, nausea, insomnia, and anemia. Drugs that are potent P-glycoprotein (P-gp) inducers significantly decrease sofosbuvir plasma concentrations and may lead to a reduced therapeutic effect. Thus, sofosbuvir should not be administered with other known inducers of P-gp, such as rifampin, carbamazepine, phenytoin or St. John's wort [62,65-77].

8.3. Ledipasvir-sofosbuvir (Harvoni®, Gilead Sciences)

The nucleotide polymerase inhibitor sofosbuvir (400 mg) has been combined with the NS5A inhibitor ledipasvir (90 mg) in a single tablet regimen (SOF/LDV) administered once daily. The combination of ledipasvir-sofosbuvir has primarily been studied as an all-oral (interferon-free) combination regimen in treatment-naive and treatment-experienced patients with genotype 1 chronic HCV infection. For patients with mild to moderate renal impairment, no dosage adjustment of ledipasvir/sofosbuvir is recommended. Severe renal impairment (estimated glomerular filtration rate <30 mL/min) does not substantially affect the pharmacokinetics of ledipasvir, but because levels of sofosbuvir and its metabolite accumulate in the setting of severe renal impairment, the combination should not be used in such settings pending further data. Thus, no dosage recommendation has been given for patients with severe renal impairment or end-stage renal disease requiring dialysis. Available data from clinical trials have shown that the combination of ledipasvir and sofosbuvir has been very well tolerated. The most commonly reported adverse effects are fatigue and headaches. Ledipasvir, like sofosbuvir, is a substrate of the P-gp drug transporter, so drugs that are potent intestinal P-gp inducers may decrease ledipasvir levels. Thus, the coadministration of ledipasvir-sofosbuvir is not recommended with rifampin, St. John's wort, carbamazepine, phenytoin, phenobarbital, oxcarbazepine, or tipranavir/ritonavir. In addition, ledipasvir is an inhibitor of P-gp and may increase absorption of P-gp substrates. The coadministration of ledipasvir with tenofovir results in increased levels of tenofovir, particularly in the presence of other boosting agents. Until further data are available, ledipasvir-sofosbuvir should not be used with the combination of elvitegravir, cobicistat, emtricitabine, and tenofovir, and should only be used cautiously with regimens that contain tenofovir and a ritonavir-boosted protease inhibitor [73,78-83].

8.4. Ombitasvir-Paritaprevir-Ritonavir and Dasabuvir (Viekira Pak®, AbbVie Inc)

The Viekira Pak is an all-oral regimen comprised of four medications: ombitasvir, paritaprevir, ritonavir, and dasabuvir. This regimen can be used with or without ribavirin. In the Viekira

http://dx.doi.org/10.5772/60949

Pak, ombitasvir, paritaprevir, and ritonavir (Viekirax®) are combined as a fixed-dose tablet and the dasabuvir (Exviera®) is a separate tablet. Ombitasvir, paritaprevir, and dasabuvir are direct-acting antivirals (DAAs) that directly interfere with HCV replication. Ombitasvir is an NS5A inhibitor with potent pan-genotypic picomolar antiviral activity, paritaprevir is an inhibitor of the NS3/4A serine protease, and dasabuvir is a nonnucleoside NS5B polymerase inhibitor. Ritonavir is a CYP3A inhibitor, and it boosts the blood levels of paritaprevir. Paritaprevir (150 mg), ritonavir (100 mg), and ombitasvir (25 mg) are coformulated in a single tablet taken as two tablets once daily. This tablet is combined with dasabuvir (250 mg) taken as one tablet twice daily. The regimen ombitasvir-paritaprevir-ritonavir plus dasabuvir is FDA approved for the treatment of chronic hepatitis C genotype 1, including those with compensated cirrhosis. The regimen ombitasvir-paritaprevir-ritonavir plus dasabuvir, with or without ribavirin, has primarily been studied as an all-oral (interferon-free) regimen in treatment-naive and treatment-experienced patients with genotype 1a or 1b chronic HCV infection, including those with compensated cirrhosis, HIV coinfection, and after receipt of liver transplantation. For patients with mild hepatic impairment (Child-Pugh A), no dosage adjustment is required for ombitasvir-paritaprevir-ritonavir and dasabuvir; however, this regimen is not recommended in patients with moderate hepatic impairment (Child-Pugh B) and is contraindicated with severe hepatic impairment (Child-Pugh C). For patients with mild, moderate, or severe renal insufficiency, no dosing adjustment is required for the regimen ombitasvir-paritaprevir-ritonavir and dasabuvir; this regimen, however, has not been adequately studied in patients with end-stage renal disease on dialysis. Available data from clinical trials have demonstrated excellent tolerance with the ombitasvir-paritaprevir-ritonavir and dasabuvir regimen. The most common (greater than 10%) adverse effects observed in clinical trials when used without ribavirin have been fatigue, nausea, pruritus, other skin reactions, insomnia, and asthenia. The concomitant use of ombitasvir-paritaprevir-ritonavir and dasabuvir with ethinyl estradiol-containing medications (e.g., oral contraceptives) can result in significant elevations in hepatic aminotransferase levels; accordingly, patients should discontinue any ethinyl estradiol-containing medications prior to starting ombitasvir-paritaprevir-ritonavir and dasabuvir. The use of ombitasvir-paritaprevir-ritonavir plus dasabuvir can potentially cause significant drug-drug interactions, primarily because of the potent ritonavir inhibition of CYP3A4 enzyme. There are a number of medications contraindicated to use concomitantly with ombitasvir-paritaprevir-ritonavir and dasabuvir, like carbamazepine, phenytoin, phenobarbital, gemfibrozil, rifampin, ergotamine, oral contraceptives containing ethinyl estradiol, lovastatin, simvastatin, sildenafil, orally administered midazolam, and St. John's wort. The efficacy of ombitasvir-paritaprevir-ritonavir plus dasabuvir is not known for patients with prior virologic failure and resistance with treatment that included another NS3/4A inhibitor, NS5A inhibitor, or NS5B inhibitor [84-90].

8.5. Daclatasvir (Daklinza®, Bristol-Myers Squibb)

The European Commission approved daclatasvir, a potent pan-genotypic NS5A replication complex inhibitor (in vitro), at the end of August 2014. Daclatasvir should be administered at the dose of 60 mg (one tablet) once per day. It is well tolerated overall. Dose adjustments are not needed in patients with Child B or C disease. Daclatasvir can be used in combination with other drugs for the treatment of chronic HCV infection genotypes 1, 2, 3, and 4 in adults. Daclatasvir, when used in combination with sofosbuvir, is an all-oral, interferon-free regimen that provided cure rates of more than 95% in clinical trials, including in patients with advanced liver disease, genotype 3, and those who have previously failed treatment with protease inhibitors. Across clinical studies, daclatasvir-based regimens have been generally well tolerated, with low discontinuation rates. The most common adverse effects with daclatasvir when used in combination with other drugs are fatigue, headaches, and nausea. Little information has been released on daclatasvir drug-drug interactions. Daclatasvir is a substrate of CYP34A and a substrate and inhibitor of P-gp. The daclatasvir dose should be adjusted to 30 mg daily in HIV-infected patients receiving atazanavir/ritonavir and to 90 mg daily in those receiving efavirenz. No dose adjustment is needed with tenofovir. No information on other antiretroviral drugs is available yet. No dose adjustments are required with cyclosporine or tacrolimus. Total daclatasvir AUC is decreased by 40% and 43% in patients with mild or moderate liver impairment, respectively. However, the unbound pharmacologically active fraction is unchanged; thus, dose adjustment is not needed in patients with liver impairment [77,91,92].

The direct acting antiviral treatment is usually used in combination for HCV treatment according to genotypes and stage of liver disease, and the patient is either naive or has previous experience of treatment.

The following recommendations can be used for treatment of HCV according to genotypes with a high response rate (>90%):

1. HCV genotype 1 [91,93]

   a. Daily fixed-dose combination of ledipasvir (90 mg)/sofosbuvir (400 mg) for 12 weeks. The addition of daily weight-based ribavirin (1000 mg [<75 kg] to 1200 mg [>75 kg]) is recommended in patients with cirrhosis. The duration of treatment extended to 24 weeks in patients with contraindications to ribavirin.

   b. Daily fixed-dose combination of paritaprevir (150 mg)/ritonavir (100 mg)/ombitasvir (25 mg) plus twice-daily dosed dasabuvir (250 mg) and daily weight-based ribavirin (1000 mg [<75 kg] to 1200 mg [>75 kg]) for 12 weeks (no cirrhosis) or 24 weeks (cirrhosis) for treatment of both naive and prior pegylated interferon and ribavirin treatment failure, in patients with HCV genotype 1a infection.

   c. Daily fixed-dose combination of paritaprevir (150 mg)/ritonavir (100 mg)/ombitasvir (25 mg) plus twice-daily dosed dasabuvir (250 mg) for 12 weeks for treatment-naive and prior pegylated interferon and ribavirin treatment failure, in patients with HCV genotype 1b infection. The addition of daily weight-based ribavirin (1000 mg [<75 kg] to 1200 mg [>75 kg]) is recommended in patients with cirrhosis.

   d. Daily fixed-dose combination of daclatasvir 60 mg and sofosbuvir 400 mg for 12 weeks. The addition of daily weight-based ribavirin (1000 mg [<75 kg] to 1200 mg [>75 kg]) is recommended in patients with cirrhosis. The duration of treatment extended to 24 weeks in patients with contraindications to ribavirin.

e. Daily sofosbuvir (400 mg) plus simeprevir (150 mg) for 12 weeks. The addition of daily weight-based ribavirin (1000 mg [<75 kg] to 1200 mg [>75 kg]) is recommended in patients with cirrhosis. The duration of treatment extended to 24 weeks in patients with contraindications to ribavirin.

f. Daily sofosbuvir (400 mg) and weight-based ribavirin (1000 mg [<75 kg] to 1200 mg [>75 kg]) plus weekly pegylated interferon for 12 weeks.

2. HCV genotype 2 [91,93]

a. Daily sofosbuvir (400 mg) and weight-based ribavirin (1000 mg [<75 kg] to 1200 mg [>75 kg]) for 12 weeks; extending duration of treatment to 16-20 weeks is recommended in patients with cirrhosis and those in whom prior pegylated interferon and ribavirin treatment has failed.

b. Daily sofosbuvir (400 mg) and daclatasvir (60 mg) for 12 weeks in cirrhotic or treatment-experienced patients.

c. Retreatment with daily sofosbuvir (400 mg) and weight-based ribavirin (1000 mg [<75 kg] to 1200 mg [≥75 kg]) plus weekly pegylated interferon for 12 weeks is an alternative in patients where prior pegylated interferon and ribavirin treatment has failed.

3. HCV genotype 3

When pegylated interferon and ribavirin was the treatment for HCV, the same regimen was administered to all subjects, and patients were defined as easy or difficult to treat according to viral genotype. HCV genotypes 1 and 4 were considered to be difficult to treat, and HCV genotypes 2 and 3 were considered to be easy to treat. The SVR rates in the latter group were above 80% with shorter treatment [94,95]. The availability of interferon-free regimens has confirmed that HCV genotype 2 patients are easy to treat, while the paradigm for HCV genotype 3 patients has been reversed compared to "older, difficult-to-treat" HCV genotype 1 patients. In fact, today, with available direct acting antiviral drugs, patients with HCV genotype 3 are the most difficult to treat patients. In large studies on HCV genotype 3 to assess the effectiveness of 12-16 weeks treatment with sofosbuvir and ribavirin, it has been shown that 12 weeks of therapy in treatment-naive patients resulted in an SVR in 61% and 34% of noncirrhotic and cirrhotic patients, respectively. Moreover, the SVR rates in experienced noncirrhotic patients were 37% at 12 weeks and were increased to 63% in patients with 16 weeks' course [70,67,95]. Extended treatments to 24 weeks of sofosbuvir and ribavirin were evaluated in the valence trial, resulting in an overall SVR rate of 83%. In particular, this was the result of higher SVR rates in treatment-naive (93% and 92% in patients without and with cirrhosis, respectively) and experienced patients without cirrhosis (87%), while rates were lower in experienced (61%) patients with cirrhosis [80,95,96]. The Lonestar-2 study tested treatment with pegylated interferon/sofosbuvir/ribavirin for 12 weeks in treatment-experienced HCV-2 and HCV-3 patients. The SVR in HCV genotype 3 patients was 83% with no difference in relation to baseline cirrhosis (SVR 83% vs. 83%, respectively) [69]. The second study tested a combination of daclatasvir/sofosbuvir, resulting in an SVR of 89% of 18 treatment-naive patients with HCV genotype 3 [97].

The following treatment options with similar efficacy can be used in genotype 3 naive patients and patients in whom prior pegylated interferon and ribavirin treatment has failed [91-93,97]:

a. Daily fixed-dose combination of daclatasvir 60 mg and sofosbuvir 400 mg for 12 weeks in patients without cirrhosis. Daily weight-based ribavirin (1000 mg [<75 kg] to 1200 mg [>75 kg]) is added to regimen to treat naive and treatment-experienced patients with cirrhosis for 24 weeks.

b. Daily sofosbuvir (400 mg) and weight-based ribavirin (1000 mg [<75 kg] to 1200 mg [>75 kg]) for 24 weeks.

c. Daily sofosbuvir (400 mg) and weight-based ribavirin (1000 mg [<75 kg] to 1200 mg [>75 kg]) plus weekly pegylated interferon for 12 weeks is an acceptable regimen for interferon-eligible, treatment-naive patients with HCV genotype 3 infection.

4. HCV genotype 4 [70,91,93,98-101]

- **a.** Daily fixed-dose combination of ledipasvir (90 mg)/sofosbuvir (400 mg) for 12 weeks. The addition of daily weight-based ribavirin (1000 mg [<75 kg] to 1200 mg [>75 kg]) is recommended in patients with cirrhosis. The duration of treatment extended to 24 weeks in patients with contraindications to ribavirin.

- **b.** Daily fixed-dose combination of paritaprevir (150 mg)/ritonavir (100 mg)/ombitasvir (25 mg) and weight-based ribavirin (1000 mg [<75 kg] to 1200 mg [>75 kg]) for 12 weeks for treatment of both naive and prior pegylated interferon and ribavirin treatment failure, and treatment can be extended to 24 weeks in patients with cirrhosis.

- **c.** Daily fixed-dose combination of daclatasvir 60 mg and sofosbuvir 400 mg for 12 weeks. The addition of daily weight-based ribavirin (1000 mg [<75 kg] to 1200 mg [>75 kg]) is recommended in patients with cirrhosis. The duration of treatment extended to 24 weeks in patients with contraindications to ribavirin.

- **d.** Daily sofosbuvir (400 mg) plus simeprevir (150 mg) for 12 weeks. The addition of daily weight-based ribavirin (1000 mg [<75 kg] to 1200 mg [>75 kg]) is recommended in patients with cirrhosis. The duration of treatment extended to 24 weeks in patients with contraindications to ribavirin.

- **e.** Daily sofosbuvir (400 mg) and weight-based ribavirin (1000 mg [<75 kg] to 1200 mg [>75 kg]) plus weekly pegylated interferon for 12 weeks.

5. HCV genotype 5 [91,93]

A few data are available to help guide decision making for patients infected with HCV genotype 5 or 6, but currently the following are the recommendations until more data are available:

- **a.** Daily sofosbuvir (400 mg) and weight-based ribavirin (1000 mg [<75 kg] to 1200 mg [>75 kg]) plus weekly pegylated interferon for 12 weeks

   b. Daily sofosbuvir (400 mg) and weight-based ribavirin (1000 mg [<75 kg] to 1200 mg [>75 kg]) for 24 weeks

   c. Weekly pegylated interferon plus weight-based ribavirin (1000 mg [<75 kg] to 1200 mg [>75 kg]) for 48 weeks is an alternative regimen for interferon-eligible, treatment-naive patients.

6. Genotype 6 [91,93]

   a. Daily fixed-dose combination of ledipasvir (90 mg)/sofosbuvir (400 mg) for 12 weeks

   b. Daily sofosbuvir (400 mg) and weight-based ribavirin (1000 mg [<75 kg] to 1200 mg [>75 kg]) plus weekly pegylated interferon for 12 weeks

   c. Daily sofosbuvir (400 mg) and weight-based ribavirin (1000 mg [<75 kg] to 1200 mg [>75 kg]) for 24 weeks

Due to the very high efficacy and the excellent tolerability of IFN-free regimens, response-guided shortening or prolongation of therapy have not been studied and, indeed, may not be needed to achieve high cure chances in the individual patient. However, given the high costs of direct antiviral drugs, HCV RNA testing during treatment may be helpful for surveillance of compliance and motivation of patients. HCV RNA should be measured at baseline, week 2 (assessment of adherence), week 4, week 12 or 24 (end of treatment), and 12 or 24 weeks after the end of therapy [102].

9. Treatment of special populations with direct acting antiviral regimens

9.1. HIV/HCV-coinfected individuals

Hepatitis C virus (HCV)-related liver disease is a major source of mortality in HIV-infected patients. Approximately one third of all patients with HIV are coinfected with HCV. Patients coinfected with HIV/HCV have shown lower rates of SVR with pegylated-interferon and weight-based ribavirin as well as more rapid progression of fibrosis than those with HCV monoinfection [103]. HIV/HCV-coinfected persons should be treated and retreated the same as persons without HIV infection, after recognizing and managing interactions with antiretroviral medications. Based on AASLD/IDSA/IAS-USA [93], the following precautions should be considered:

a. Antiretroviral treatment interruption in patients with HIV/HCV is not recommended to allow HCV therapy.

b. Fixed-dose combination of ledipasvir (90 mg)/sofosbuvir (400 mg) should not be used with cobicistat and elvitegravir, pending further data.

c. Sofosbuvir or ledipasvir/sofosbuvir should not be used with tipranavir because of the potential of this antiretroviral drug to induce P-gp.

d. Fixed-dose combination of paritaprevir (150 mg)/ritonavir (100 mg)/ombitasvir (25 mg) plus twice-daily dosed dasabuvir (250 mg) should not be used with efavirenz, rilpivirine, darunavir, or ritonavir-boosted lopinavir.

e. Paritaprevir/ritonavir/ombitasvir with or without dasabuvir should not be used in HIV/HCV-coinfected individuals who are not taking antiretroviral therapy.

f. Simeprevir should not be used with efavirenz, etravirine, nevirapine, cobicistat, or any HIV protease inhibitors.

g. Ribavirin should not be used with didanosine, stavudine, or zidovudine.

The management of HIV/HCV patients should take place in collaboration with an HIV practitioner. Special precautions should be taken when prescribing DAAs in patient on AIDS treatment to avoid under- or overdose in such patients as a result of drug-drug interactions. For example, ledipasvir increases tenofovir levels, concomitant use needs to be avoided in patients with CrCl below 60 mL/min. Because potentiation of this effect is expected when tenofovir is used with ritonavir-boosted HIV protease inhibitors, ledipasvir should be avoided with this combination. Paritaprevir/ritonavir/ombitasvir plus dasabuvir should be used with antiretroviral drugs with which it does not have substantial interactions like atazanavir, enfuvirtide, lamivudine, emtricitabine, tenofovir, and raltegravir (and probably dolutegravir) [93].

The dose of ritonavir used for boosting of HIV protease inhibitors may need to be adjusted (or held) when administered with paritaprevir/ritonavir/ombitasvir plus dasabuvir, and then restored when HCV treatment is completed. The HIV protease inhibitor should be administered at the same time as the fixed-dose HCV combination. Simeprevir should only be used with antiretroviral drugs, with which it does not have clinically significant interactions like raltegravir (and probably dolutegravir), rilpivirine, maraviroc, enfuvirtide, tenofovir, emtricitabine, lamivudine, and abacavir [93].

9.2. Patients with decompensated cirrhosis

In patients with Child-Pugh B or C cirrhosis awaiting transplantation, antiviral therapy may be offered on an individual basis in experienced centers, pending the presentation of more data in this population. It is possible that patients with decompensated cirrhosis who are not on a transplant list could benefit from an interferon-free treatment regimen. However, the safety and efficacy of an interferon-free regimen in patients with decompensated cirrhosis not on a transplant waiting list is unknown, and the impact on mortality in this group is not yet established. According to AASLD/IDSA/IAS-USA [93] and EASL recommendations on treatment of hepatitis C 2015 [91], the following medications can be used with high virological response >90%:

a. Decompensated cirrhosis: genotypes 1 and 4

- Daily fixed-dose combination of ledipasvir (90 mg)/sofosbuvir (400 mg) and ribavirin (initial dose of 600 mg, increased as tolerated) for 12 weeks is recommended for patients with decompensated cirrhosis.

- For patients with decompensated cirrhosis and anemia or ribavirin intolerance, daily fixed-dose combination of ledipasvir (90 mg)/sofosbuvir (400 mg) for 24 weeks is recommended.
- For patients with decompensated cirrhosis in whom prior sofosbuvir-based treatment has failed, daily fixed-dose combination of ledipasvir (90 mg)/sofosbuvir (400 mg) and ribavirin (initial dose of 600 mg, increased as tolerated) for 24 weeks is an alternative regimen.
- Daily fixed-dose combination of sofosbuvir (400 mg), ribavirin (initial dose of 600 mg, increased as tolerated), and daclatasvir 60 mg for 12 weeks before liver transplantation is recommended for patients with decompensated cirrhosis.

b. Decompensated cirrhosis: genotypes 2 and 3

- Daily sofosbuvir (400 mg) and weight-based ribavirin (1000 mg [<75 kg] to 1200 mg [>75 kg]) (doses need to be adjusted according to the patient's creatinine clearance rate and hemoglobin level) for up to 48 weeks is recommended for patients with HCV genotype 2 or 3 who have decompensated cirrhosis.

9.3. Patients with HCV recurrence post liver transplantation

Patients with posttransplant recurrence of HCV infection should be considered for therapy. Significant fibrosis or portal hypertension 1 year after transplantation could predict rapid disease progression and graft loss and could indicate the need for more urgent antiviral treatment. Interferon-free DAA can cure most liver transplant recipients with recurrent hepatitis C, including a majority of those with severe post-transplant liver disease. In addition to viral suppression, treatment also improves liver function. DAA treatment is generally safe and well tolerated, certainly more so than interferon-based therapy, although anemia remains a concern for people taking ribavirin. Drug-drug interactions may be important in the posttransplant setting. No clinically significant drug-drug interactions have been found between sofosbuvir, simeprevir, or daclatasvir on the one hand, and cyclosporine and tacrolimus on the other hand.

The following options proved to be useful in post-liver transplantation patients according to genotypes, with high virological response, waiting more data in near future [91,93,104,105]:

a. Daily fixed-dose combination of ledipasvir (90 mg)/sofosbuvir (400 mg) with weight-based ribavirin (1000 mg [<75 kg] to 1200 mg [>75 kg]) for 12 weeks is recommended for patients with HCV genotype 1 or 4 infection in the allograft, including compensated cirrhosis.

b. Patients who are ribavirin intolerant or ineligible, ledipasvir (90 mg)/sofosbuvir (400 mg) usually extended for 24 weeks in patients with HCV genotype 1 or 4 infection.

c. Daily sofosbuvir (400 mg) plus simeprevir (150 mg) with or without weight-based ribavirin (1000 mg [<75 kg] to 1200 mg [>75 kg]) for 12 to 24 weeks in patients with genotype 1 or 4 infection in the allograft, including compensated cirrhosis.

d. Daily fixed-dose combination of paritaprevir (150 mg)/ritonavir (100 mg)/ombitasvir (25 mg) plus twice-daily dosed dasabuvir (250 mg) and weight-based ribavirin (1000 mg [<75 kg] to 1200 mg [>75 mg]), in the allograft, without cirrhosis, for 24 weeks in patients with HCV genotype 1 infection.

e. Daily sofosbuvir (400 mg) plus daclatasvir (60 mg) with or without weight-based ribavirin (1000 mg [<75 kg] to 1200 mg [>75 kg]) for 24 weeks for patients with HCV genotypes 1, 3, 4, 5, and 6 in the allograft, including those with compensated and decompensated cirrhosis is another combination with high virological response and improvement of liver function.

f. Daily sofosbuvir (400 mg) and weight-based ribavirin (1000 mg [<75 kg] to 1200 mg [>75 kg]) for 24 weeks is recommended for patients with HCV genotype 2 in the allograft, including compensated cirrhosis.

g. Daily sofosbuvir (400 mg) and weight-based ribavirin (1000 mg [<75 kg] to 1200 mg [>75 kg]) for 24 weeks is recommended as alternative for treatment patients with HCV genotype 3 infection in the allograft, including compensated and decompensated cirrhosis.

9.4. Patients with renal impairments

For patients with creatinine clearance of >30 mL/min, no dosage adjustment is required when using simeprevir, sofosbuvir, daclatasvir, fixed-dose combination of ledipasvir (90 mg)/sofosbuvir (400 mg), or fixed-dose combination of paritaprevir (150 mg)/ritonavir (100 mg)/ombitasvir (25 mg) plus twice-daily dosed dasabuvir (250 mg) to treat patients with HCV infection. Simeprevir, daclatasvir, and the combination of paritaprevir, ritonavir, ombitasvir and dasabuvir are cleared by hepatic metabolism and can be used in patients with severe renal impairment [91].

EASL Recommendations on Treatment of Hepatitis C 2015 and AASLD/IDSA/IAS-USA 2014 guidelines on HCV treatment do not recommend sofosbuvir in patients with creatinine clearance of <30 mL/min or with ESRD until more data are available [91,93].

9.5. Patients with acute HCV infection

When the efficacy of the treatment of acute HCV infection was superior to the treatment of chronic infection, there was a strong impetus to identify and treat acute HCV infection with interferon [106]. The current availability of interferon-sparing HCV treatments that have high safety and efficacy reduces the advantage of early treatment of HCV infection. Until data documenting the efficacy and safety of treatment of acute hepatitis C with direct acting antiviral drugs are available, monitoring for spontaneous clearance for minimum of 6 months before initiating treatment is required. When a decision is made to treat patients after 6 months of acute infection, then the patient can be treated as described for chronic HCV [93].

http://dx.doi.org/10.5772/60949

10. Conclusion

Chronic hepatitis C in the presence of the new direct-acting antiviral drugs became a curable disease, with a sustained virological response of more than 90%. The second-generation protease inhibitors that have been approved for treatment of HCV and are available in the market are simeprevir, sofosbuvir, ledipasvir/sofosbuvir, daclatasvir, and the combination of ombitasvir-paritaprevir-ritonavir and dasabuvir. The cost of these new agents prevents universal delivery of medications and prioritization of treatment should be given to patients who are in need of immediate care like those with advanced liver disease and extrahepatic complications. Trials are still ongoing with other new products, many of which are expected to appear in the market soon.

Author details

Abdullah Saeed Gozai Al-Ghamdi

Address all correspondence to: asgalghamdi@hotmail.com

Gastroenterology Unit, Medical Department, King Fahad Hospital, Jeddah, Saudi Arabia

References

[1] WHO. Guidelines for the Screening, Care and Treatment of Persons with Hepatitis C Infection. April 2014. ISBN: 978 92 4 154875 5

[2] Lavanchy D. The global burden of hepatitis C. Liver International 2009;29:74-81.

[3] Mohd Hanafiah K, Groeger J, et al. Global epidemiology of hepatitis C virus infection: new estimates of age-specific antibody to HCV seroprevalence. Hepatology 2013;57:1333-1342.

[4] Gower E, Estes C, et al. Global epidemiology and genotype distribution of the hepatitis C virus infection. J Hepatol 2014;61(1S):S45-S57.

[5] Kim CW, Chang KM. Hepatitis C virus: virology and life cycle. Clin Mol Hepatol 2013;19(1):17-25.

[6] Choo QL, Kuo G, et al. Isolation of a cDNA clone derived from a blood-borne non-A, non-B viral hepatitis genome. Science 1989;244:359-362.

[7] Bartenschlager R, Penin F, et al. Assembly of infectious hepatitis C virus particles. Trends Microbiol 2011;19:95-103.

[8] Neumann AU, Lam NP, et al. Hepatitis C viral dynamics in vivo and the antiviral efficacy of interferon-alpha therapy. Science 1998;282:103-107.

[9] Xu Z, Choi J, et al. Hepatitis C virus F protein is a short-lived protein associated with the endoplasmic reticulum. J Virol 2003, 77:1578-1583.

[10] McLauchlan J, Lemberg MK, et al. Intramembrane proteolysis promotes trafficking of hepatitis C virus core protein to lipid droplets. EMBO J 2002, 21:3980-3988.

[11] Carrere-Kremer S, Montpellier-Pala C, et al. Subcellular localization and topology of the p7 polypeptide of hepatitis C virus. J Virol 2002;76:3720-3730.

[12] Yamaga AK, Ou JH. Membrane topology of the hepatitis C virus NS2 protein. J Biol Chem 2002;277:33228-33234.

[13] Egger D, Wolk B, et al. Expression of hepatitis C virus proteins induces distinct membrane alterations including a candidate viral replication complex. J Virol 2002;76:5974-5984

[14] Mottola G, Cardinali G, et al. Hepatitis C virus nonstructural proteins are localized in a modified endoplasmic reticulum of cells expressing viral subgenomic replicons. Virology 2002;293:31-43.

[15] Tu H, Gao L, et al. Hepatitis C virus RNA polymerase and NS5A complex with a SNARE-like protein. Virology 1999;263:30-41.

[16] Hoofnagle JH. Hepatitis C: the clinical spectrum of disease. Hepatology. 1997;26(3 Suppl 1):15S-20S.

[17] Marcellin P. Hepatitis C: the clinical spectrum of the disease. J Hepatol. 1999;31(Suppl 1):9-16

[18] Alberti A, Chemello L, Benvegnù L. Natural history of hepatitis C. J Hepatol. 1999;31(Suppl 1):17-24.

[19] Seeff LB. Natural history of hepatitis C. Hepatology. 1997;26(3 Suppl 1):21S-28S.

[20] Leone N, Rizzetto M. Natural history of hepatitis C virus infection: from chronic hepatitis to cirrhosis, to hepatocellular carcinoma. Minerva Gastroenterol Dietol. 2005;51(1):31-46.

[21] Nelson PK, Mathers BM, et al. Global epidemiology of hepatitis B and hepatitis C in people who inject drugs: results of systematic reviews. Lancet. 2011;378(9791):571-83.

[22] Wasley A, Alter M. Epidemiology of hepatitis C: geographic differences and temporal trends. Semin Liver Dis. 2000;20:1-16.

[23] Medhat A, Shehata M, et al. Hepatitis C in a community in Upper Egypt: risk factors for infection. Am J Trop Med Hyg. 2002;66:633-638.

[24] Simonsen L, Kane A, et al. Unsafe injections in the developing world and transmission of bloodborne pathogens: a review. Bull World Health Organ. 1999;77:789-800.

[25] Kane A, Lloyd J, et al. Transmission of hepatitis B, hepatitis C and human immunodeficiency viruses through unsafe injections in the developing world: model-based regional estimates. Bull World Health Organ.1999;77:801-807.

[26] Kidney disease: improving global outcomes. KDIGO clinical practice guidelines for the prevention, diagnosis, evaluation, and treatment of hepatitis C in chronic kidney disease. Kidney Int 2008;73 (Suppl 109): S1-S99.

[27] Mast EE, Hwang LY, et al. Risk factors for perinatal transmission of hepatitis C virus (HCV) and the natural history of HCV infection acquired in infancy. J Infect Dis. 2005;192(11):1880-1889.

[28] Thomas DL, Villano SA, et al. Perinatal transmission of hepatitis C virus from human immunodeficiency virus type 1-infected mothers. Women and Infants Transmission Study. J Infect Dis. 1998;177(6):1480-1488.

[29] van de Laar TJW, Matthews GV, et al. Acute hepatitis C in HIV infected men who have sex with men: an emerging sexually transmitted infection. AIDS 2010;24:1799-1812.

[30] Mele A, Corona R, et al. Beauty treatments and risk of parenterally transmitted hepatitis: results from the hepatitis surveillance system in Italy. Scand J Infect Dis 1995;27:441-444.

[31] Mansell CJ, Locarnini SA. Epidemiology of hepatitis C in the East. Semin Liver Dis 1995;15:15

[32] Pawlotsky JM. Use and interpretation of virological tests for hepatitis C. Hepatology. 2002;36(Suppl 1):S65-S73.

[33] Pawlotsky JM, Lonjon I, et al. What strategy should be used for diagnosis of hepatitis C virus infection in clinical laboratories? Hepatology. 1998;27:1700-1702.

[34] Blatt LM, Mutchnick MG, et al. Assessment of hepatitis C virus RNA and genotype from 6807 patients with chronic hepatitis C in the United States. J Viral Hepat. 2000;7:196-202.

[35] AnsaldiF, Torre F, et al. Evaluation of a new hepatitis C virus sequencing assay as a routine method for genotyping. J Med Virol. 2001;63:17-21.

[36] Wiesner R, Edwards E, et al. Model for end-stage liver disease (MELD) and allocation of donor livers. Gastroenterology. 2003;124:91.

[37] http://optn.transplant.hrsa.gov/resources/MeldPeldCalculator.asp?index=98. Accessed January 24, 2014.

[38] Ravaioli M, Grazi GL, et al. Liver transplantation with the Meld system: a prospective study from a single European center. Am J Transplant. 2006;6:1572.

[39] Asrani SK, Kim WR. Model for end-stage liver disease: end of the first decade. Clin Liver Dis. 2011;15:685.

[40] National Medical Policy. FIBROSpect, FIBROSURE, ActiTest and Other Non-invasive Testing for Liver Fibrosis. 2014, health net.

[41] Al-Ghamdi AS. Fibroscan®: a noninvasive test of liver fibrosis assessment. Saudi J Gastroenterol 2007;13:147-149.

[42] Verveer C, de Knegt RJ. Non-invasive measurement of liver fibrosis: application of the FibroScan® in hepatology. Scand J Gastroenterol Suppl. 2006;243:85-8.

[43] Bedossa P, Poynard T. An algorithm for the grading of activity in chronic hepatitis C. The METAVIR Cooperative Study Group. Hepatology 1996;24:289-93.

[44] Ziol M, Handra-Luca A, et al. Non-invasive assessment of liver fibrosis by measurement of stiffness in patients with chronic hepatitis C. Hepatology. 2005;41:48-54.

[45] Palacios PA, Salmerón EJ. Role of liver biopsy in the diagnosis and management of chronic hepatitis C. Gastroenterol Hepatol. 2007;30(7):402-407.

[46] Foster GR. A Guide to PEGylation, Pharmacokinetics and Pegylated Interferons. Roche; Basel, Switzerland: 2003. Better by Design.

[47] Glue P, Fang JWS, et al. Pegylated interferon-[alpha]2b: pharmacokinetics, pharmacodynamics, safety, and preliminary efficacy data. Clin Pharmacol Ther. 2000;68:556-67.

[48] Jacobson IM, McHutchison JG, et al. Telaprevir for previously untreated chronic hepatitis C virus infection. N Engl J Med. 2011;364:2405-2416.

[49] Sherman KE, Flamm SL, et al. Response-guided telaprevir combination treatment for hepatitis C virus infection. N Engl J Med. 2011;365:1014-1024.

[50] Zeuzem S, Andreone P, et al. Telaprevir for retreatment of HCV infection. N Engl J Med. 2011;364:2417-2428.

[51] Poordad F, McCone J, Jr., Bacon BR, et al. Boceprevir for untreated chronic HCV genotype 1 infection. N Engl J Med. 2011;364:1195-1206.

[52] Bacon BR, Gordon SC, et al. Boceprevir for previously treated chronic HCV genotype 1 infection. N Engl J Med. 2011;364:1207-1217.

[53] Myers RP, Ramji A, Bilodeau M, Wong S, Feld JJ. An update on the management of hepatitis C: consensus guidelines from the Canadian Association for the Study of the Liver. Can J Gastroenterol.2012;26:359-375.

[54] Prescribing Information for OLYSIOTM (simeprevir): Janssen Therapeutics, Division of Janssen Products, LP, Titusville NJ 08560. Issued November 2013.

[55] FDA. Olysio U.S. prescribing information http://www.accessdata.fda.gov/drugsatfda. Accessed on October 15, 2014.

[56] Jacobson IM, Dore GJ, et al. Simeprevir with pegylated interferon alfa 2a plus ribavirin in treatment-naive patients with chronic hepatitis C virus genotype 1 infection (QUEST-1): a phase 3, randomised, double-blind, placebo-controlled trial. Lancet. 2014;384:403-413.

[57] Manns M, Marcellin P, et al. Simeprevir with pegylated interferon alfa 2a or 2b plus ribavirin in treatment-naive patients with chronic hepatitis C virus genotype 1 infection (QUEST-2): a randomised, double-blind, placebo-controlled phase 3 trial. Lancet. 2014;384:414-426.

[58] Dieterich D, Rockstroh JK, et al. Simeprevir (TMC435) with pegylated interferon/ribavirin in patients coinfected with HCV genotype 1 and HIV-1: a phase 3 study. Clin Infect Dis. 2014;59:1579-1587.

[59] Zeuzem S, Berg T, et al. Simeprevir increases rate of sustained virologic response among treatment-experienced patients with HCV genotype-1 infection: a phase IIb Trial. Gastroenterology. 2014;146:430-441.

[60] Forns X, Lawitz E, et al. Simeprevir with peginterferon and ribavirin leads to high rates of SVR in patients with HCV genotype 1 who relapsed after previous therapy: a phase 3 trial. Gastroenterology. 2014;146:1669-1679.e3.

[61] Kiser JJ, Burton JR Jr, Everson GT. Drug-drug interactions during antiviral therapy for chronic hepatitis C. Nat Rev Gastroenterol Hepatol. 2013;10:596-606.

[62] Lawitz E, Sulkowski MS, et al. Simeprevir plus sofosbuvir, with or without ribavirin, to treat chronic infection with hepatitis C virus genotype 1 in non-responders to pegylated interferon and ribavirin and treatment-naive patients: the COSMOS randomised study. Lancet. 2014;384:1756-1765.

[63] Sulkowski M, Jacobson IM, et al. Once-daily simeprevir (TMC435) plus sofosbuvir (GS-7977) with or without ribavirin in HCV genotype 1 prior null responders with METAVIR F0-2: COSMOS study subgroup analysis. 49th Annual Meeting of the EASL; April 9-13, 2014; London, England. Abstract 07.

[64] Flanagan S, Crawford-Jones A, Orkin C. Simeprevir for the treatment of hepatitis C and HIV/hepatitis C co-infection. Expert Rev Clin Pharmacol. 2014;7:691-704.

[65] Sovaldi-Gilead Sciences, Inc.https://www.gilead.com/~/media/Files/pdfs/medicines/liver-disease/sovaldi/sovaldi_pi.pdf.

[66] Gane EJ, Stedman CA, et al. Nucleotide polymerase inhibitor sofosbuvir plus ribavirin for hepatitis C. N Engl J Med. 2013;368:34-44.

[67] Jacobson IM, Gordon SC, et al. Sofosbuvir for hepatitis C genotype 2 or 3 in patients without treatment options. N Engl J Med. 2013;368:1867-77.

[68] Kowdley KV, Lawitz E, et al. Sofosbuvir with pegylated interferon alfa-2a and ribavirin for treatment-naive patients with hepatitis C genotype-1 infection (ATOMIC): an open-label, randomised, multicentre phase 2 trial. Lancet. 2013;381:2100-2107.

[69] Lawitz E, Poordad F, et al. Sofosbuvir with peginterferon-ribavirin for 12 weeks in previously treated patients with hepatitis C genotype 2 or 3 and cirrhosis. Hepatology. 2015;769-775.

[70] Lawitz E, Mangia A, et al. Sofosbuvir for previously untreated chronic hepatitis C infection. N Engl J Med. 2013;368:1878-87.

[71] Svarovskaia ES, Dvory-Sobol H, et al. Infrequent development of resistance in genotype 1-6 hepatitis C virus-infected subjects treated with sofosbuvir in phase 2 and 3 clinical trials. Clin Infect Dis. 2014;15:1666-1674.

[72] Osinusi A, Meissner EG, et al. Sofosbuvir and ribavirin for hepatitis C genotype 1 in patients with unfavorable treatment characteristics: a randomized clinical trial. JAMA. 2013;310:804-11.

[73] Lawitz E, Poordad FF, et al. Sofosbuvir and ledipasvir fixed-dose combination with and without ribavirin in treatment-naive and previously treated patients with genotype 1 hepatitis C virus infection (LONESTAR): an open-label, randomised, phase 2 trial. Lancet. 2014;383:515-523.

[74] Sulkowski MS, Naggie S, et al. Sofosbuvir and ribavirin for hepatitis C in patients with HIV coinfection. JAMA. 2014;312:353-361.

[75] Yoshida EM, Sulkowski MS, et al. Concordance of sustained virologic response 4, 12, and 24 weeks post-treatment with sofosbuvir-containing regimens for hepatitis C virus. Hepatology. 2014;61:41-45.

[76] Zeuzem S, Dusheiko GM, et al. Sofosbuvir and ribavirin in HCV genotypes 2 and 3. N Engl J Med. 2014;370:1993-2001.

[77] Sulkowski MS, Gardiner DF, et al. Daclatasvir plus sofosbuvir for previously treated or untreated chronic HCV infection. N Engl J Med. 2014;370:211-221.

[78] HARVONI® (ledipasvir and sofosbuvir)-Gilead Sciences, Inc. http://www.gilead.com/~/media/Files/pdfs/medicines/liver-disease/harvoni/harvoni_pi.pdf.

[79] Afdhal N, Reddy KR, et al. Ledipasvir and sofosbuvir for previously treated HCV genotype 1 infection. N Engl J Med. 2014;370:1483-1493.

[80] Afdhal N, Zeuzem S, et al. Ledipasvir and sofosbuvir for untreated HCV genotype 1 infection. N Engl J Med. 2014;370:1889-1898.

[81] Gane EJ, Stedman CA, et al. Efficacy of nucleotide polymerase inhibitor sofosbuvir plus the NS5A inhibitor ledipasvir or the NS5B non-nucleoside inhibitor GS-9669 against HCV genotype 1 infection. Gastroenterology. 2014;146:736-743.

[82] Kowdley KV, Gordon SC, et al. Ledipasvir and sofosbuvir for 8 or 12 weeks for chronic HCV without cirrhosis. N Engl J Med. 2014;370:1879-1888.

[83] Osinusi A, Kohli A, et al. Re-treatment of chronic hepatitis C virus genotype 1 infection after relapse: an open-label pilot study. Ann Intern Med. 2014;161:634-638.

[84] VIEKIRA PAK (ombitasvir, paritaprevir, and ritonavir tablets; dasabuvir tablets)-AbbVie Inc. http://www.rxabbvie.com/pdf/viekirapak_pi.pdf.

[85] Feld JJ, Kowdley KV, et al. Treatment of HCV with ABT-450/r-ombitasvir and dasabuvir with ribavirin. N Engl J Med. 2014;370:1594-1603.

[86] Ferenci P, Bernstein D, et al. ABT-450/r-ombitasvir and dasabuvir with or without ribavirin for HCV. N Engl J Med. 2014;370:1983-1992.

[87] Zeuzem S, Jacobson IM, et al. Retreatment of HCV with ABT-450/r-ombitasvir and dasabuvir with ribavirin. N Engl J Med. 2014;370:1604-1614.

[88] Andreone P, Colombo MG, et al. ABT-450, ritonavir, ombitasvir, and dasabuvir achieves 97% and 100% sustained virologic response with or without ribavirin in treatment-experienced patients with HCV genotype 1b infection. Gastroenterology. 2014;147:359-365.

[89] Poordad F, Hezode C, Trinh R, et al. ABT-450/r-ombitasvir and dasabuvir with ribavirin for hepatitis C with cirrhosis. N Engl J Med. 2014;370:1973-1982.

[90] Kwo PY, Mantry PS, et al. An interferon-free antiviral regimen for HCV after liver transplantation. N Engl J Med. 2014;371:2375-2382.

[91] EASL Recommendations on Treatment of Hepatitis C, April 2015. http://www.easl.eu/research/our-contributions/clinical-practice-guidelines/detail/recommendations-on-treatment-of-hepatitis-c-2015.

[92] Asselah T. Daclatasvir plus sofosbuvir for HCV infection: an oral combination therapy with high antiviral efficacy. J Hepatol. 2014;61:435-438.

[93] AASLD/IDSA/IAS-USA. Recommendations for testing, managing, and treating hepatitis C. http://www.hcvguidelines.org. Accessed April 24, 2014.

[94] EASL Clinical Practice Guidelines: management of hepatitis C virus infection. J Hepatol. 2011;55:245-64.

[95] Petta S, Craxì A. Current and future HCV therapy—do we still need other anti-HCV drugs? Liver Int. 2015;35(s1):4-10.

[96] Zeuzem S, Dusheiko G, et al. Sofosbuvir þ ribavirin for 12 or 24 weeks for patients with HCV genotype 2 or 3: the VALENCE trial. Hepatology. 2013;58 (Suppl 1):733A.

[97] Sulkowski MS, Gardiner DF, et al. Daclatasvir plus sofosbuvir for previously treated or untreated chronic HCV infection. N Engl J Med. 2014;370:211-221.

[98] Molina JM, Orkin C, Iser DM, et al. All-oral therapy with sofosbuvir plus ribavirin for the treatment of HCV genotypes 1, 2, 3 and 4 infection in patients co-infected with HIV (PHOTON-2). 20th International AIDS Conference; July 20-25, 2014; Melbourne, Australia. Abstract MOAB0105LB.

[99] Pol S, Reddy KR, Baykal T et al. Interferon-free regimens of ombitasvir and ABT-450/r with or without ribavirin in patients with HCV genotype 4 infection: PEARL-I study results. [Abstract 1928.] 65th Annual Meeting of the AASLD. November 7-11, 2014; Boston, MA.

[100] Esmat GE, Shiha G, et al. Sofosbuvir plus ribavirin in the treatment of Egyptian patients with chronic genotype 4 HCV infection. [Abstract 959.] 65th Annual Meeting of the AASLD. November 7-11, 2014; Boston, MA.

[101] Kapoor R, Kohli A, Sidharthan S et al. All oral treatment for genotype 4 chronic hepatitis C infection with sofosbuvir and ledipasvir: interim results from the NIAID SYNERGY trial. [Abstract 240.] 65th Annual Meeting of the AASLD. November 7-11, 2014; Boston, MA.

[102] Maasoumy B, Hunyady B, et al. Performance of two HCV RNA assays during protease inhibitor-based triple therapy in patients with advanced liver fibrosis and cirrhosis. PLOS ONE. 2014 Nov;9(11):e110857.

[103] Martel-Laferrière V, Bichoupan K, et al. Hepatitis C direct-acting antiviral agents: changing the paradigm of hepatitis C treatment in HIV-infected patients. J Clin Gastroenterol. 2014 Feb;48(2):106-112.

[104] R Fontana, R Bahirwani, R Reddy, et al. High efficacy and favorable safety profile of daclatasvir based all oral antiviral therapy in liver transplant recipients with severe recurrent HCV. AASLD Liver Meeting. Boston, November 7-12, 2014. AbstractLB-22.

[105] V Leroy, J Dumortier, et al. High rates of virological response and major clinical improvement during sofosbuvir and daclatasvir-based regimens for the treatment of fibrosing cholestatic HCV-recurrence after liver transplantation: the ANRS CO23 CUPILT Study. AASLD Liver Meeting. Boston, November 7-12, 2014. Abstract21.

[106] Ghany MG, Strader DB, et al. Diagnosis, management, and treatment of hepatitis C: an update. Hepatology.2009;49(4):1335-1374

Chapter 5

Past, Present, and Future Perspectives on the Systemic Therapy for Advanced Hepatocellular Carcinoma (HCC) — A Comprehensive Review

Ahmed Abu-Zaid, Lynn Alkhatib, Judie Noemie Hoilat, Sana Samer Kadan, Abdulaziz Mohammed Eshaq, Ahmed Mubarak Fothan, Abdulrahman Mohammed Bakather, Mohammed Abuzaid, Daniah Saud Aloufi, Abdulhadi A. Alamodi and Ayman Azzam

Additional information is available at the end of the chapter

http://dx.doi.org/10.5772/60991

Abstract

Hepatocellular carcinoma (HCC) is the fifth most frequent cancer, the third leading cause of cancer-related mortality, and the first leading cause of death in patients with cirrhosis. Management of primary locally advanced, inoperable, recurrent or metastatic HCC is very challenging and continues to be a topic of controversy. Herein, we shed light on the past, present, and future perspectives on the systemic therapy (hormonal therapy, cytotoxic chemotherapy, and novel molecularly targeted therapy) for management of patients with advanced HCC.

Keywords: Hepatocellular Carcinoma

1. Introduction

Globally, hepatocellular carcinoma (HCC) is the fifth most frequent cancer, the third leading cause of cancer-related mortality, and the first leading cause of death in patients with cirrhosis. The incidence of HCC has doubled in developing and developed countries over the recent decades [3]. HCC generally takes place in the setting of variable underlying hepatic conditions, such as autoimmune hepatitis, nonalcoholic steatohepatitis (NASH), hepatitis B, hepatitis C, alcohol-associated liver disease, hemochromatosis, alpha-1 antitrypsin deficiency, Wilson's disease, primary sclerosing cholangitis (PSC), primary biliary cirrhosis (PBC), and other liver diseases [4]. Therefore, the patient population is varied, accounting for the intricacy of studying this neoplasm, and how to effectively manage it.

Therapeutic modalities for management of HCC can be largely categorized into three main types: surgical and nonsurgical therapies [5, 6]. Surgical therapies include surgical resection, cryosurgery, and living/deceased donor liver transplantation. Nonsurgical therapies can be divided into liver-directed and systemic. Liver-directed therapies include percutaneous ethanol/acetic acid injection, percutaneous microwave coagulation therapy, radiofrequency ablation, microwave coagulation therapy, interstitial laser photo-coagulation, targeted cryoablation therapy, high-intensity focused ultrasound, transcatheter arterial therapy, and radiation therapy. Systemic therapy includes hormonal therapy, cytotoxic chemotherapy, and novel molecularly targeted therapy.

At the time of clinical diagnosis, roughly 60%-70% of HCC patients present with primary advanced, inoperable, recurrent, or metastatic disease [7]. Moreover, tumor relapse (recurrence) following curative surgical management continues to be a substantial dilemma and is documented as high as approximately 70% at 5 years postoperatively [8]. The standard of care management for recurrent HCC remains undefined [8].

The management of primary locally advanced, inoperable, recurrent, or metastatic HCC is very challenging and continues to be a topic of controversy. Herein, we shed light on the past, present, and future perspectives on the systemic therapy (hormonal therapy, cytotoxic chemotherapy, and novel molecularly targeted therapy) for the management of patients with advanced HCC.

2. Hormonal therapy

Several HCCs express sex-hormone receptors such as estrogen (ER), progesterone (PR), and androgen receptors [9] as well as somatostatin receptors [10, 11]. Hence, hormonal therapies (hormone receptor blockers) can be initiated as practical therapeutic choices in patients with hormone receptor-positive HCC [5]. The most frequently employed hormonal agents for the management of HCC include tamoxifen, megestrol, octreotide, and lanreotide.

2.1. Tamoxifen

Multiple studies including single-center and multicenter prospective randomized controlled trials, systematic reviews, and meta-analyses investigated the role of tamoxifen for the management of patients with advanced unresectable HCC [12-16]. These studies were unsatisfactory and failed to demonstrate improved survival advantages (disease-free survival [DFS] and overall survival [OS] rates) or enhanced quality of life (functional status).

One plausible explanation for absence of survival efficacy could be attributed to the existence of variant estrogen receptors (ERs) in a subset of these HCC lesions leading to more hostile biological behavior and insensitivity to tamoxifen therapy [17, 18].

Tamoxifen has been shown to function as a potential multidrug resistance (MDR)-reversing remedy in the chemoresistant HCC [19]. Subsequently, several clinical trials have been conducted exploring the clinical benefits of combining tamoxifen with diverse cytotoxic chemotherapeutics.

The cellular (molecular) potentiation of doxorubicin-induced apoptosis of HCC cells by tamoxifen has been confirmed in a bench laboratory work by Cheng et al. [20]. Subsequently, in 1998, a prospective phase II study by the same authors [21] enrolled 36 patients with advanced HCC. Patients received high-dose tamoxifen (120 mg/m^2 per day) plus doxorubicin. Only 12 patients (33.3%) attained partial remission with a median PFS of roughly 7 months.

Another randomized controlled study by Melia et al. [22] enrolled around 60 advanced inoperable HCC patients who were then randomized to two groups: (1) doxorubicin alone (60 mg/m^2 at 3-week intervals) and (2) combined doxorubicin plus tamoxifen (10 mg twice daily). Drug response happened only in 3 (11%) and 4 (16%) patients of the above-mentioned groups, respectively, without statistical significant difference.

Moreover, Lu et al. [23] studied the combination therapy of high-dose tamoxifen, doxorubicin, and interferon alpha [IFNα] in 25 patients with advanced unresectable HCC. Partial remission was achieved in five patients (20%) with median PFS of 7 months. Overall, median OS was 6 months, whereas the 1-year survival rate was roughly 16%. The study concluded that this triple combination (high-dose tamoxifen, doxorubicin plus IFNα) is effective but not superior to the double therapy (high-dose tamoxifen plus doxorubicin).

Furthermore, the combination of tamoxifen with oral etoposide [24] and epirubicin [25] have been conducted with only modest antitumor outcomes.

2.2. Megestrol

In 1997, Chao et al. [26] (phase II study) explored the role of megestrol acetate (160 mg/day, orally) in 46 patients with advanced unresectable HCC. Thirty-two patients were included in the analysis. No single patient attained partial or complete response. Twenty patients (62%) experienced disease progression, and a similar percentage (62%) experienced improved symptoms/functional status. Twelve patients (38%) attained stable disease. Glucocorticoid receptor-positive HCC (n = 4/5) experienced stable disease, whereas glucocorticoid receptor-negative HCC (n = 5/5) experienced disease progression. The study concluded that while megestrol acetate does not exhibit noteworthy anticancer activities against HCC, it is very beneficial as palliative treatment to improve quality of life. Also, the stable disease status may be attributed to glucocorticoid receptor-positive HCC. Further research is needed.

In 2001, Villa et al. [18] studied 45 patients with variant ER HCC. Twenty-one (n = 21) and twenty-four (n = 24) patients were randomized to receive megestrol 160 mg daily and only best supportive care (BSC), respectively. In comparison with the BSC group, the megestrol-treated group achieved higher statistically significant median survival (18 vs. 7 months; $P = 0.0090$) and decelerated tumor growth ($P = 0.0212$).

More recently in 2011, Chow et al. [27] studied 204 patients with therapy-naive advanced HCC across six Asia-Pacific countries. Patients were randomized to two groups: (1) treated group with megestrol acetate (320 mg daily) and (2) placebo group. Placebo group had higher (statistically insignificant) OS than the treated group (2.14 vs. 1.88 months, respectively). The treated group had lower frequencies of nausea, vomiting, and anorexia but experienced a worse (statistically insignificant) global health status. The study concluded that megestrol acetate does not extend OS in patients with advanced treatment-naive HCC.

Most importantly, the noticeably dissimilar OS intervals in the Chow et al. [27] placebo group versus the supportive care group in the Villa et al. [18] study (2.14 vs. 7 months, respectively) propose that therapeutic results may be largely dependent on different aspects, for example, baseline liver function (Child-Pugh score [CPS]) and performance status (Eastern Cooperative Oncology Group performance status).

2.3. Octreotide

In 1998, Kouroumalis et al. [11] studied the role of octreotide in 58 patients with advanced unresectable HCC. Patients were randomized to two groups: (1) treated group with somatostatin analog, i.e., octreotide (250 mg twice daily subcutaneously) and (2) placebo-controlled group. Numerous quantities of somatostatin receptors were recognized in the liver tissue of all patients with HCC. The treated group achieved higher statistically significant median OS rates than the control group (13 vs. 4 months, respectively; $P = 0.002$), but without objective responses rates (ORR). Moreover, the treated group achieved higher cumulative survival rates than the placebo-controlled group at 6 and 12 months (75% vs. 37% and 56% vs. 13%, respectively). At 6 months post octreotide administration, the treated group had significantly decreased alpha-fetoprotein (AFP) levels. The study concluded that octreotide administration substantially offers survival advantages and is a plausible substitute in the management of advanced unresectable HCC.

However, the above-mentioned findings [11] could not be validated and reproduced in 2 successive randomized placebo-controlled trials employing sandostatin—a long-acting analog of octreotide [28, 29]. The two studies were conducted in 2002 and 2007.

In 2011, Ji et al. [30] conducted an updated systematic review and meta-analysis of 11 randomized controlled trials (total of 802 patients) exploring the role of somatostatin analogs in advanced HCC. Only nine studies were incorporated into the meta-analysis and revealed higher statistically significant 6-month and 12-month survival rates in the treated octreotide group versus the control/placebo group. This meta-analysis concluded that octreotide administration could provide survival benefits in patients with advanced HCC.

2.4. Lanreotide

Previous nonrandomized studies have shown inadequate antineoplastic effects of lanreotide for the management of patients with advanced inoperable HCC [10, 31].

In 2000, Raderer et al. [31] administered lanereotide (30 mg once intramuscularly every 2-week period) in 21 treatment-naive patients with advanced HCC. The object response rate (ORR) and the stable disease rates were 5% and 38%, respectively, whereas the median OS and the time to progression (TTP) were 4.2 months and 2.5 months, respectively.

In 2006, Cebon et al. [10] administered lanereotide (20 mg once intramuscularly every 4-week period) in 63 patients with advanced HCC. Only one patient (2%) experienced partial objective response and median OS was 8 months.

In 2009, Barbare et al. [32] conducted a multicenter, phase III, randomized, double-blind placebo-controlled study investigating the role of lanreotide in 272 patients with primary advanced or recurrent HCC. Patients were randomized to two groups: (1) treated group with lanreotide (intramuscular injection of 30 mg once every 4 weeks for up to 2-year interval) and (2) placebo-controlled group. The median OS and the disease-free survival (DFS) were comparable and did not differ significantly between both groups. Four and zero objective responses were achieved in the placebo and treated groups, respectively. Objective response and disease stabilization were achieved in 0% and 33% of the lanreotide-treated group, respectively. The treated group had faster global heath deterioration that the control group. The study concluded that lanreotide has fairly a well-tolerated toxicity profile, negative influence on functional status, and nonbeneficial OS outcomes.

2.5. Conclusion

All studies examining the role of single-agent tamoxifen or in combination with diverse chemotherapeutic drugs were unsatisfactory and failed to yield substantial worthy survival advantages. Similar discouraging results occurred with megestrol administration as well as somatostatin analogs (octreotide and lanreotide). It can be concluded that the use of hormonal therapy for the management of advanced inoperable HCC is not recommended. Its use may be only recommended within the context of clinical trials. Further research is needed.

3. Systemic cytotoxic chemotherapy

Several nonrandomized and phase I, II, and III clinical trials have been conducted to investigate the role of systemic cytotoxic chemotherapy (monotherapy or combination therapy) for the management of advanced inoperable HCC.

3.1. Monotherapy (single-agent) systemic chemotherapy

Several single-agent systemic chemotherapies have been tested in patients with advanced HCC, such as: doxorubicin, pegylated liposomal doxorubicin (PLD), epirubicin, mitoxantrone, 5-fluorouracil (5-FU), etoposide, capecitabine, gemcitabine, irinotecan, and thalidomide.

3.1.1. Doxorubicin

Single-agent doxorubicin is the most frequently investigated systemic chemotherapeutic agent in patients with locally advanced unresectable HCC [33].

In 1975, Olweny et al. [34] (phase II clinical trial) studied the role of doxorubicin (75 mg/m^2 intravenously once every 3 weeks) in 14 patients with primary advanced inoperable HCC. Eleven patients (78.5%) achieved objective responses (78.5%). However, successive studies (from 1977 to 2005) failed to validate Olweny et al. [34] study and rather exhibited that the actual objective response rate with single-agent doxorubicin (dose: 75 mg/m^2) was roughly equal to or less than 20% [35-40]. Additional large-sized subsequent randomized trials employing lower doses of single-agent doxorubicin (dose: equals to or less than 60 mg/m^2 per schedule) were shown to yield even lower objective response rates ranging from 4% to 10.1% [41-42].

In 1988, Lai et al. [39] (prospective randomized trial) studied the efficacy of doxorubicin (60-75 mg/m^2) versus the best supportive care (no chemotherapy) in 60 and 46 patients, respectively. The doxorubicin-treated group achieved higher statistically significant median OS than the no chemotherapy group (10.6 vs. 7.6 weeks; P = 0.036). However, life-threatening toxicities (cardiotoxicity and septicemia) occurred in the doxorubicin-treated group (25%). The study concluded that despite the minimal survival advantages of doxorubicin, it was associated with serious complications and should not be recommended for the management of inoperable HCC.

In 2007, Gish et al. [42] (phase III randomized controlled trial) examined the efficacy of doxorubicin versus nolatrexed in 445 patients. The doxorubicin-treated group achieved a higher statistically significant OS than nolatrexed-treated group (32.3 vs. 22.3 weeks; P = 0.0068). The objective response rates for doxorubicin-treated and nolatrexed-treated groups were 4% and 1.4%, respectively. The most frequently observed toxicities for doxorubicin-treated and nolatrexed-treated groups were alopecia and grade 3/4 (thrombocytopenia, vomiting, diarrhea, and stomatitis), respectively.

In conclusion, single-agent doxorubicin can be effective in 20% of patients; however, OS advantages are uncertain. Moreover, its cardiotoxicity is a major limiting adverse event. Combination therapy with other systemic cytotoxic chemotherapeutics and novel molecularly targeted therapies are in progress.

3.1.2. Pegylated liposomal doxorubicin (PLD)

The efficacy of single-agent PLD has been studied in a pilot study [43] and two phase II trials [44, 45] as an initial therapy in patients with advanced inoperable HCC. The research outcomes were discouraging. Combination chemotherapeutic remedies containing PLD are elaborated below.

3.1.3. Epirubicin and mitoxantrone

In comparison with doxorubicin, previous retrospective studies and phase II trials demonstrated that single-agent epirubicin [46, 47] and mitoxantrone [48, 49] share relatively comparable antineoplastic activity as well as relatively equal or slightly higher objective response rates (epirubicin, range: 9.1%-23%; mitoxantrone, range: 23.7%-27.2%). Cardiotoxicity is a major limiting adverse event. Both chemotherapeutics are not commonly used.

3.1.4. 5-Fluorouracil (5-FU)

In one prospective randomized controlled trial by Choi et al. [37], there were higher objective response rates and median OS in HCC patients receiving doxorubicin versus those patients receiving 5-fluorouracil-containg quadruple therapy (5-fluorouracil, methotrexate, cyclophosphamide, and vincristin) therapy (24% vs. 0%, respectively; 14.4 vs. 6.5 weeks, respectively).

In 1995, Porta et al. [50] (preliminary results of a phase II study) explored the role of 5-FU (370 mg/m^2) plus racemic leucovorin (200 mg/m^2) for 5 successive days in 25 patients with advanced inoperable HCC. The regimen cycle was continual every 28 days until disease progression took place. Seven objective responses (28%) were achieved as follows: 6 partial (24%) and 1 complete (4%) responses. Only 5 patients (20%) displayed stable disease, whereas 13 patients exhibited disease progression. Regimen-related adverse events were mild and no grade 4 toxicity occurred. Specifically, 1 patient (4%) experienced grade 1 skin toxicity, 2 patients (8%) grade 3 granulocytopenia, 7 patients (28%) grade 2 nausea, 10 patients (40%) grade 2 diarrhea, and 11 patients (44%) grade 2/3 mucositis. The study concluded that (5-FU plus racemic leucovorin) chemotherapeutic schedule could provide objective responses in patients with advanced unresectable HCCs, which are frequently regarded as chemoresistant neoplasms.

In 1995, Tetef et al. [51] (phase II trial) examined the role of 5-FU (250-450 mg/m^2/day for 5 days by means of an intravenous [IV] bolus) in combination with calcium leucovorin (500 mg/m^2/day for 5 days by means of continuous IV infusion) in 15 patients with advanced unresectable HCC. The regimen was given on a 28-day schedule. Overall, 8 (53%), 6 (40%), and 1 (7%) patients experienced stable disease, disease progression, and partial response, respectively. The median duration of stable disease was 5.7 months, whereas the median TTP was 2.7 months and the partial response persisted only for 2.4 months. Overall, the median OS was roughly 4 months. Regarding regimen-related adverse events, only 9% and 10% of chemotherapeutic schedules were impacted negatively by grade 3/4 hematological toxicity and grade 3/4 gastrointestinal toxicity, respectively. The study concluded that (5-FU plus calcium leucovorin) chemotherapeutic schedule is ineffective highlighting the chemoresistant characteristic of HCC to the modulated 5-FU.

In conclusion, objective response rates with single-agent 5-FU have been frequently low despite the addition of modulating agents such as leucovorin. Advantageously, despite the widespread hepatic metabolism, satisfactory doses of 5-FU can be often administered in HCC patients with hepatic insufficiency or jaundice.

3.1.5. Etoposide

An early prospective randomized controlled trial demonstrated higher ORR (however no survival advantages) when single-agent doxorubicin was contrasted to single-agent etoposide (28% vs. 18%, respectively)[52].

Further trials are underway to test its true efficacy both singly and in combination with other drugs in the management of HCC.

3.1.6. Capecitabine

In 2004, Patt et al. [53] (retrospective analysis) studied the role of single-agent oral capecitabine (1000 mg/m^2 twice daily for 2 weeks; treatment was repeated every 3 weeks) in 37 patients with advanced inoperable HCC. Of the 37 patients, 22 patients had not received any previous treatment. Objective responses were attained in 9 patients (24.3%), comprising 1 complete response. The median OS was 10.1 months. Grade 3 thrombocytopenia happened in 3 patients. The study concluded that capecitabine is well tolerated and offers only minimal antitumor activities against HCC.

In 2013, Brandi et al. [54] (single-center phase II study) examined the role of single-agent metronomic capecitabine (500 mg twice daily) in 90 patients with advanced HCC. The patients were divided into two groups. The first group consisted of 59 patients who had received no prior therapy. Three objective responses (1 partial and 2 complete) were attained whereas 30 patients experienced stable disease. The median PFS and OS were 6.03 and 14.47 months, respectively. The second group consisted of 31 patients who received prior therapy with sorafenib. No objective responses (neither partial nor complete) were attained whereas 10 patients experienced stable disease. The median PFS and OS were 3.27 and 9.77 months, respectively. The first group (capecitabine-treated) was matched to untreated HCC patients from the Italian Liver Cancer group. The capecitabine-treated group achieved a higher statistically significant median OS than the matched untreated patients (15.6 months vs. 8.0 months; $P = 0.043$). The study concluded that metronomic capecitabine seems to offer anti-neoplastic activities in therapy-naive and sorafenib-treated patients.

The superiority of single-agent sorafenib over capecitabine was confirmed in a single-center, open-label, phase II trial by Abdel-Rahman et al. [55]. The study enrolled 52 treatment-naive HCC patients who were randomized to get administered sorafenib (400 mg twice daily) or capecitabine (100 mg mg/m^2 twice daily). In comparison with the capecitabine-treated group, the sorafenib-treated group achieved higher statistically significant median PFS (6 months vs. 4 months; $P < 0.005$) and OS (7.05 vs. 5.07 months; $P < 0.016$). Four objective responses (3 partial and 1 complete) were achieved in sorafenib-treated group; only 1 partial response was achieved in capecitabine-treated group. The most commonly observed toxicities in sorafenib-treated and capecitabine-treated groups were hand-foot skin reaction and hyperbilirubinemia, respectively. The study concluded that (1) sorafenib is superior to capecitabine in patients with HCC and (2) capecitabine should not be employed as a single-agent therapy; instead, combination regimens with sorafenib should be attempted.

In conclusion, the DFS and OS advantages of single-agent fluoropyrimidines (5-FU and capecitabine) are uncertain, partly due to inconsistent study participants (treatment naive and previously treated). Combination regimens with other chemotherapeutic agents should be examined in phase II/III clinical trials.

3.1.7. Gemcitabine

Single-agent gemcitabine chemotherapy has showed varied modest results in 3 phase II clinical trials [56-58].

In 2000, Yang et al. [56] studied the role of gemcitabine (intravenous 1250 mg/m^2 once weekly for 3 weeks followed by a 1-week rest) in 28 chemotherapy-naive patients with inoperable, nonembolizable, locally advanced or metastatic HCC. All study patients received 6 cycles of gemcitabine, as follows: 1250 mg/m^2 once weekly for 3 weeks followed by a 1-week rest. Partial response was attained in 5 of 28 patients (overall response rate: 17.8%). Stable disease was attained in 7 patients (25%). Disease progression occurred in 16 patients (57.2%). The median OS in all the 28 patients and those 5 patients who had partial response was 18.7 and 34.7 weeks, respectively. The median TTP was roughly 12 weeks. Grade 3/4 adverse events mainly comprised equally thrombocytopenia and leucopenia (10.7%) as well as equally anemia and hepatotoxicity (14.3%).

In 2001, Kubicka et al. [57] studied the role of gemcitabine in 20 patients with advanced unresectable HCC. The median number of gemcitabine administration was 7.6 (range: 3-21). The overall response rate was attained in 1 patient (5%), and gemcitabine did not ameliorate the cancer-related symptoms. Grade 3/4 thrombocytopenia was the most commonly observed adverse event (30%).

In 2002, Fuchs et al. [58] studied the role of gemcitabine (intravenous 1000 mg/m^2 once weekly for 3 weeks followed by 1 resting week) in 30 patients with advanced unresectable metastatic HCC. The enrolled patients had received at least one prior modality of systemic therapy in the past. The median number of gemcitabine administration was 2 (range: 1-8). Neither complete nor partial responses were attained. Only 9 patients (30%) attained stable disease (median interval: 7.4 months). The median OS was 6.9 months, whereas the overall 1-year survival was 40%. One patient (3%) suffered grade 3 thrombocytopenia whereas another one patient (3%) suffered hemolytic-uremic syndrome. Additionally, 2 patients (7%) developed grade 4 neutropenia.

In conclusion, although gemcitabine is largely well tolerated, phase II clinical trials of gemcitabine exhibited minimal effects in patients with advanced unresectable HCC and therefore is not recommended. Gemcitabine-based combination therapies are interesting therapeutic targets.

3.1.8. Thalidomide

Single-agent thalidomide chemotherapy has been investigated in 3 early phase II clinical trials -61]. Thalidomide showed lower rates of antineoplastic effects; however, disease stabilization was achieved in up to 33% of patients.

In 2003, Hsu et al. studied the role of low-dose thalidomide (starting dose of 200 mg per day; the dose was gradually upgraded in 100-mg phases up to maximum tolerated dose or 600 mg per day) in 68 patients with advanced unresectable HCC. Four patients (6.3%) attained chemotherapy responses (1 complete and 3 partial), and their AFP levels fell greatly. Moreover, an additional 6 patients experienced more than 50% reduction in their AFP levels post treatment with thalidomide. In total, 10 patients achieved objective response to thalidomide with a median OS of 62.4 weeks (range: 31.2-93.6). For all patients, the median OS was 18.7

weeks, whereas the overall 1-year survival was 27.6%. Only 6 and none patients developed grade 3 and grade 4 thalidomide-related adverse events, respectively.

In 2005, Lin et al. studied the role of thalidomide (starting dose of 200 mg per day; the dose was gradually upgraded in 100-mg phases up to maximum tolerated dose or 800 mg per day) in 27 patients with advanced unresectable HCC. The median daily dose was 300 mg. Only 1 patient achieved near-complete drug response (expressed as reduced AFP level) as well as partial radiological response on computed tomography (CT) imaging. Stable disease of 16-week interval was attained in 2 patients. The median DFS was 6 weeks, whereas the overall OS was 17.6 weeks. Fatigue (81%) and somnolence (62%) were the two most frequent thalidomide-related adverse events. Three patients suffered grade 4 hyperbilirubinemia.

In 2005, Patt et al. [61] studied the role of thalidomide (starting dose of 200 mg per day; the dose was gradually upgraded from 400 mg during the first week to 1000 mg during the fifth week) in 37 patients with advanced unresectable HCC. Overall, 1 (5%), 1 (5%), and 10 (31.3%) patients attained partial response, minor response, and stable disease, respectively. Twenty patients (62.5%) experienced disease progression. The overall OS was roughly 6.8 months. The most frequently observed drug-related adverse events were grade 2/3/4 somnolence in 65% whereas grade 3/4 reactions occurred in 20% of patients.

In conclusion, with gradual dose escalation, thalidomide exhibited well-tolerated toxicity profile. While thalidomide demonstrated lower response rates, it offered disease stabilization in one-third of patients. Future studies should be targeted toward exploring different thalidomide analogs and doses as well as trial of combination therapy with other systemic management modalities. As of now, thalidomide use in the management of advanced HCC is not recommended.

3.1.9. Irinotecan

Single-agent irinotecan chemotherapy has been investigated in two phase II clinical trials for the management of patients with advanced unresectable HCC [62,.

In 2001, O'Reilly et al. (phase II) studied the role of irinotecan (starting dose of 125 mg once weekly for 4 weeks followed by a 2-week rest) in 14 patients with advanced unresectable HCC. The median number of irinotecan cycle administration was 1 (range: 1-6). Partial response was attained in only 1 patient (7%), which lasted for 7 weeks. Transient stable disease was attained in 1 patient (7%). Disease progression occurred in all the 12 remaining patients (86%). Significant irinotecan-related adverse events were noted, mainly nausea, vomiting, diarrhea, fatigue, and neutropenia.

In 2006, Boige et al. (multicenter phase II study) studied the role of irinotecan (dose was adjusted according to total bilirubin level) in 29 patients with advanced unresectable HCC. In total, 0, 1, and 12 patients experienced objective response, minor response, and disease stabilization, respectively. Median TTP was 3.1 months whereas the OS was 7.4 months. Grade 3/4 toxicities primarily compromised diarrhea (17%), anemia (24%), and neutropenia (47%).

In conclusion, irinotecan had considerable drug-related toxicities (adverse events) and very minimal antitumor effects against advanced unresectable HCC. Single-agent irinotecan chemotherapy is not recommended.

3.2. Combination systemic cytotoxic chemotherapy

Various combinations of systemic cytotoxic chemotherapeutics have been investigated in patients with advanced HCC, such as cisplatin-based, gemcitabine-based, and oxaliplatin-based regimens.

Table 1 exhibits a summary of major phase I to II studies on combination systemic cytotoxic chemotherapy in patients with advanced inoperable HCC.

Overall, cisplatin-based combination chemotherapeutic schedules seem to yield greater objective response rates than non-cisplatin-based combination chemotherapeutic schedules. However, no single combination systemic chemotherapy regimen definitely appeared to offer superior or valuable survival advantages such as TTP, PFS, OS, and disease stabilization.

Regimens containing oxaliplatin plus short-term infusional 5-FU and leucovorin are most frequently utilized in the management of advanced colorectal cancer with hepatic metastases.

In 2013, Qin et al. (multicenter open-label, phase III randomized trial) examined the efficacy of single-agent doxorubicin (50 mg/m^2 once every three weeks) versus modified FOLFOX4 regimen (infusional 5-fluorouracil, leucovorin, and oxaliplatin) in 371 Asian patients with primary locally advanced, inoperable, or metastatic HCC. Of note, 90 of all enrolled 371 patients (24.3%) had cirrhosis secondary to hepatitis B virus infection. In comparison with the doxorubicin group, the modified FOLFOX4 achieved slightly higher PFS (2.93 vs. 1.77 months, respectively), median OS (6.40 vs. 4.97 months, respectively), ORR (8.15%, vs. 2.67%, respectively), and DCR (52% vs. 32%, respectively). On continual follow-up, there was a statistically significant sustainable tendency toward improved OS with FOLFOX4 regimen versus doxorubicin ($P = 0.04$). Modified FOLFOX4-related adverse events were comparable to earlier studies. Both treated groups experienced similar grade 3/4 drug-related toxicities. The study concluded that the propensity toward enhanced OS, PFS, and ORR with modified FOLFOX4 regimen may offer some palliative advantages to the Asian HCC patients; however, a definite OS advantage cannot be deduced from their study, and further research was suggested.

3.3. Interferon alpha (IFNα)

Interferon alpha (IFNα) is an immunomodulatory cytokine (immunotherapy/biotherapy) that has exhibited antineoplastic effects against many neoplasms counting HCC.

3.3.1. IFNα monotherapy

As a minimum, three controlled trials have examined single-agent IFNα therapy in patients with far-advanced unresectable HCC; however, research outcomes were contradictory.

Regimen	Reference	Authors	Year	Combination systemic chemotherapy	*n*	RR (%)	DS (%)	TTP (mon)	PFS (mon)	OS (mon)
Cisplatin-based regimen	[134]	Lee et al.	2004	Cisplatin plus doxorubicin	42	18.9	16.2	6.6	NR	7.3
		Yang et al.	2004	Cisplatin, mitoxantrone, plus continuous infusion 5-FU	63	23.8	NR	2.5	NR	4.9
		Ikeda et al.	2005	Cisplatin, mitoxantrone, plus continuous infusion 5-FU	51	27	NR	NR	4	11.6
	[137]	Boucher et al.	2002	Cisplatin, epirubicin plus infusional 5-FU	21	14.5	NR	5.9	NR	10
	[138]	Park et al.	2006	Cisplatin, doxorubicin plus capecitabine	29	24	20.7	3.7	NR	7.7
	[139]	Shim et al.	2009	Cisplatin plus capecitabine	178	19.7	45	NR	2.8	10.5
	[140]	Lee et al.	2009	Cisplatin plus capecitabine	32	6.3	34.3	2	NR	12.2
Gemcitabine-based regimen	[141]	Parikh et al.	2005	Gemcitabine and cisplatin	30	20	43	4.5	NR	5.3
	[142]	Chia et al.	2008	Gemcitabine and cisplatin	15	6.7	20	NR	1.5	4.5
	[143]	Lombardi et al.	2011	Gemcitabine plus pegylated liposomal doxorubicin	41	NR	24	NR	5.8	22.5
Oxaliplatin-based regimen	[144]	Louafi et al.	2007	Gemcitabine plus oxaliplatin (GEMOX)	34	18	58	NR	6.3	11.5
	[145]	Mir et al.	2012	Gemcitabine plus oxaliplatin (GEMOX)	18	18.8	18.8	NR	3.2	4.7
	[146]	Zaanan et al.	2013	Gemcitabine plus oxaliplatin (GEMOX)	204	22	66	NR	4.5	11
	[147]	Boige et al.	2007	Gapecitabine plus oxaliplatin (XELOX)	50	6	72	NR	4.1	9.3

n: sample size; RR: response rate; DS: disease stabilization; TTP: time to progression; PFS: progression-free survival; OS: overall survival; NR: not reported; mon: months

Table 1. Summary of major phases I and II studies on combination systemic chemotherapy in patients with advanced inoperable HCC

In 1989, Lai et al. (Chinese prospective randomized trial) explored the efficacy of single-agent IFNα versus single-agent doxorubicin in 75 patients with advanced unresectable HCC. The IFNα group achieved a higher median OS than the doxorubicin group (8.3 months vs. 4.8 months), although it was not statistically significant. Doxorubicin-related adverse events included neutropenia and cardiotoxicity in approximately 25% of patients. Conversely, IFNα-related adverse events included adrenal gland failure and dementia in roughly 3.8% of patients. Overall, IFNα achieved statistically significant robust cancer regression ($P = 0.00199$), less worsening cancers ($P = 0.00017$), less life-threatening long-lasting bone marrow suppression ($P = 0.01217$), and less severe drug-related adverse events ($P = 0.01383$) when compared to doxorubicin group. The study concluded that IFNα was superior to doxorubicin in terms of cancer control as well as less lethal bone marrow suppression and adverse events.

In 1993, Lai et al. [66] (randomized controlled trial) examined the efficacy of IFNα (intramuscular 50×10^6 IU/m^2 3 times weekly) and no anticancer treatment in 35 and 36 advanced unresectable HCC Chinese patients, respectively. The IFNα group achieved a higher median OS than no anticancer group (14.5 vs. 7.5 months; $P = 0.0471$), as well as significant robust cancer regression ($P < 0.0001$) and less worsening (progressive) cancers ($P = 0.001$). Despite the IFNα dose was comparatively high, it was well tolerated; roughly 34% of patients had one-third to one-half dosage decreases as a result of continuous generalized weakness. Moreover, type 2 diabetes mellitus patients experienced mental worsening that could be related to IFNα treatment. The study concluded that IFNα was beneficial in a subset of Chinese patients with advanced unresectable HCC, in terms of cancer control (tumor regression) and extended disease-related survival expectancy.

However, the above-mentioned results of Lia et al. [66] were not validated and reciprocated in a second randomized clinical trial by Llovet et al. in 58 advanced HCC patients with ineligibility to undergo surgery, transplantation, or other treatment modalities. The study took place in year 2000 and randomized patients to receive either IFNα ($n = 30$) or BSC ($n = 28$). Of the 30 IFNα-treated patients, only 2 patients (6.6%) achieved objective partial responses. Although the 1-year and 2-year survival rates were higher in IFNα-treated vs. BSC groups (58% vs. 38% and 36% vs. 12%, respectively), there were no statistical significant differences. Although IFNα dose was greatly decreased, 23 (76.7%) of 30 patients experienced severe unbearable drug-related adverse events (toxicities) resulting in drug suspension in exactly 13 patients. The study concluded that IFNα was not appropriately endured by advanced HCC patients, and its administration did not yield beneficial advantages in the context of cancer progression and OS rates.

In conclusion, studies on single-agent IFNα therapy showed conflicting outcomes. Additionally, dose-related toxicities were frequent despite lower doses were administered. Clear-cut clinical benefits are uncertain and further research is needed.

3.3.2. IFNα-based combination therapy

There are two major IFN-based combination chemotherapeutic regimens: PIAF regimen and (5-FU plus IFNα) regimen.

3.3.2.1. PIAF regimen

PIAF regimen is composed of cisplatin, IFNα, doxorubicin, and infusional 5-FU. PIAF regimen has been shown to exhibit active antitumor effects despite its significantly lethal drug-related toxic adverse events in patients with advanced HCC 8-. For example, in 1999, Leung et al. administered PIAF regimen in 50 patients. Around 13 patients (26%) experienced a partial response. The median OS was 8.9 months. The most frequent toxicities were mucositis and myelosuppression. There were two events of drug-related mortality as a result of neutropenic sepsis.

In 2005, Yeo et al. (multinational randomized phase III study) examined the efficacy of single-agent doxorubicin (60 mg/m^2 every three weeks) versus PIAF regimen (cisplatin: 20 mg/m^2 on days 1-4; IFNα: 5 MU/m^2 subcutaneously on days 1-4; doxorubicin: 40 mg/m^2 on day 1; and 5-FU 400 mg/m^2 on days 1-4) in 188 chemotherapy-naive patients with inoperable HCC. Although not statistically significant, the PIAF-treated group achieved higher ORR and median OS than the single-agent doxorubicin group (20.9% vs. 10.5% and 8.7 months vs. 6.8 months, respectively). However, as expected, drug-related adverse events were more noticeable and statistically significant in the PIAF-treated group than in doxorubicin-treated group, as follows: grade 3/4 hypokalemia (7% vs. 0%, respectively), grade 3/4 neutropenia (82% vs. 63%, respectively), and grade 3/4 thrombocytopenia (57% vs. 24%, respectively). The study concluded that although the PIAF-treated group achieved higher overall ORR and beneficial survival outcomes, the difference was statistically insignificant and not worthwhile. Additionally, PIAF regimen incurred far greater statistically significant drug-related adverse events.

One potential clarification for the Yeo et al. study's failure to demonstrate a survival advantage may be attributed to the improper patient selection. Subsequently, the correlation significance between results of PIAF regimen and baseline liver function was exhibited in a retrospective analysis by Leung et al.. The study analyzed a series of roughly 150 patients with advanced inoperable HCC who received prior therapy with PIAF regimen. The study concluded that good risk patients (normal baseline total bilirubin levels and noncirrhotic liver) achieved higher statistically significant objective responses (50% vs. 6%) and prolonged survival rates than bad risk patients (total serum bilirubin level >0.6 mg/dL and cirrhotic liver) when medicated with systemic PIAF regimen.

In short, the role of PIAF chemotherapeutic schedule in the management of advanced inoperable HCC remains unclear. Bearing in mind the lethal drug-related toxicity profile, it should be indicated only for physically and biochemically fit patients who possess appropriate performance status and minimal hepatic insufficiency.

3.3.2.2. 5-FU plus IFNα

Stuart et al. and Patt et al. had conflicting results. In 1996, Stuart et al. administered 5-FU (750 mg/m^2 weekly) plus IFNα (9 MU three times weekly) in 10 patients with advanced HCC. The ORR and the OS were 0% and 10 months, respectively. It was concluded that the 5-FU plus IFNα regimen was not effective and drug-related toxicities were highly significant.

Moreover, in 2003, Patt et al. (phase II) administered 5-FU (200 mg/m^2/day for 3 weeks every 4-week interval) plus IFNα2b (4 million U/m^2 for three times weekly) in 43 patients with advanced HCC. Liver cirrhosis was present among 71% of HCC. ORR was evaluable in only 28 patients, and it was 14% (all were partial responses). For all patients, the OS was 15.5 months. The study concluded that 5-FU plus IFNα is effective and can be tolerated by cirrhotic patients.

http://dx.doi.org/10.5772/60991

Of note, several studies by Sakon et al., Ota et al., and Nagano et al. have examined the combination of systemic IFNα with intrahepatic arterial 5-FU in patients with primary advanced inoperable HCC complicated by major portal vein thrombosis. Interestingly, ORRs ranging from 33% to 73% were achieved. More specifically, chemotherapy responsiveness, TTP, and OS rates were higher in IFN-alpha type 2 receptor (IFNAR2)-positive HCC versus IFNAR2-negative HCC. It was concluded that chemotherapy responsiveness, TTP, and OS are significantly linked to expression of IFNAR2 in HCC patients receiving 5 FU plus IFNα combined chemotherapeutic regimen.

In conclusion, combinations of chemotherapeutics with interferon alpha (IFNα) seem to be active. However, definitive survival benefits are not clear.

3.4. Conclusion

The employment of systemic chemotherapy has been accompanied by low ORRs, no survival advantages, and high incidences of drug-related toxicities and adverse events. Moreover, there are no adequate data to endorse or approve any single-agent or combined chemotherapeutic regimens for the management of patients with advanced inoperable HCC [76].

Recently, chemotherapy is not being employed routinely for patients with advanced inoperable HCC. This tendency can be attributed to three major rationales:

1. First, HCC is largely a chemoresistant neoplasm. This may be related to expression of several drug resistance genes, such as heat shock proteins, p53 mutations, glutathione-S-transferase, p-glycoprotein, and multidrug resistance gene (MDR-1) -81].

2. Second, the status of underlying liver cirrhosis and its associated complications (for example, hepatic encephalopathy, portal hypertension, hypoalbuminemia, coagulopathies, portal venous thrombosis, ascites, hypersplenism, platelet sequestration, varices and gastrointestinal bleeding, discrepant drug binding, altered biochemical distribution, and disrupted pharmacokinetics) in the vast majority of patients precludes the choice and effective dosing administration of substantial proportions of anticancer chemotherapeutics. Systemic chemotherapeutics are generally not well tolerated by patients with substantial underlying hepatic insufficiencies, and this is a major limitation. In one study by Nagahama et al. [82], there were no objective responses among HCC patients with bilateral disease (2 hepatic lobes), 50% or more of hepatic involvement, ascites, total serum bilirubin >2.0 mg/dL, portal venous thrombosis, and poor functional status of 2-3.

3. Third, the vast majority of studies have been conducted in diverse patient populations with various clinicopathological factors such as old vs. young, cirrhosis due to hepatitis B or C virus vs. cirrhosis due to alcoholism, chemotherapy-naive patients vs. previously chemotherapy-treated patients, etc. Such population diversity is expected to result in inconsistent enrolling criteria and study outcomes among the various controlled trials. Moreover, almost all controlled clinical trials are negatively impacted by insufficient sample size, improper study controls, and inappropriate study primary/secondary end points.

The arrival of novel molecularly targeted therapy (specifically sorafenib) is rapidly emerging as the standard of care in patients with advanced inoperable HCC.

That being said, systemic chemotherapy may still be regarded in patients whom their HCC get worse while on sorafenib and whom baseline liver function and performance status are adequate enough to endure it.

The chemotherapy-related adverse events of any single-agent or combined regimen should be deliberated cautiously in patients with progressive inoperable HCC, multiple comorbidities, and very short life expectancy. Generally speaking, systemic chemotherapy should be selectively administered to physically and medically fit patients who possess appropriate hepatic functional reserve. Moreover, such administration should be ideally considered only within the context of phase II and III clinical trials.

The choice of systemic chemotherapy should be guided by patients' functional hepatic reserve, physical fitness, prognosis, life expectancy, and most importantly availability of the best evidence-based medicine (randomized controlled phase III clinical trials).

Lastly, the reactivation of viral hepatitis may take place in HCC patients receiving aggressively exhaustive systemic chemotherapeutic regimens. Accordingly, it is crucial and greatly recommended to maintain antiviral therapies, whenever deemed necessarily.

4. Novel molecularly targeted therapy

These therapies are targeted against specific molecular signaling pathways involved in HCC carcinogenesis. Several nonrandomized and phase I, II, and III clinical trials have been conducted to examine the role of novel molecularly targeted therapy (monotherapy or combination therapy) for the management of advanced inoperable HCC.

4.1. Sorafenib

Sorafenib is the official first Food and Drug Administration (FDA)-approved monotherapy drug for the management of patients with advanced unresectable HCC, ineligible for surgical resection, liver transplantation, and loco-regional therapies. Several prospective studies have evaluated the efficacy of sorafenib as single-agent (monotherapy) and combination therapy with systemic cytotoxic chemotherapy and loco-regional therapy.

4.1.1. Sorafenib monotherapy

A total of 7 studies have been conducted on single-agent sorafenib with a sum of 1072 patients.

Table 2 exhibits a summary of major phase I and III studies on single-agent sorafenib for the management of patients with advanced inoperable HCC.

Ref.	Authors	Year	Phase	*n*	Age (yr)	Gender (%)		CPS (%)			Hepatitis		DCR (%)	TTP (mon)	OS (mon)	Toxicities		
						Male	Female	A	B	C	HBV	HCV				Diarrhea	Fatigue	HFS
[88]	Furuse et al.	2008	I	27	70	93	17	48	52	0	15	74	83	4.9	15.6	0	0	27
[148]	Castroagudin et al.	2008	I	13	64	100	0	92	NR	NR	0	23	62	NR	2	82	91	18
[149]	Abou-Alfa et al.	2006	II	137	69	88	12	72	28	0	17	48	36	4.2	9.2	8	10	5
[150]	Massa et al.	2008	II	16	72	88	12	NR	NR	NR	NR	NR	64	3	15	6	6	6
[87]	Yau et al.	2008	II	51	56	93	7	71	26	3	90	6	26	3	5	16	20	8
[84]	Llovet et al.	2008	III (sorafenib)	299	65	87	13	95	5	0	19	29	43	5.6	10.7	1	3	3
			III (placebo)	303	66	87	13	98	2	0	18	27	32	2.8	7.9	1	0.6	0.3
[85]	Cheng et al.	2009	III (sorafenib)	150	51	85	15	97	3	0	71	11	35	2.8	6.5	6	3	11
			III (placebo)	76	52	87	13	97	3	0	78	4	16	1-4	4.2	1	0	0

n: sample size; yr: year; CPS: Child-Pugh score; HBV: hepatitis B virus; HCV: hepatitis C virus; DCR: disease control rate; TTP: time to progression; OS: overall survival; HFS: hand-foot syndrome; NR: not reported; mon: months.

Table 2. Summary of major phases I-III studies on single-agent sorafenib for the management of patients with advanced inoperable HCC

The numbers of phase I, II, and III studies were 2, 3, and 2, respectively. Overall, the vast majority of patients were elderly (above 50 years), males, CPS-A/CPS-B, and HBV/HCV positive. The DCR ranged from as low as 26% to as high as 82%. TTP ranged from 3 to 5.5 months, whereas OS ranged from 3 to 15.6 months. The most frequent sorafenib-related toxicities were fatigue (range: 0-91%), diarrhea (range: 0-82%), and hand-foot syndrome [HFS] (range: 3-27%).

The two high-quality, large-sized, randomized placebo-controlled phase III trials were the SHARP and Asia-Pacific reports. In both reports, the greater proportions of patients had CPS-A cirrhosis, and these proportions were almost similar (95% and 97%, respectively). However, the occurrence of hepatitis B infection (HBV) was different (19% vs. 71%, respectively). In the SHARP report, in comparison with placebo groups, the sorafenib group achieved higher statistically significant median TTP (5.5 vs. 2.8 months, respectively; $P < 0.05$) and OS (10.7 vs. 7.9 months, respectively; $P < 0.05$). Conversely, in the Asia-Pacific report, in comparison with the placebo groups, the sorafenib group achieved higher statistically significant median TTP (2.8 vs. 1.4 months, respectively; $P < 0.05$) and OS (6.5 vs. 4.2 months, respectively; $P < 0.05$).

The noted differences between TTP and OS between SHARP and Asia-Pacific trials were contemplated, and a question was raised as whether etiology of cirrhosis (HBV vs. HCV) influences the therapeutic response to sorafenib. Subsequently, Bruix et al. conducted sub-analyses of SHARP study and showed that the median OS (sorafenib vs. placebo) was highest in patients with HCV cirrhosis (14 vs. 7.4 months; difference: 6.6 months), followed by patients with HBV cirrhosis (9.7 vs. 6.1 months; difference: 3.6 months), and then by patients with underlying alcohol-related liver disease (10.3 vs. 8 months; difference: 2.3 months). The study concluded that HCV (as opposed to HBV) positively influences therapeutic response to sorafenib. Similar conclusions were attained elsewhere in other studies in Korea and Japan.

Exploring prognostic biomarkers of therapeutic responses is necessary. Several molecular (for example, FGF3/FGF4, MET, VEGF/VEGFR, pERK), biochemical (for example, elevated AST) -, and clinical (for example, diarrhea, high blood pressure) [94, 95] factors have been proposed to forecast therapeutic response; however, none has been confirmed and definitely established for employment in clinical practice.

In summary, based on the findings of SHARP and Asia-Pacific phase III trials, sorafenib is the official first Food and Drug Administration (FDA)-approved monotherapy drug for the management of patients with advanced unresectable HCC, ineligible for surgical resection, liver transplantation, and loco-regional therapies [83]. Table 2 exhibits that single-agent sorafenib therapy yields statistically significant, although moderate, clinical improvements in the contexts of DCR, TTP, and OS in males younger than 70 years and have CPS-A cirrhosis. Not much information are existing regarding the effects of single-agent sorafenib therapy in females and in patient populations older than 70 years of age and having advanced CPS-B/ CPS-C cirrhosis. Patients with HCV-related cirrhosis have longer OS and higher DCR rates, whereas patients with HBV-related cirrhosis have shorter OS and lower DCR rates in patients receiving sorafenib. The most frequent sorafenib-related adverse events include fatigue, diarrhea, and HFS.

4.1.2. *Sorafenib-based combination therapy*

Several studies have combined sorafenib with loco-regional and systemic therapies in patients with advanced unresectable HCC. Loco-regional therapies mainly include transarterial chemoembolization (TACE), transarterial radioemobolization (TARE), radiation, and others. Systemic therapies mainly include cytotoxic chemotherapeutics, hormonal (somatostatin analog) therapies, and others.

The most frequently studied sorafenib-based combination regimen is sorafenib plus TACE. A recently published meta-analysis in 2014 by Zhang et al. [96] examined six studies published from 2011 to 2013 (n = 1254 patients) about the efficacy and safety of sorafenib plus TACE versus TACE alone in patients with intermediate to advanced unresectable HCC. The meta-analysis concluded that the combination therapy of sorafenib plus TACE was associated with higher statistically significant ORR (P = 0.021), TTP (P = 0.003), and OS (P = 0.007); however, greater frequency of grade 3/4 adverse events than in the TACE group.

Prete et al. [97] examined the safety and efficacy of sorafenib plus octreotide in 50 patients with advanced HCC; 16 patients (*n* = 16) were treatment naive (34%), whereas the rest underwent prior local and/or systemic management. Partial response, stable disease, and disease progression occurred in 10%, 66%, and 24% of patients, respectively. The median TTP and OS were 7 months and 12 months, respectively. Regimen therapy was generally well endured, and hypertension (4%) and diarrhea (6%) were the most common grade 3/4 drug-related adverse side effects. The study concluded that sorafenib plus octreotide regimen is active and well tolerated and signifies a potential therapeutic choice in such patient population with advanced HCC.

Hsu et al. [98] examined the safety and efficacy of sorafenib plus metronomic tegafur/uracil in 53 patients with advanced HCC, all of which (100%) and 72% were CPS-A and Hepatitis B surface antigen positive. Partial response and stable disease occurred in 8% and 49% of patients, respectively. The median TTP and OS were 3.7 months and 7.4 months, respectively. The most common grade 3/4 drug-related adverse side effects included bleeding (8%), HFS (9%), elevated serum lipase enzyme (10%), deranged liver function tests (13%), and generalized weakness (15%).

Petrini et al. [99] investigated the safety and efficacy of sorafenib plus 5-FU in 38 patients with advanced HCC. DCR was 48%, whereas the median TTP and OS were 7.6 months and 12.2 months, respectively. The most common drug-related adverse side effects were HFS (55%) and diarrhea (13%).

Yau et al. [100] investigated the safety and efficacy of sorafenib plus capecitabine plus oxaliplatin in 51 patients with advanced or metastatic HCC (phase II trial). The vast majority of patients had CPS-A (98%) and HBV infection (84%). DCR was 75%, whereas the median TTP and OS were 7.1 months and 10.2 months, respectively. The most common drug-related adverse side effects were HFS (73%) and diarrhea (69%).

Richly et al. [101] investigated the safety and efficacy of sorafenib plus doxorubicin in 47 patients with advanced or metastatic HCC (phase II trial). All patients had CPS-A (100%). DCR was 62%, whereas the median TTP and OS were 6.4 months and 13.7 months, respectively. The most common drug-related adverse side effects were HFS (6%), diarrhea (11%), and generalized weakness (6%).

There was only one randomized, placebo-controlled, phase III trial that examined the efficacy of doxorubicin plus sorafenib (*n* = 47) versus doxorubicin plus placebo (*n* = 49) in patients with advanced unresectable HCC [102]. In contrast to the doxorubicin plus placebo group, the doxorubicin plus sorafenib group achieved higher statistically significant DCR (62% vs. 29%, respectively), TTP (6.4 vs. 2.8 months, respectively), and OS (13.7 vs. 6.5 months, respectively). The frequencies of drug-related adverse events were comparable to those for monotherapies. Despite the survival benefits associated with doxorubicin plus sorafenib, the combination of doxorubicin plus sorafenib is not yet indicated for routine clinical use.

In summary, studies of sorafenib-based combination therapy report better DCR, TTP, and OS benefits when compared to single-agent sorafenib therapy, without increased frequencies of excessive treatment-related toxicities and adverse events. However, the vast majority of the conducted sorafenib-based combination therapy studies were quite small-sized case series reporting preliminary findings, and comprehensive data about patient characteristics and clinical outcomes were not often provided. Thus, it is improper to compare such studies. Moreover, in the only phase III trial by Abou-Alfa et al. [102], it was demonstrated that sorafenib plus doxorubicin regimen is more efficacious than doxorubicin alone but does not automatically deliberate that combination therapy (doxorubicin plus sorafenib) is better than single-agent doxorubicin alone. Further research is needed.

4.1.3. Safety and efficacy of sorafenib in hepatic dysfunction

The safety of sorafenib in patients with hepatic dysfunction, as determined by Child-Pugh score (CPS), has been explored.

In 2011, Abou-Alfa et al. [103] explored the efficacy and safety of sorafenib in HCC patients with CPS-A (n = 98) and CPS-B (n = 38). In comparison with CPS-A patients, CPS-B patients achieved lower statistically significant median duration of therapy (1.8 vs. 4 months, respectively) and OS (3.2 vs. 9.5 months, respectively). Moreover, grade 3/4 adverse events took place in both CPS-A and CPS-B patients and encompassed encephalopathy (3% vs. 13%, respectively), ascites (3% vs. 5%, respectively), and hyperbilirubinemia (14% vs. 53%, respectively).

Moreover, Pinter et al. [104] examined the efficacy and safety of sorafenib in HCC patients with CPS-A (n = 26), CPS-B (n = 23), and CPS-C (n = 10). Respectively, the median OS was 8.3, 4.3, and 1.5 months. It was concluded that sorafenib is questionable to offer survival advantages in patients with CPS-C cirrhosis.

Furthermore, Lencioni et al. [105] examined the safety and efficacy of sorafenib in 1586 patients with liver dysfunction in their first interim analysis of the Global Investigation of Therapeutic Decisions in Hepatocellular Carcinoma and of its Treatment with Sorafenib (GIDEON). CPS-B patients experienced more serious adverse events than CPS-A patients (60% vs. 3%, respectively), higher rates of treatment termination (40% vs. 25%, respectively), and higher frequencies of mortality during treatment up to 1 month from the latest sorafenib dose administration (37% vs. 18%, respectively).

However, Raoul et al. [106] in a subanalysis of SHARP trial concluded that sorafenib was safe and effective in patients with mild to moderate liver dysfunction (equal to or greater than 1.8 times the upper limit of normal) without events of increased hepatic toxicities.

In conclusion, sorafenib has better efficacy and safety profiles in HCC patients with CPS-A than CPS-B and CPS-C. For HCC patients with CPS-B, standard dosing should be initiated and then doses can be adjusted accordingly, whenever deemed necessary. Sorafenib is not recommended for HCC patients with CPS-C. Further research is needed.

4.1.4. Safety and efficacy of sorafenib post liver transplantation

There are minimal data regarding the safety and efficacy of sorafenib plus immunosuppressive therapies (such as mammalian target of rapamycin [mTOR] or calcineurin inhibitors) in patients with recurrent HCC post orthotopic liver transplantation (OLT).

The largest experienced was reported by Gomez-Martin et al. [107]. Twenty-six patients had recurrent HCC post OLT. Ten and sixteen patients received sorafenib doses at 800 mg and 400 mg daily, respectively, in addition to anti-mTOR as an immunosuppresive therapy post OLT. The overall DCR was 54%, whereas the overall TTP and OS were 6.8 and 19.3 months, respectively. Diarrhea (13%, probably due to sorafenib treatment) and mucositis (8%, probably due to anti-mTOR treatment) were the most frequent adverse events.

However, higher frequencies of therapy-related toxicities and adverse events were documented in other studies combining sorafenib and anti-mTOR [108-110]. For instance, Staufer et al. [109] reported grade 3/4 adverse events in 92% of patients, 77% of whom terminated sorafenib therapy. However, partial response and stable disease were attained in 1 and 4 patients, respectively.

In summary, the combination of sorafenib plus anti-mTOR is feasible in recurrent HCC patients following OLT. However, therapy should be carefully checked due to the probability of severe adverse events. Dose modification may be needed.

4.2. Antiangiogenic agents

HCCs are largely vascular neoplasms as increased expressions of micro-vessel concentration and vascular endothelial growth factor (VEGF) have been identified [111-114]. The increased expression of VEGF has been linked to poorer survival outcomes [115-117]. Thus, the inhibition of angiogenesis denotes a highly desired therapeutic target in patients with advanced inoperable HCC. Numerous antiangiogenic drugs have already been introduced in clinical studies in monotherapies and combined therapies. Such drugs include bevacizumab, sunitinib, brivanib, pazopanib, inifanib (ABT-869), cediranib (AZD2171), selumetinib (AZD6244), orantinib (TSU-68), ramucirumab, vatalanib (PTK787/ZK 222584), tivantinib, and others.

In a randomized, placebo-controlled, double-blind, phase III trial (BRISK-PS study) by Llovet et al. [118], a total of 395 HCC patients—who failed sorafenib treatment (during or after therapy) or who were ineligible for sorafenib treatment in the first place—were enrolled in the study. Patients were randomized to receive brivanib (800 mg orally once per day) plus best supportive care (BSC) or placebo plus BSC. In brivanib versus placebo groups, the median OS was 9.4 months vs. 8.2 months ($P = 0.3307$), respectively, whereas TTP was 4.2 months vs. 2.7 months ($P < 0.001$), respectively. Treatment-related study termination occurred in 23% and 7% of brivanib and placebo groups, respectively. Grade 3/4 decreased appetite (10%), hyponatremia (11%), fatigue (13%), and hypertension (17%) were the most common drug-related harmful frequencies. The study concluded that patients who were previously managed with sorafenib, brivanib therapy did not substantially improve OS.

Tivantinib (ARQ 187) is a selective oral inhibitor of c-Met (tyrosine kinase receptor) with multiple roles in neoplastic cell proliferation, migration, invasion, and angiogenesis [33]. Santoro et al. [119] conducted a randomized placebo-controlled phase II trial and examined the role of tivantinib as a second-line novel molecularly targeted therapy in patients with advanced HCC. Major DCR, TTP and DFS advantages were attained in Met+ patients, with an initial OS inclination favoring tivantinib (HR = 0.47) and no negative effects in Met- patients.

For Met+ patients, tivantinib achieved higher DCR (50% vs. 20%) and OS (7.2 months vs. 3.8 weeks) than placebo-treated group [33, 119]. Four drug-related mortalities happened in tivantinib group. Grade 3/4 adverse events in tivantinib group included: neutropenia (14%) and anaemia (11%); none occurred in the placebo groups. The study concluded that tivantinib (compared to placebo) substantially benefited second-line HCC patients, particularly if Met+ patients with well-tolerated drug safety dosing at 240 mg twice daily. There is an ongoing prospective, randomized, double-blind, phase III study of tivantinib in Met-high advanced unresectable HCC patients with one previous administration of systemic therapy [33].

Table 3 exhibits a summary of major phase I and II studies on antiangiogenesis monotherapies in patients with advanced HCC. Among the antiangiogenic drugs, bevacizumab stands out as the most effective single-agent novel molecularly targeted therapy. Objective response and disease stabilization rates can be achieved in 7%-13% and 54%-57%, respectively, whereas PFS and OS durations can achieve durations of 3.5-6.9 months and 12.4 months, respectively. However, the drug-related toxicities of hypertension as well as major bleeding and thrombo-embolic events are major limiting factors [120-122].

	Reference	Authors	Year	Phase	Single-agent therapy	n	RR (%)	DS (%)	TTP (mon)	PFS (mon)	OS (mon)
Antiangiogenic agents	[122]	Schwartz et al.	2006	II	Bevacizumab	30	6.7	57	6.4	NR	NR
	[120]	Malka et al.	2007	II	Bevacizumab	30	12.5	54	NR	3.5	NR
	[121]	Siegel et al.	2008	II	Bevacizumab	46	13	NR	NR	6.9	12.4
	[151]	Hoda et al.	2008	II	Sunitinib	23	6	35	NR	NR	NR
	[152]	Zhu et al.	2009	II	Sunitinib	34	2.9	47	4.1	3.9	9.8
	[153]	Faivre et al.	2009	II	Sunitinib	37	2.7	35	5.3	3.7	8
	[154]	Koeberle et al.	2010	II	Sunitinib	45	2	40	2.8	2.8	9.3
	[155]	Finn et al.	2012	II	Brivanib	46	4.3	41.3	2.7	NR	9.79
	[156]	Yau et al.	2009	I	Pazopanib	27	7	41	4.6	NR	NR
	[157]	Toh et al.	2009	II	Inifanib (ABT-869)	44	8.7	NR	3.7	3.7	9.8
	[158]	Alberts et al.	2007	II	Cediranib (AZD2171)	28	0	NR	2.8	NR	5.8
	[159]	O'Neil et al.	2009	II	Selumetinib (AZD6244)	19	0	37.5	2	NR	NR
	[160]	Kanai et al.	2010	I/II	Orantinib (TSU-68)	35	8.6	42.8	2.1	NR	13.1
	[161]	Zhu et al.	2010	II	Ramucirumab	42	NR	50	NR	4.3	NR
	[162]	Koch et al.	2007	I	Vatalanib (PTK787)	18	0	50	NR	NR	7.3
Anti-EGFR agents	[128]	Philip et al.	2005	II	Erlotinib	38	7.9	59	NR	3.2	13
	[129]	Thomas et al.	2007	II	Erlotinib	40	0	43	NR	3.1	11
	[163]	O'Dwyer et al.	2006	II	Gefitinib	31	3	22.5	NR	2.8	6.5
	[164]	Ramanathan et al.	2009	II	Lapatinib	57	5	35	NR	2.3	6.2

	Reference	Authors	Year	Phase	Single-agent therapy	*n*	RR (%)	DS (%)	TTP (mon)	PFS (mon)	OS (mon)
	[165]	Lin et al.	2008	II	Imatinib	15	0	13.3	NR	NR	NR
	[166]	Zhu et al.	2007	II	Cetuximab	30	0	17	NR	1.4	9.6
	[167]	Gruenwald et al.	2007	II	Cetuximab	32	0	44	1.9	2	NR
Anti-mTOR agents	[168]	Blaszkowsky et al.	2011	I/II	Everolimus	28	4	44	NR	3.8	8.4
	[169]	Rizell et al.	2008	II	Sirolimus	21	4.8	23.8	NR	NR	6.5

n: sample size; RR: response rate; DS: disease stabilization; TTP: time to progression; PFS: progression-free survival; OS: overall survival; NR: not reported; mon: months

Table 3. Summary of major phases I and II studies on single-agent novel molecularly targeted therapy in advanced HCC patients

In summary, the inhibition of angiogenesis appears to be feasible and promising. The combination of antiangiogenic drugs (particularly bevacizumab) and other local/systemic therapies may further enhance survival outcomes in patients with advanced inoperable HCC. Additional research is needed and many randomized controlled trials are already in place.

4.3. Epidermal growth factor receptor (EGFR) inhibitors

The expression of numerous EGF family members (such as EGF, EGFR, transforming growth factor-alpha [TGF-α], heparin-binding epidermal growth factor, and others) has been confirmed in many HCC cell tissues [123-127]. Thus, disrupting the EGFR signaling pathway denotes a highly desired therapeutic target in patients with advanced inoperable HCC. Subsequently, two major categories of anti-EGFR have been created: EGFR tyrosine kinase inhibitors and monoclonal antibodies against EGFR. Numerous anti-EGFR drugs have already been introduced in clinical studies in monotherapies and combined therapies. Examples of EGFR tyrosine kinase inhibitors include erlotinib, gefitinib, lapatinib, and imatinib. The most commonly used monoclonal antibody against EGFR is cetuximab.

Among the anti-EGFR drugs, erlotinib stands out the most effective single-agent novel molecularly targeted therapy. In two randomized controlled trials [128, 129] examining the role of erlotinib in patients with advanced unresectable HCC, a total of 78 patients were enrolled. Although ORR ranged from 0% to 9%, the average disease stabilization rate reached 51%, whereas average PFR and OS achieved durations of 3 and 12 months, respectively. However, the most frequent drug-related toxicities were skin-related reactions and diarrhea. Apart from the fairly moderate antitumor effects associated with erlotinib, the remaining drugs belonging to EGFR inhibitors have failed to demonstrate any substantial antineoplastic effects as monotherapies in patients with advanced HCC [33].

Table 3 exhibits a summary of major phase I and II studies on single-agent EGFR inhibitors (novel molecularly targeted therapy) in patients with advanced HCC.

In summary, interfering with EGFR signaling pathway appears to be feasible, promising, and an exciting area for future research. The combination of anti-EGFR drugs (particularly erlotinib) and other local/systemic therapies may further enhance survival outcomes in patients with advanced inoperable HCC. Additional research is needed and many randomized controlled trials are already in place.

4.4. Mammalian target of rapamycin (mTOR) inhibitors

The significance of the mTOR signaling pathway in HCC pathogenesis was explored in a large-sized research study involving 314 HCC and 37 noncancerous tissues that utilized a variety of molecular-based laboratory techniques [130]. The major study findings were abnormal mTOR signaling (p-RPS6) in 50% of patients, chromosomal gains in rapamycinin-sensitive companion of mTOR (RICTOR) in 25% of patients, and direct correlation between positive p-RPS6 immunohistochemical staining and HCC recurrence post surgical excision. Thus, disrupting the mTOR signaling pathway designates a highly potential therapeutic target in patients with advanced inoperable HCC. Numerous anti-mTOR drugs have already been introduced in clinical studies in monotherapies and combined therapies. Examples of mTOR inhibitors include everolimus, sirolimus, and temsirolimus.

Among the anti-mTOR drugs, everolimus stands out as the most effective single-agent novel molecularly targeted therapy despite the modest antitumor activities. Dose-limiting adverse events are common and include infection, diarrhea, elevated alanine aminotransferase, elevated total bilirubin, cardiac ischemia, and reactivation of HBV/HCV [131].

Table 3 exhibits a summary of major phase I and II studies on single-agent mTOR inhibitors (novel molecularly targeted therapy) in patients with advanced HCC.

In view of the modest antitumor activities of everolimus, Zhu et al. [132] conducted a multi-center, randomized, double-blind, phase III trial (EVOLVE-1) in 546 adult HCC patients who failed sorafenib treatment (during or after therapy) or who were ineligible for sorafenib treatment in the first place. Patients were randomized to everolimus plus best supportive care (BSC) (n = 362) and placebo plus BSC (n = 184) groups. No statistically significant differences in median TTP and OS were achieved among both treatment groups. However, a statistically significant DCR was achieved in everolimus versus placebo group (56.1% vs. 45.1%, respectively; P = 0.01), and mortality rate was comparable (83.7% vs. 82.1%, respectively). The most frequent grade 3/4 toxicities observed in everolimus versus placebo groups were generalized weakness (7.8% vs. 5.5%, respectively), diminished appetite (6.1% vs. 0.5%, respectively), and anemia (7.8% vs. 3.3%, respectively). No single patient encountered HCV flare-up, however, HBV reactivation was encountered by 29 everolimus and 10 placebo (n = 39 patients; overall 7%); all of which were symptom free. The study concluded that administration of everolimus did not improve OS in patients with advanced HCC whose cancer progressed during or after receiving sorafenib or who were intolerant of sorafenib.

4.5. Combination therapy with novel molecularly targeted therapy and systemic chemotherapy

Table 4 exhibits a summary of phases I and II on combined novel molecularly targeted therapy and systemic chemotherapy in patients with advanced HCC.

Reference	Authors	Year	Phase	Combined Therapy	n	RR (%)	DS (%)	TTP (mon)	PFS (mon)	OS (mon)
[144]	Louafi et al.[1]	2007	II	Cetuximab plus gemcitabine plus oxaliplatin	35	24	4.5	NR	NR	9.2
[170]	Asnacios et al.[1]	2008	II	Cetuximab plus gemcitabine plus oxaliplatin	45	20	40	NR	4.7	9.5
[171]	Sanoff et al.	2011	II	Cetuximab plus capecitabine plus oxaliplatin	24	12.5	71	4.5	NR	4.4
[172]	Zhu et al.	2006	II	Bevacizumab plus gemcitabine plus oxaliplatin	33	20	27	NR	5.3	9.6
[173]	Sun et al.	2007	II	Bevacizumab plus capecitabine plus oxaliplatin	29	11	78	NR	4.5	NR
[174]	Hsu et al.	2008	II	Bevacizumab plus capecitabine	45	9	41	NR	4.1	10.7
[175]	Thomas et al.	2009	II	Bevacizumab plus erlotinib	40	25	42.5	NR	9	15.7
[176]	Kaseb et al.	2012	II	Bevacizumab plus erlotinib	59	24	56	NR	7.2	13.7
[177]	Philip et al.	2012	II	Bevacizumab plus erlotinib	27	3.7	48	3	NR	9.5
[178]	Berlin et al.	2008	II	Bortezomib plus doxorubicin	39	2.3	25.6	NR	2.4	5.7
[179]	Knox et al.[2]	2008	II	Oblimersen (G3139) plus doxorubicin	17	0	35	1.8	NR	5.4

n: sample size; RR: response rate; DS: disease stabilization; TTP: time to progression; PFS: progression-free survival; OS: overall survival; NR: not reported; mon: months

[1] Overlap of patient cohorts cannot be excluded from abstracts.

[2] Terminated secondary to absence of efficacy.

Table 4. Summary of phase II studies on combined novel molecularly targeted therapy and systemic chemotherapy in advanced HCC

Several combination therapy regimens exist, such as bevacizumab based, cetuximab based, and others. Among all, bevacizumab-based regimens appear to have the most effective antitumor effects with ORR achieving 3.7%-25%, disease stabilization 27%-48%, PFS 4.1-7.2 months, and OS 9.5-15.7 months. Future studies comparing sorafenib-based versus bevacizumab-based combination therapies are needed.

4.6. Conclusion

Sorafenib remains the first-line standard of care management in patients with advanced unresectable HCC. Multimodal therapy with sorafenib and other local/systemic therapy is an exciting area for future exploration. Absolute advantages of combining novel molecularly targeted therapy (sorafenib or bevacizumab) and cytotoxic chemotherapy is not yet surely defined. Much more research is needed about efficacy of existing combination systemic therapy (cytotoxic chemotherapy plus novel molecularly targeted therapy) versus sorafenib alone (the first-line therapy so far) for the management of patients with advanced unresectable HCC. Such studies should be addressed through large-sized randomized controlled phase II and III trials; some of which are already ongoing.

Several genetic and epigenetics take place during hepatocarcinogenesis. These signaling pathways include the Wnt-b-catenin pathway, the hepatocyte growth factor/c-Met pathway, IGF and IGF-R pathways, and PI3 K/Akt/mTOR pathway. Several drugs targeting these significant pathways are currently undergoing early-stage assessment in patients with HCC [33, 133].

5. Summary and final remarks

- Hepatocellular carcinoma (HCC) is a largely aggressive neoplasm that commonly takes place in the setting of chronic liver disease and cirrhosis.
- At the time of clinical diagnosis, roughly 60%-70% of HCC patients present with primary advanced inoperable, recurrent, or metastatic disease [7]. Moreover, tumor relapse (recurrence) following curative surgical management continues to be a substantial dilemma and is documented as high as approximately 70% at 5 years postoperatively [8].
- Systemic therapy is the most appropriate choice for patients with primary advanced, inoperable, recurrent, or metastatic disease who were inappropriate candidates for other local or loco-regional therapies.
- Systemic therapy is a rapidly developing area of research. Options of systemic therapy mainly include hormonal therapy, cytotoxic therapy, and novel molecularly targeted therapy.
- Single-agent tamoxifen or in combination with diverse chemotherapeutic drugs was unsatisfactory and failed to yield substantial worthy survival advantages. Similar discouraging results occurred with megestrol administration as well as somatostatin analogs (octreotide and lanreotide). It can be concluded that the use of hormonal therapy for the management of advanced inoperable HCC is not recommended. Its use may be only recommended in the context of clinical trials.
- HCC is largely a chemoresistant neoplasm [77]. The employment of systemic cytotoxic chemotherapy has been accompanied by low objective response rates, no survival advantages, and high frequencies of drug-related toxicities and adverse events. Moreover, there are no adequate data to endorse or approve any single-agent or combined chemotherapeutic cytotoxic regimens for the management of patients with advanced inoperable HCC [76].
- Systemic chemotherapy may still be regarded in patients whom their HCC get worse while on sorafenib and whom baseline liver function and performance status are adequate enough to endure it. The chemotherapy-related toxicities and adverse events should be carefully

anticipated in such patients. This selection of cytotoxic chemotherapy should be guided by the available best evidence-based medicine.

- By far, sorafenib is the first-line standard of care therapy for patients with advanced unresectable HCC. Studies have shown feasibility and safety profiles in patients with hepatic dysfunction (CPS-A and CPS-B, but not CPS-C).
- The combination of sorafenib and anti-mTOR is feasible in recurrent HCC patients following orthotopic liver transplantation. However, therapy should be carefully checked due to the probability for severe adverse events. Dose modification may be needed.
- Studies of sorafenib-based combination therapy report better DCR, TTP, and OS benefits when compared to single-agent sorafenib therapy, without increased frequencies of excessive treatment-related toxicities and adverse events. However, such studies cannot be appropriately compared, and definitive conclusions are yet to be established.
- Multimodal therapy with sorafenib and other local/systemic therapy is an exciting area for future exploration.
- Absolute advantages of combining molecularly targeted therapy (sorafenib or bevacizumab) and cytotoxic chemotherapy are not yet surely defined.
- Further prospective research should continue to discover the mechanism of hepatocarcinogenesis and subsequently recognize significant molecular targets for therapeutic interventions.

Author details

Ahmed Abu-Zaid[1*], Lynn Alkhatib[1], Judie Noemie Hoilat[1], Sana Samer Kadan[1], Abdulaziz Mohammed Eshaq[1], Ahmed Mubarak Fothan[1], Abdulrahman Mohammed Bakather[1], Mohammed Abuzaid[2], Daniah Saud Aloufi[3], Abdulhadi A. Alamodi[4] and Ayman Azzam[1,5,6]

*Address all correspondence to: aabuzaid@live.com

1 College of Medicine, Alfaisal University, Riyadh, Saudi Arabia

2 Faculty of Medicine, Khartoum University, Khartoum, Sudan

3 College of Medicine, Taiba University, Madinah, Saudi Arabia

4 University of Mississippi Medical Center, Jackson, Mississippi, United States of America

5 Faculty of Medicine, Alexandria University, Alexandria, Egypt

6 King Faisal Oncology Centre, King Faisal Specialist Hospital & Research Centre, Riyadh, Saudi Arabia

References

[1] Bosch FX, Ribes J, Cleries R, Diaz M. Epidemiology of hepatocellular carcinoma. Clin Liver Dis. 2005;9:191-211, v.

[2] Torre LA, Bray F, Siegel RL, Ferlay J, Lortet-Tieulent J, Jemal A. Global cancer statistics, 2012. CA Cancer J Clin. 2015.

[3] Venook AP, Papandreou C, Furuse J, de Guevara LL. The incidence and epidemiology of hepatocellular carcinoma: a global and regional perspective. Oncologist. 2010;15(Suppl 4):5-13.

[4] Tinkle CL, Haas-Kogan D. Hepatocellular carcinoma: natural history, current management, and emerging tools. Biologics. 2012;6:207-19.

[5] Chen X, Liu HP, Li M, Qiao L. Advances in non-surgical management of primary liver cancer. World J Gastroenterol. 2014;20(44):16630-8.

[6] Lin S, Hoffmann K, Schemmer P. Treatment of hepatocellular carcinoma: a systematic review. Liver Cancer. 2012;1(3-4):144-58.

[7] Llovet JM, Bruix J. Novel advancements in the management of hepatocellular carcinoma in 2008. J Hepatol. 2008;48(Suppl 1):S20-37.

[8] Llovet JM, Fuster J, Bruix J. Intention-to-treat analysis of surgical treatment for early hepatocellular carcinoma: resection versus transplantation. Hepatology. 1999;30(6): 1434-40.

[9] Boonyaratanakornkit V, Edwards DP. Receptor mechanisms mediating non-genomic actions of sex steroids. Semin Reprod Med. 2007;25(3):139-53.

[10] Cebon J, Findlay M, Hargreaves C, Stockler M, Thompson P, Boyer M, et al. Somatostatin receptor expression, tumour response, and quality of life in patients with advanced hepatocellular carcinoma treated with long-acting octreotide. Br J Cancer. 2006;95(7):853-61.

[11] Kouroumalis E, Skordilis P, Thermos K, Vasilaki A, Moschandrea J, Manousos ON. Treatment of hepatocellular carcinoma with octreotide: a randomised controlled study. Gut. 1998;42(3):442-7.

[12] Castells A, Bruix J, Bru C, Ayuso C, Roca M, Boix L, et al. Treatment of hepatocellular carcinoma with tamoxifen: a double-blind placebo-controlled trial in 120 patients. Gastroenterology. 1995;109(3):917-22.

[13] Tamoxifen in treatment of hepatocellular carcinoma: a randomised controlled trial. CLIP Group (Cancer of the Liver Italian Programme). Lancet. 1998;352(9121):17-20.

[14] Chow PK, Tai BC, Tan CK, Machin D, Win KM, Johnson PJ, et al. High-dose tamoxifen in the treatment of inoperable hepatocellular carcinoma: a multicenter randomized controlled trial. Hepatology. 2002;36(5):1221-6.

[15] Nowak A, Findlay M, Culjak G, Stockler M. Tamoxifen for hepatocellular carcinoma. Cochrane Database Syst Rev. 2004(3):Cd001024.

[16] Barbare JC, Bouche O, Bonnetain F, Raoul JL, Rougier P, Abergel A, et al. Randomized controlled trial of tamoxifen in advanced hepatocellular carcinoma. J Clin Oncol. 2005;23(19):4338-46.

[17] Villa E, Dugani A, Fantoni E, Camellini L, Buttafoco P, Grottola A, et al. Type of estrogen receptor determines response to antiestrogen therapy. Cancer Res. 1996;56(17):3883-5.

[18] Villa E, Ferretti I, Grottola A, Buttafoco P, Buono MG, Giannini F, et al. Hormonal therapy with megestrol in inoperable hepatocellular carcinoma characterized by variant oestrogen receptors. Br J Cancer. 2001;84(7):881-5.

[19] Lavie Y, Cao H, Volner A, Lucci A, Han TY, Geffen V, et al. Agents that reverse multidrug resistance, tamoxifen, verapamil, and cyclosporin A, block glycosphingolipid metabolism by inhibiting ceramide glycosylation in human cancer cells. J Biol Chem. 1997;272(3):1682-7.

[20] Cheng AL, Chuang SE, Fine RL, Yeh KH, Liao CM, Lay JD, et al. Inhibition of the membrane translocation and activation of protein kinase C, and potentiation of doxorubicin-induced apoptosis of hepatocellular carcinoma cells by tamoxifen. Biochem Pharmacol. 1998;55(4):523-31.

[21] Cheng AL, Yeh KH, Fine RL, Chuang SE, Yang CH, Wang LH, et al. Biochemical modulation of doxorubicin by high-dose tamoxifen in the treatment of advanced hepatocellular carcinoma. Hepatogastroenterology. 1998;45(24):1955-60.

[22] Melia WM, Johnson PJ, Williams R. Controlled clinical trial of doxorubicin and tamoxifen versus doxorubicin alone in hepatocellular carcinoma. Cancer Treat Rep. 1987;71(12):1213-6.

[23] Lu YS, Hsu C, Li CC, Kuo SH, Yeh KH, Yang CH, et al. Phase II study of combination doxorubicin, interferon-alpha, and high-dose tamoxifen treatment for advanced hepatocellular carcinoma. Hepatogastroenterology. 2004;51(57):815-9.

[24] Cheng AL, Chen YC, Yeh KH, Chuang SE, Chen BR, Chen DS. Chronic oral etoposide and tamoxifen in the treatment of far-advanced hepatocellular carcinoma. Cancer. 1996;77(5):872-7.

[25] Raderer M, Pidlich J, Muller C, Pfeffel F, Kornek GV, Hejna M, et al. A phase I/II trial of epirubicin and high dose tamoxifen as a potential modulator of multidrug resistance in advanced hepatocellular carcinoma. Eur J Cancer. 1996;32a(13):2366-8.

[26] Chao Y, Chan WK, Wang SS, Lai KH, Chi CW, Lin CY, et al. Phase II study of megestrol acetate in the treatment of hepatocellular carcinoma. J Gastroenterol Hepatol. 1997;12(4):277-81.

[27] Chow PK, Machin D, Chen Y, Zhang X, Win KM, Hoang HH, et al. Randomised double-blind trial of megestrol acetate vs placebo in treatment-naive advanced hepatocellular carcinoma. Br J Cancer. 2011;105(7):945-52.

[28] Yuen MF, Poon RT, Lai CL, Fan ST, Lo CM, Wong KW, et al. A randomized placebo-controlled study of long-acting octreotide for the treatment of advanced hepatocellular carcinoma. Hepatology. 2002;36(3):687-91.

[29] Becker G, Allgaier HP, Olschewski M, Zahringer A, Blum HE. Long-acting octreotide versus placebo for treatment of advanced HCC: a randomized controlled double-blind study. Hepatology. 2007;45(1):9-15.

[30] Ji XQ, Ruan XJ, Chen H, Chen G, Li SY, Yu B. Somatostatin analogues in advanced hepatocellular carcinoma: an updated systematic review and meta-analysis of randomized controlled trials. Med Sci Monit. 2011;17:Ra169-76.

[31] Raderer M, Hejna MH, Muller C, Kornek GV, Kurtaran A, Virgolini I, et al. Treatment of hepatocellular cancer with the long acting somatostatin analog lanreotide in vitro and in vivo. Int J Oncol. 2000;16(6):1197-201.

[32] Barbare JC, Bouche O, Bonnetain F, Dahan L, Lombard-Bohas C, Faroux R, et al. Treatment of advanced hepatocellular carcinoma with long-acting octreotide: a phase III multicentre, randomised, double blind placebo-controlled study. Eur J Cancer. 2009;45(10):1788-97.

[33] Germano D, Daniele B. Systemic therapy of hepatocellular carcinoma: current status and future perspectives. World J Gastroenterol. 2014;20(12):3087-99.

[34] Olweny CL, Toya T, Katongole-Mbidde E, Mugerwa J, Kyalwazi SK, Cohen H. Treatment of hepatocellular carcinoma with adriamycin. Preliminary communication. Cancer. 1975;36(4):1250-7.

[35] Ihde DC, Kane RC, Cohen MH, McIntire KR, Minna JD. Adriamycin therapy in American patients with hepatocellular carcinoma. Cancer Treat Rep. 1977;61(7):1385-7.

[36] Chlebowski RT, Brzechwa-Adjukiewicz A, Cowden A, Block JB, Tong M, Chan KK. Doxorubicin (75 mg/m2) for hepatocellular carcinoma: clinical and pharmacokinetic results. Cancer Treat Rep. 1984;68(3):487-91.

[37] Choi TK, Lee NW, Wong J. Chemotherapy for advanced hepatocellular carcinoma. Adriamycin versus quadruple chemotherapy. Cancer. 1984;53(3):401-5.

[38] Nerenstone SR, Ihde DC, Friedman MA. Clinical trials in primary hepatocellular carcinoma: current status and future directions. Cancer Treat Rev. 1988;15(1):1-31.

[39] Lai CL, Wu PC, Chan GC, Lok AS, Lin HJ. Doxorubicin versus no antitumor therapy in inoperable hepatocellular carcinoma. A prospective randomized trial. Cancer. 1988;62(3):479-83.

[40] Yeo W, Mok TS, Zee B, Leung TW, Lai PB, Lau WY, et al. A randomized phase III study of doxorubicin versus cisplatin/interferon alpha-2b/doxorubicin/fluorouracil (PIAF) combination chemotherapy for unresectable hepatocellular carcinoma. J Natl Cancer Inst. 2005;97(20):1532-8.

[41] Sciarrino E, Simonetti RG, Le Moli S, Pagliaro L. Adriamycin treatment for hepatocellular carcinoma. Experience with 109 patients. Cancer. 1985;56(12):2751-5.

[42] Gish RG, Porta C, Lazar L, Ruff P, Feld R, Croitoru A, et al. Phase III randomized controlled trial comparing the survival of patients with unresectable hepatocellular carcinoma treated with nolatrexed or doxorubicin. J Clin Oncol. 2007;25(21):3069-75.

[43] Schmidinger M, Wenzel C, Locker GJ, Muehlbacher F, Steininger R, Gnant M, et al. Pilot study with pegylated liposomal doxorubicin for advanced or unresectable hepatocellular carcinoma. Br J Cancer. 2001;85(12):1850-2.

[44] Halm U, Etzrodt G, Schiefke I, Schmidt F, Witzigmann H, Mossner J, et al. A phase II study of pegylated liposomal doxorubicin for treatment of advanced hepatocellular carcinoma. Ann Oncol. 2000;11(1):113-4.

[45] Lind PA, Naucler G, Holm A, Gubanski M, Svensson C. Efficacy of pegylated liposomal doxorubicin in patients with advanced hepatocellular carcinoma. Acta Oncol. 2007;46(2):230-3.

[46] Hochster HS, Green MD, Speyer J, Fazzini E, Blum R, Muggia FM. 4'Epidoxorubicin (epirubicin): activity in hepatocellular carcinoma. J Clin Oncol. 1985;3(11):1535-40.

[47] Pohl J, Zuna I, Stremmel W, Rudi J. Systemic chemotherapy with epirubicin for treatment of advanced or multifocal hepatocellular carcinoma. Chemotherapy. 2001;47(5): 359-65.

[48] Colleoni M, Buzzoni R, Bajetta E, Bochicchio AM, Bartoli C, Audisio R, et al. A phase II study of mitoxantrone combined with beta-interferon in unresectable hepatocellular carcinoma. Cancer. 1993;72(11):3196-201.

[49] Dunk AA, Scott SC, Johnson PJ, Melia W, Lok AS, Murray-Lyon I, et al. Mitozantrone as single agent therapy in hepatocellular carcinoma. A phase II study. J Hepatol. 1985;1(4):395-404.

[50] Porta C, Moroni M, Nastasi G, Arcangeli G. 5-Fluorouracil and d, l-leucovorin calcium are active to treat unresectable hepatocellular carcinoma patients: preliminary results of a phase II study. Oncology. 1995;52(6):487-91.

[51] Tetef M, Doroshow J, Akman S, Coluzzi P, Leong L, Margolin K, et al. 5-Fluorouracil and high-dose calcium leucovorin for hepatocellular carcinoma: a phase II trial. Cancer Invest. 1995;13(5):460-3.

[52] Melia WM, Johnson PJ, Williams R. Induction of remission in hepatocellular carcinoma. A comparison of VP 16 with adriamycin. Cancer. 1983;51(2):206-10.

[53] Patt YZ, Hassan MM, Aguayo A, Nooka AK, Lozano RD, Curley SA, et al. Oral capecitabine for the treatment of hepatocellular carcinoma, cholangiocarcinoma, and gallbladder carcinoma. Cancer. 2004;101(3):578-86.

[54] Brandi G, de Rosa F, Agostini V, di Girolamo S, Andreone P, Bolondi L, et al. Metronomic capecitabine in advanced hepatocellular carcinoma patients: a phase II study. Oncologist. 2013;18(12):1256-7.

[55] Abdel-Rahman O, Abdel-Wahab M, Shaker M, Abdel-Wahab S, Elbassiony M, Ellithy M. Sorafenib versus capecitabine in the management of advanced hepatocellular carcinoma. Med Oncol. 2013;30(3):655.

[56] Yang TS, Lin YC, Chen JS, Wang HM, Wang CH. Phase II study of gemcitabine in patients with advanced hepatocellular carcinoma. Cancer. 2000;89(4):750-6.

[57] Kubicka S, Rudolph KL, Tietze MK, Lorenz M, Manns M. Phase II study of systemic gemcitabine chemotherapy for advanced unresectable hepatobiliary carcinomas. Hepatogastroenterology. 2001;48(39):783-9.

[58] Fuchs CS, Clark JW, Ryan DP, Kulke MH, Kim H, Earle CC, et al. A phase II trial of gemcitabine in patients with advanced hepatocellular carcinoma. Cancer. 2002;94(12):3186-91.

[59] Hsu C, Chen CN, Chen LT, Wu CY, Yang PM, Lai MY, et al. Low-dose thalidomide treatment for advanced hepatocellular carcinoma. Oncology. 2003;65(3):242-9.

[60] Lin AY, Brophy N, Fisher GA, So S, Biggs C, Yock TI, et al. Phase II study of thalidomide in patients with unresectable hepatocellular carcinoma. Cancer. 2005;103(1):119-25.

[61] Patt YZ, Hassan MM, Lozano RD, Nooka AK, Schnirer, II, Zeldis JB, et al. Thalidomide in the treatment of patients with hepatocellular carcinoma: a phase II trial. Cancer. 2005;103(4):749-55.

[62] O'Reilly EM, Stuart KE, Sanz-Altamira PM, Schwartz GK, Steger CM, Raeburn L, et al. A phase II study of irinotecan in patients with advanced hepatocellular carcinoma. Cancer. 2001;91(1):101-5.

[63] Boige V, Taieb J, Hebbar M, Malka D, Debaere T, Hannoun L, et al. Irinotecan as first-line chemotherapy in patients with advanced hepatocellular carcinoma: a multicenter phase II study with dose adjustment according to baseline serum bilirubin level. Eur J Cancer. 2006;42(4):456-9.

[64] Qin S, Bai Y, Lim HY, Thongprasert S, Chao Y, Fan J, et al. Randomized, multicenter, open-label study of oxaliplatin plus fluorouracil/leucovorin versus doxorubicin as palliative chemotherapy in patients with advanced hepatocellular carcinoma from Asia. J Clin Oncol. 2013;31(28):3501-8.

[65] Lai CL, Wu PC, Lok AS, Lin HJ, Ngan H, Lau JY, et al. Recombinant alpha 2 interferon is superior to doxorubicin for inoperable hepatocellular carcinoma: a prospective randomised trial. Br J Cancer. 1989;60(6):928-33.

[66] Lai CL, Lau JY, Wu PC, Ngan H, Chung HT, Mitchell SJ, et al. Recombinant interferon-alpha in inoperable hepatocellular carcinoma: a randomized controlled trial. Hepatology. 1993;17(3):389-94.

[67] Llovet JM, Sala M, Castells L, Suarez Y, Vilana R, Bianchi L, et al. Randomized controlled trial of interferon treatment for advanced hepatocellular carcinoma. Hepatology. 2000;31(1):54-8.

[68] Leung TW, Patt YZ, Lau WY, Ho SK, Yu SC, Chan AT, et al. Complete pathological remission is possible with systemic combination chemotherapy for inoperable hepatocellular carcinoma. Clin Cancer Res. 1999;5(7):1676-81.

[69] Leung TW, Tang AM, Zee B, Yu SC, Lai PB, Lau WY, et al. Factors predicting response and survival in 149 patients with unresectable hepatocellular carcinoma treated by combination cisplatin, interferon-alpha, doxorubicin and 5-fluorouracil chemotherapy. Cancer. 2002;94(2):421-7.

[70] Lau WY, Ho SK, Yu SC, Lai EC, Liew CT, Leung TW. Salvage surgery following downstaging of unresectable hepatocellular carcinoma. Ann Surg. 2004;240(2): 299-305.

[71] Stuart K, Tessitore J, Huberman M. 5-Fluorouracil and alpha-interferon in hepatocellular carcinoma. Am J Clin Oncol. 1996;19(2):136-9.

[72] Patt YZ, Hassan MM, Lozano RD, Brown TD, Vauthey JN, Curley SA, et al. Phase II trial of systemic continuous fluorouracil and subcutaneous recombinant interferon Alfa-2b for treatment of hepatocellular carcinoma. J Clin Oncol. 2003;21(3):421-7.

[73] Sakon M, Nagano H, Dono K, Nakamori S, Umeshita K, Yamada A, et al. Combined intraarterial 5-fluorouracil and subcutaneous interferon-alpha therapy for advanced hepatocellular carcinoma with tumor thrombi in the major portal branches. Cancer. 2002;94(2):435-42.

[74] Ota H, Nagano H, Sakon M, Eguchi H, Kondo M, Yamamoto T, et al. Treatment of hepatocellular carcinoma with major portal vein thrombosis by combined therapy with subcutaneous interferon-alpha and intra-arterial 5-fluorouracil; role of type 1 interferon receptor expression. Br J Cancer. 2005;93(5):557-64.

[75] Nagano H, Miyamoto A, Wada H, Ota H, Marubashi S, Takeda Y, et al. Interferon-alpha and 5-fluorouracil combination therapy after palliative hepatic resection in pa-

tients with advanced hepatocellular carcinoma, portal venous tumor thrombus in the major trunk, and multiple nodules. Cancer. 2007;110(11):2493-501.

[76] Nowak AK, Chow PK, Findlay M. Systemic therapy for advanced hepatocellular carcinoma: a review. Eur J Cancer. 2004;40(10):1474-84.

[77] Huang M, Liu G. The study of innate drug resistance of human hepatocellular carcinoma Bel7402 cell line. Cancer Lett. 1999;135(1):97-105.

[78] Kato A, Miyazaki M, Ambiru S, Yoshitomi H, Ito H, Nakagawa K, et al. Multidrug resistance gene (MDR-1) expression as a useful prognostic factor in patients with human hepatocellular carcinoma after surgical resection. J Surg Oncol. 2001;78(2):110-5.

[79] Huang CC, Wu MC, Xu GW, Li DZ, Cheng H, Tu ZX, et al. Overexpression of the MDR1 gene and P-glycoprotein in human hepatocellular carcinoma. J Natl Cancer Inst. 1992;84(4):262-4.

[80] Soini Y, Virkajarvi N, Raunio H, Paakko P. Expression of P-glycoprotein in hepatocellular carcinoma: a potential marker of prognosis. J Clin Pathol. 1996;49(6):470-3.

[81] Caruso ML, Valentini AM. Overexpression of p53 in a large series of patients with hepatocellular carcinoma: a clinicopathological correlation. Anticancer Res. 1999;19(5B):3853-6.

[82] Nagahama H, Okada S, Okusaka T, Ishii H, Ikeda M, Nakasuka H, et al. Predictive factors for tumor response to systemic chemotherapy in patients with hepatocellular carcinoma. Jpn J Clin Oncol. 1997;27(5):321-4.

[83] Xie B, Wang DH, Spechler SJ. Sorafenib for treatment of hepatocellular carcinoma: a systematic review. Dig Dis Sci. 2012;57(5):1122-9.

[84] Llovet JM, Ricci S, Mazzaferro V, Hilgard P, Gane E, Blanc JF, et al. Sorafenib in advanced hepatocellular carcinoma. N Engl J Med. 2008;359(4):378-90.

[85] Cheng AL, Kang YK, Chen Z, Tsao CJ, Qin S, Kim JS, et al. Efficacy and safety of sorafenib in patients in the Asia-Pacific region with advanced hepatocellular carcinoma: a phase III randomised, double-blind, placebo-controlled trial. Lancet Oncol. 2009;10(1):25-34.

[86] Bruix J, Raoul JL, Sherman M, Mazzaferro V, Bolondi L, Craxi A, et al. Efficacy and safety of sorafenib in patients with advanced hepatocellular carcinoma: subanalyses of a phase III trial. J Hepatol. 2012;57(4):821-9.

[87] Yau T, Chan P, Ng KK, Chok SH, Cheung TT, Fan ST, et al. Phase 2 open-label study of single-agent sorafenib in treating advanced hepatocellular carcinoma in a hepatitis B-endemic Asian population: presence of lung metastasis predicts poor response. Cancer. 2009;115(2):428-36.

[88] Furuse J, Ishii H, Nakachi K, Suzuki E, Shimizu S, Nakajima K. Phase I study of sorafenib in Japanese patients with hepatocellular carcinoma. Cancer Sci. 2008;99(1): 159-65.

[89] Personeni N, Rimassa L, Pressiani T, Destro A, Ligorio C, Tronconi MC, et al. Molecular determinants of outcome in sorafenib-treated patients with hepatocellular carcinoma. J Cancer Res Clin Oncol. 2013;139(7):1179-87.

[90] Arao T, Ueshima K, Matsumoto K, Nagai T, Kimura H, Hagiwara S, et al. FGF3/FGF4 amplification and multiple lung metastases in responders to sorafenib in hepatocellular carcinoma. Hepatology. 2013;57(4):1407-15.

[91] Scartozzi M, Faloppi L, Svegliati Baroni G, Loretelli C, Piscaglia F, Iavarone M, et al. VEGF and VEGFR genotyping in the prediction of clinical outcome for HCC patients receiving sorafenib: the ALICE-1 study. Int J Cancer. 2014;135(5):1247-56.

[92] Pinter M, Sieghart W, Hucke F, Graziadei I, Vogel W, Maieron A, et al. Prognostic factors in patients with advanced hepatocellular carcinoma treated with sorafenib. Aliment Pharmacol Ther. 2011;34(8):949-59.

[93] Llovet JM, Pena CE, Lathia CD, Shan M, Meinhardt G, Bruix J. Plasma biomarkers as predictors of outcome in patients with advanced hepatocellular carcinoma. Clin Cancer Res. 2012;18(8):2290-300.

[94] Estfan B, Byrne M, Kim R. Sorafenib in advanced hepatocellular carcinoma: hypertension as a potential surrogate marker for efficacy. Am J Clin Oncol. 2013;36(4): 319-24.

[95] Bettinger D, Schultheiss M, Knuppel E, Thimme R, Blum HE, Spangenberg HC. Diarrhea predicts a positive response to sorafenib in patients with advanced hepatocellular carcinoma. Hepatology. 2012;56(2):789-90.

[96] Zhang L, Hu P, Chen X, Bie P. Transarterial chemoembolization (TACE) plus sorafenib versus TACE for intermediate or advanced stage hepatocellular carcinoma: a meta-analysis. PLoS One. 2014;9(6):e100305.

[97] Prete SD, Montella L, Caraglia M, Maiorino L, Cennamo G, Montesarchio V, et al. Sorafenib plus octreotide is an effective and safe treatment in advanced hepatocellular carcinoma: multicenter phase II So.LAR. study. Cancer Chemother Pharmacol. 2010;66(5):837-44.

[98] Hsu CH, Shen YC, Lin ZZ, Chen PJ, Shao YY, Ding YH, et al. Phase II study of combining sorafenib with metronomic tegafur/uracil for advanced hepatocellular carcinoma. J Hepatol. 2010;53(1):126-31.

[99] Petrini ILM, et al. A phase II trial of sorafenib in combination with 5-fluorouracil continuous infusion in patients with advanced hepatocellular carcinoma: preliminary data. Journal of clinical oncology. 2009;27(Suppl 15):4592.

[100] Yau TCP, et al. Phase II trial of sorafenib with capecitabine and oxaliplatin (SECOX) in patients with locally advanced or metastatic hepatocellular carcinoma. EJC supplements. 2009;7(3):20-21.

[101] Richly H, Schultheis B, Adamietz IA, Kupsch P, Grubert M, Hilger RA, et al. Combination of sorafenib and doxorubicin in patients with advanced hepatocellular carcinoma: results from a phase I extension trial. Eur J Cancer. 2009;45(4):579-87.

[102] Abou-Alfa GK, Johnson P, Knox JJ, Capanu M, Davidenko I, Lacava J, et al. Doxorubicin plus sorafenib vs doxorubicin alone in patients with advanced hepatocellular carcinoma: a randomized trial. JAMA. 2010;304:2154-60.

[103] Abou-Alfa GK, Amadori D, Santoro A, Figer A, De Greve J, Lathia C, et al. Safety and efficacy of sorafenib in patients with hepatocellular carcinoma (HCC) and Child-Pugh A versus B cirrhosis. Gastrointest Cancer Res. 2011;4(2):40-4.

[104] Pinter M, Sieghart W, Graziadei I, Vogel W, Maieron A, Konigsberg R, et al. Sorafenib in unresectable hepatocellular carcinoma from mild to advanced stage liver cirrhosis. Oncologist. 2009;14(1):70-6.

[105] Lencioni R, Kudo M, Ye SL, Bronowicki JP, Chen XP, Dagher L, et al. First interim analysis of the GIDEON (Global Investigation of therapeutic decisions in hepatocellular carcinoma and of its treatment with sorafeNib) non-interventional study. Int J Clin Pract. 2012;66(7):675-83.

[106] Raoul JL, Bruix J, Greten TF, Sherman M, Mazzaferro V, Hilgard P, et al. Relationship between baseline hepatic status and outcome, and effect of sorafenib on liver function: SHARP trial subanalyses. J Hepatol. 2012;56(5):1080-8.

[107] Gomez-Martin C, Bustamante J, Castroagudin JF, Salcedo M, Garralda E, Testillano M, et al. Efficacy and safety of sorafenib in combination with mammalian target of rapamycin inhibitors for recurrent hepatocellular carcinoma after liver transplantation. Liver Transpl. 2012;18(1):45-52.

[108] Kim R, El-Gazzaz G, Tan A, Elson P, Byrne M, Chang YD, et al. Safety and feasibility of using sorafenib in recurrent hepatocellular carcinoma after orthotopic liver transplantation. Oncology. 2010;79(1-2):62-6.

[109] Staufer K, Fischer L, Seegers B, Vettorazzi E, Nashan B, Sterneck M. High toxicity of sorafenib for recurrent hepatocellular carcinoma after liver transplantation. Transpl Int. 2012;25(11):1158-64.

[110] Zavaglia C, Airoldi A, Mancuso A, Vangeli M, Vigano R, Cordone G, et al. Adverse events affect sorafenib efficacy in patients with recurrent hepatocellular carcinoma after liver transplantation: experience at a single center and review of the literature. Eur J Gastroenterol Hepatol. 2013;25(2):180-6.

[111] Miura H, Miyazaki T, Kuroda M, Oka T, Machinami R, Kodama T, et al. Increased expression of vascular endothelial growth factor in human hepatocellular carcinoma. J Hepatol. 1997;27(5):854-61.

[112] Yamaguchi R, Yano H, Iemura A, Ogasawara S, Haramaki M, Kojiro M. Expression of vascular endothelial growth factor in human hepatocellular carcinoma. Hepatology. 1998;28(1):68-77.

[113] Yamaguchi R, Yano H, Nakashima Y, Ogasawara S, Higaki K, Akiba J, et al. Expression and localization of vascular endothelial growth factor receptors in human hepatocellular carcinoma and non-HCC tissues. Oncol Rep. 2000;7(4):725-9.

[114] Messerini L, Novelli L, Comin CE. Microvessel density and clinicopathological characteristics in hepatitis C virus and hepatitis B virus related hepatocellular carcinoma. J Clin Pathol. 2004;57(8):867-71.

[115] Chao Y, Li CP, Chau GY, Chen CP, King KL, Lui WY, et al. Prognostic significance of vascular endothelial growth factor, basic fibroblast growth factor, and angiogenin in patients with resectable hepatocellular carcinoma after surgery. Ann Surg Oncol. 2003;10(4):355-62.

[116] Jeng KS, Sheen IS, Wang YC, Gu SL, Chu CM, Shih SC, et al. Prognostic significance of preoperative circulating vascular endothelial growth factor messenger RNA expression in resectable hepatocellular carcinoma: a prospective study. World J Gastroenterol. 2004;10(5):643-8.

[117] Poon RT, Ho JW, Tong CS, Lau C, Ng IO, Fan ST. Prognostic significance of serum vascular endothelial growth factor and endostatin in patients with hepatocellular carcinoma. Br J Surg. 2004;91(10):1354-60.

[118] Llovet JM, Decaens T, Raoul JL, Boucher E, Kudo M, Chang C, et al. Brivanib in patients with advanced hepatocellular carcinoma who were intolerant to sorafenib or for whom sorafenib failed: results from the randomized phase III BRISK-PS study. J Clin Oncol. 2013;31(28):3509-16.

[119] Santoro A, Rimassa L, Borbath I, Daniele B, Salvagni S, Van Laethem JL, et al. Tivantinib for second-line treatment of advanced hepatocellular carcinoma: a randomised, placebo-controlled phase 2 study. Lancet Oncol. 2013;14(1):55-63.

[120] Malka D, Dromain C, Farace F, Horn S, Pignon J, Ducreux M, Boige V. Bevacizumab in patients (pts) with advanced hepatocellular carcinoma (HCC): preliminary results of a phase II study with circulating endothelial cell (CEC) monitoring. J Clin Oncol. 2007;25(18S):4570.

[121] Siegel AB, Cohen EI, Ocean A, Lehrer D, Goldenberg A, Knox JJ, et al. Phase II trial evaluating the clinical and biologic effects of bevacizumab in unresectable hepatocellular carcinoma. J Clin Oncol. 2008;26(18):2992-8.

[122] Schwartz JD, Schwartz M, Sung M, Lehrer D, Cohen E, Kinkhabwala M, Holloway SB, Siegel A, Ocean A, Wadler S. Bevacizumab in unresectable hepatocellular carci-

noma (HCC) for patients without metastasis and without invasion of the portal vein. Gastrointestinal Cancers Symposium. 2006:A210. 2006.

[123] Yeh YC, Tsai JF, Chuang LY, Yeh HW, Tsai JH, Florine DL, et al. Elevation of transforming growth factor alpha and its relationship to the epidermal growth factor and alpha-fetoprotein levels in patients with hepatocellular carcinoma. Cancer Res. 1987;47(3):896-901.

[124] Carlin CR, Simon D, Mattison J, Knowles BB. Expression and biosynthetic variation of the epidermal growth factor receptor in human hepatocellular carcinoma-derived cell lines. Mol Cell Biol. 1988;8(1):25-34.

[125] Kiss A, Wang NJ, Xie JP, Thorgeirsson SS. Analysis of transforming growth factor (TGF)-alpha/epidermal growth factor receptor, hepatocyte growth Factor/c-met, TGF-beta receptor type II, and p53 expression in human hepatocellular carcinomas. Clin Cancer Res. 1997;3(7):1059-66.

[126] Kira S, Nakanishi T, Suemori S, Kitamoto M, Watanabe Y, Kajiyama G. Expression of transforming growth factor alpha and epidermal growth factor receptor in human hepatocellular carcinoma. Liver. 1997;17(4):177-82.

[127] Ito Y, Takeda T, Higashiyama S, Sakon M, Wakasa KI, Tsujimoto M, et al. Expression of heparin binding epidermal growth factor-like growth factor in hepatocellular carcinoma: an immunohistochemical study. Oncol Rep. 2001;8(4):903-7.

[128] Philip PA, Mahoney MR, Allmer C, Thomas J, Pitot HC, Kim G, et al. Phase II study of erlotinib (OSI-774) in patients with advanced hepatocellular cancer. J Clin Oncol. 2005;23:6657-63.

[129] Thomas MB, Chadha R, Glover K, Wang X, Morris J, Brown T, et al. Phase 2 study of erlotinib in patients with unresectable hepatocellular carcinoma. Cancer. 2007;110(5): 1059-67.

[130] Villanueva A, Chiang DY, Newell P, Peix J, Thung S, Alsinet C, et al. Pivotal role of mTOR signaling in hepatocellular carcinoma. Gastroenterology. 2008;135(6):1972-83, 83 e1-11.

[131] Chen L, Shiah HS, Chen CY. Randomized, phase I, and pharmacokinetic (PK) study of RAD001, an mTOR inhibitor, in patients (pts) with advanced hepatocellular carcinoma (HCC) J Clin Oncol. 2009;27(Suppl):4587.

[132] Zhu AX, Kudo M, Assenat E, Cattan S, Kang YK, Lim HY, et al. Effect of everolimus on survival in advanced hepatocellular carcinoma after failure of sorafenib: the EVOLVE-1 randomized clinical trial. JAMA. 2014;312(1):57-67.

[133] Tazi el M, Essadi I, M'Rabti H, Touyar A, Errihani PH. Systemic treatment and targeted therapy in patients with advanced hepatocellular carcinoma. N Am J Med Sci. 2011;3(4):167-75.

[134] Lee J, Park JO, Kim WS, Park SH, Park KW, Choi MS, et al. Phase II study of doxorubicin and cisplatin in patients with metastatic hepatocellular carcinoma. Cancer Chemother Pharmacol. 2004;54(5):385-90.

[135] Yang TS, Chang HK, Chen JS, Lin YC, Liau CT, Chang WC. Chemotherapy using 5-fluorouracil, mitoxantrone, and cisplatin for patients with advanced hepatocellular carcinoma: an analysis of 63 cases. J Gastroenterol. 2004;39(4):362-9.

[136] Ikeda M, Okusaka T, Ueno H, Takezako Y, Morizane C. A phase II trial of continuous infusion of 5-fluorouracil, mitoxantrone, and cisplatin for metastatic hepatocellular carcinoma. Cancer. 2005;103(4):756-62.

[137] Boucher E, Corbinais S, Brissot P, Boudjema K, Raoul JL. Treatment of hepatocellular carcinoma (HCC) with systemic chemotherapy combining epirubicin, cisplatinum and infusional 5-fluorouracil (ECF regimen). Cancer Chemother Pharmacol. 2002;50(4):305-8.

[138] Park SH, Lee Y, Han SH, Kwon SY, Kwon OS, Kim SS, et al. Systemic chemotherapy with doxorubicin, cisplatin and capecitabine for metastatic hepatocellular carcinoma. BMC Cancer. 2006;6:3.

[139] Shim JH, Park JW, Nam BH, Lee WJ, Kim CM. Efficacy of combination chemotherapy with capecitabine plus cisplatin in patients with unresectable hepatocellular carcinoma. Cancer Chemother Pharmacol. 2009;63(3):459-67.

[140] Lee JO, Lee KW, Oh DY, Kim JH, Im SA, Kim TY, et al. Combination chemotherapy with capecitabine and cisplatin for patients with metastatic hepatocellular carcinoma. Ann Oncol. 2009;20(8):1402-7.

[141] Parikh PM, Fuloria J, Babu G, Doval DC, Awasthy BS, Pai VR, et al. A phase II study of gemcitabine and cisplatin in patients with advanced hepatocellular carcinoma. Trop Gastroenterol. 2005;26(3):115-8.

[142] Chia WK, Ong S, Toh HC, Hee SW, Choo SP, Poon DY, et al. Phase II trial of gemcitabine in combination with cisplatin in inoperable or advanced hepatocellular carcinoma. Ann Acad Med Singapore. 2008;37(7):554-8.

[143] Lombardi G, Zustovich F, Farinati F, Cillo U, Vitale A, Zanus G, et al. Pegylated liposomal doxorubicin and gemcitabine in patients with advanced hepatocellular carcinoma: results of a phase 2 study. Cancer. 2011;117(1):125-33.

[144] Louafi S, Boige V, Ducreux M, Bonyhay L, Mansourbakht T, de Baere T, et al. Gemcitabine plus oxaliplatin (GEMOX) in patients with advanced hepatocellular carcinoma (HCC): results of a phase II study. Cancer. 2007;109(7):1384-90.

[145] Mir O, Coriat R, Boudou-Rouquette P, Ropert S, Durand JP, Cessot A, et al. Gemcitabine and oxaliplatin as second-line treatment in patients with hepatocellular carcinoma pre-treated with sorafenib. Med Oncol. 2012;29(4):2793-9.

[146] Zaanan A, Williet N, Hebbar M, Dabakuyo TS, Fartoux L, Mansourbakht T, et al. Gemcitabine plus oxaliplatin in advanced hepatocellular carcinoma: a large multicenter AGEO study. J Hepatol. 2013;58(1):81-8.

[147] Boige V, Raoul JL, Pignon JP, Bouche O, Blanc JF, Dahan L, et al. Multicentre phase II trial of capecitabine plus oxaliplatin (XELOX) in patients with advanced hepatocellular carcinoma: FFCD 03-03 trial. Br J Cancer. 2007;97(7):862-7.

[148] Castroagudin JF, Molina E, Otero E, Tome S, Lopez R, Varo E. Short-term efficacy and safety of treatment of advanced hepatocellular carcinoma with sorafenib. Journal of Hepatology. 2008;48(362 Suppl 2):s141-s142.

[149] Abou-Alfa GK, Schwartz L, Ricci S, Amadori D, Santoro A, Figer A, et al. Phase II study of sorafenib in patients with advanced hepatocellular carcinoma. J Clin Oncol. 2006;24(26):4293-300.

[150] Massa ESC, et al. Efficacy, safety and impact on quality of life of a treatment with sorafenib in elderly cancer patients with advanced hepatocellular carcinoma. Result of a phase II study. Ann Oncol. 2009;20 (Suppl 8):s65.

[151] Hoda D, Catherine C, Strosberg J, Valone T, Jump H, Campos T, Halina G, Wood G, Hoffe S, Garrett CR. Phase II study of sunitinib malate in adult pts (pts) with metastatic or surgically unresectable hepatocellular carcinoma (HCC). Proceedings of the 2008 Gastrointestinal Cancers Symposium. Abstract: 267.

[152] Zhu AX, Sahani DV, Duda DG, di Tomaso E, Ancukiewicz M, Catalano OA, et al. Efficacy, safety, and potential biomarkers of sunitinib monotherapy in advanced hepatocellular carcinoma: a phase II study. J Clin Oncol. 2009;27(18):3027-35.

[153] Faivre S, Raymond E, Boucher E, Douillard J, Lim HY, Kim JS, et al. Safety and efficacy of sunitinib in patients with advanced hepatocellular carcinoma: an open-label, multicentre, phase II study. Lancet Oncol. 2009;10(8):794-800.

[154] Koeberle D, Montemurro M, Samaras P, Majno P, Simcock M, Limacher A, et al. Continuous sunitinib treatment in patients with advanced hepatocellular carcinoma: a Swiss Group for Clinical Cancer Research (SAKK) and Swiss Association for the Study of the Liver (SASL) multicenter phase II trial (SAKK 77/06). Oncologist. 2010;15(3):285-92.

[155] Finn RS, Kang YK, Mulcahy M, Polite BN, Lim HY, Walters I, et al. Phase II, open-label study of brivanib as second-line therapy in patients with advanced hepatocellular carcinoma. Clin Cancer Res. 2012;18:2090-8.

[156] Yau CC, Chen PJ, Curtis CM, Murphy PS, Suttle AB, Arumugham T, Hodge JP, Dar MM, Poonet R. A phase I study of pazopanib in patients with advanced hepatocellular carcinoma. J Clin Oncol. 2009;27(Suppl):3561.

[157] Toh H, Chen P, Carr BI, Knox J, Gill S, Steinberg J, Carlson DM, Qian J, Qin Q, Yong W. A phase II study of ABT-869 in hepatocellular carcinoma (HCC): interim analysis. J Clin Oncol. 2009;27(Suppl):4581.

[158] Alberts SR, Fitch TR, Kim GP, Morlan BW, Dakhil SR, Gross HM, et al. Cediranib (AZD2171) in patients with advanced hepatocellular carcinoma: a phase II North Central Cancer Treatment Group Clinical Trial. Am J Clin Oncol. 2012;35(4):329-33.

[159] O'Neil BH, Williams-Goff LW, Kauh J, Bekaii-Saab T, Strosberg JR, Lee R, Deal AM, Sullivan D, Sebti SM. A phase II study of AZD6244 in advanced or metastatic hepatocellular carcinoma. J Clin Oncol. 2009;27(Suppl):Ae15574.

[160] Kanai F, Yoshida H, Tateishi R, Sato S, Kawabe T, Obi S, et al. A phase I/II trial of the oral antiangiogenic agent TSU-68 in patients with advanced hepatocellular carcinoma. Cancer Chemother Pharmacol. 2011;67(2):315-24.

[161] Zhu AX, Finn RS, Mulcahy MF, Gurtler JS, Sun W, Schwartz, P Rojas, A.Dontabhaktuni, H. Youssoufian, Stuart KE. A phase II study of ramucirumab as first-line monotherapy in patients (pts) with advanced hepatocellular carcinoma (HCC). J Clin Oncol. 2010;28(15s):4083.

[162] Koch I, Baron A, Roberts S. Influence of hepatic dysfunction on safety, tolerability, and pharmacokinetics (PK) of PTK787/ZK 222584 in patients (pts) with unresectable hepatocellular carcinoma (HCC). J Clin Oncol. 2007;23(Suppl):4134.

[163] O'Dwyer, O'Neil BH, Williams-Goff LW, Kauh J, Bekaii-Saab T, Strosberg JR, Lee R, Deal AM, Sullivan D, Sebti SM. A phase II study of AZD6244 in advanced or metastatic hepatocellular carcinoma. J Clin Oncol. 2009;27(Suppl):Ae15574. 2006.

[164] Ramanathan RK, Belani CP, Singh DA, Tanaka M, Lenz HJ, Yen Y, et al. A phase II study of lapatinib in patients with advanced biliary tree and hepatocellular cancer. Cancer Chemother Pharmacol. 2009;64:777-783.

[165] Lin AY, Fisher GA, So S, Tang C, Levitt L. Phase II study of imatinib in unresectable hepatocellular carcinoma. Am J Clin Oncol. 2008;31(1):84-8.

[166] Zhu AX, Stuart K, Blaszkowsky LS, Muzikansky A, Reitberg DP, Clark JW, et al. Phase 2 study of cetuximab in patients with advanced hepatocellular carcinoma. Cancer. 2007;110(3):581-9.

[167] Gruenwald V, Wilkens LGM, Greten TF, Kubicka S, Ganser A, Manns MP, Malek NP. A phase II open-label study of cetuximab in unresectable hepatocellular carcinoma: final results. J Clin Oncol. 2007;(Suppl 15S):25 [18S], 4598.

[168] Blaszkowsky LS, Abrams TA, Miksad RA, Zheng H, Meyerhardt JA, Schrag D, Kwak EL, Fuchs C, Ryan DP, Zhu AX. Phase I/II study of everolimus in patients with advanced hepatocellular carcinoma (HCC) J Clin Oncol. 2010;28(Suppl 15S):Ae14542.

[169] Rizell M, Andersson M, Cahlin C, Hafstrom L, Olausson M, Lindner P. Effects of the mTOR inhibitor sirolimus in patients with hepatocellular and cholangiocellular cancer. Int J Clin Oncol. 2008;13(1):66-70.

[170] Asnacios A, Fartoux L, Romano O, Tesmoingt C, Louafi SS, Mansoubakht T, et al. Gemcitabine plus oxaliplatin (GEMOX) combined with cetuximab in patients with progressive advanced stage hepatocellular carcinoma: results of a multicenter phase 2 study. Cancer. 2008;112(12):2733-9.

[171] Sanoff HK, Bernard S, Goldberg RM, Morse MA, Garcia R, Woods L, et al. Phase II study of capecitabine, oxaliplatin, and cetuximab for advanced hepatocellular carcinoma. Gastrointest Cancer Res. 2011;4(3):78-83.

[172] Zhu AX, Blaszkowsky LS, Ryan DP, Clark JW, Muzikansky A, Horgan K, et al. Phase II study of gemcitabine and oxaliplatin in combination with bevacizumab in patients with advanced hepatocellular carcinoma. J Clin Oncol. 2006;24(12):1898-903.

[173] Sun W, Sohal D, Haller DG, Mykulowycz K, Rosen M, Soulen MC, et al. Phase 2 trial of bevacizumab, capecitabine, and oxaliplatin in treatment of advanced hepatocellular carcinoma. Cancer. 2011;117(14):3187-92.

[174] Hsu C, Yang T, Hsu C, Toh H, Epstein R, Hsiao L, Cheng A. Phase II study of bevacizumab (A) plus capecitabine (X) in patients (pts) with advanced/metastatic hepatocellular carcinoma (HCC): final report. J Clin Oncol. 2008;26(Suppl 15S):A4603.

[175] Thomas MB, Morris JS, Chadha R, Iwasaki M, Kaur H, Lin E, et al. Phase II trial of the combination of bevacizumab and erlotinib in patients who have advanced hepatocellular carcinoma. J Clin Oncol. 2009;27:843-50.

[176] Kaseb AO, Garrett-Mayer E, Morris JS, Xiao L, Lin E, Onicescu G, et al. Efficacy of bevacizumab plus erlotinib for advanced hepatocellular carcinoma and predictors of outcome: final results of a phase II trial. Oncology. 2012;82(2):67-74.

[177] Philip PA, Mahoney MR, Holen KD, Northfelt DW, Pitot HC, Picus J, et al. Phase 2 study of bevacizumab plus erlotinib in patients with advanced hepatocellular cancer. Cancer. 2012;118(9):2424-30.

[178] Berlin JD, Powell ME, Su Y, Horton L, Short S, Richmond A, Kauth JS, Staley CA, Mulchay M, Benson AB. Bortezomib (B) and doxorubicin (dox) in patients (pts) with hepatocellular cancer (HCC): a phase II trial of the Eastern Cooperative Oncology Group (ECOG 6202) with laboratory correlates. J Clin Oncol. 2008;26(Suppl 20S):A4592.

[179] Knox JJ, Chen XE, Feld R, Nematollahi M, Cheiken R, Pond G, et al. A phase I-II study of oblimersen sodium (G3139, Genasense) in combination with doxorubicin in advanced hepatocellular carcinoma (NCI # 5798). Invest New Drugs. 2008;26(2): 193-4.

Chapter 6

LAPTM4B Targeting as Potential Therapy for Hepatocellular Carcinoma

Rou Li Zhou, Mao Jin Li, Xuan Hui Wei, Hua Yang, Yi Shan, Ly Li and Xin Rong Liu

Additional information is available at the end of the chapter

http://dx.doi.org/10.5772/61345

Abstract

HCC is one of the most common cancers worldwide with high prevalence, recurrence, and lethality. The curative rate is not satisfactory. *LAPTM4B* is a novel driver gene of HCC first indentified by our group. It is over-expressed in 87.3% of HCC. The expression levels of the encoded LAPTM4B-35 protein in HCC is also over-expressed in 86.2% of HCC and shows a significant positive correlation with pathological grade, metastasis, and recurrence, and a negative correlation with postoperative overall- and cancer free-survival of HCC patients. Moreover, HCC cells showing high expression of LAPTM4B-35 show a strong tendency to metastasize and enhanced drug resistance. Overexpression of this gene promotes tumorigenesis, faster growth of human HCC xenografts and metastasis in nude mice, and leads to anti-apoptosis, deregulation of proliferation, enhancement of migration and invasion, as well as multi-drug resistance. In addition, overexpression of LAPTM4B-35 leads to accumulation of a number of oncoproteins and to down-regulation of a number of tumor suppressing proteins. By contrary, knockdown of endogenous LAPTM4B-35 via RNAi results in remarkable inhibition of xenograft growth and metastasis of human HCC in nude mice. Also, RNAi knockdown of LAPTN4B-35 can reverse the cellular and molecular malignant phenotypes noted above.

Therefore, it is suggested that to down-regulate over-expression of *LAPTM4B* gene and LAPTM4B-35 in HCC cells may provide novel strategy for HCC treatment. Moreover, the extensive effects caused by LAPTM4B-35 overexpression are based on its critical function in signaling network. Overexpression of LAPTM4B-35 activates at least 4 signaling pathways that are commonly known to be associated with tumorigenesis. Taken together, it is suggests that *LAPTM4B* is a HCC driver gene and LAPTM4B-35 is a key protein which functions in the upstream of cancer-associated signaling network and plays a critical role in tumorigenesis, progression, metastasis, multi-drug resistance and recurrence. Therefore, it may be worth considering the *LAPTM4B* gene and the LAPTM4B-35 protein a novel target in cancer therapy.

In recent years, we identified small chemicals that target LAPTM4B-35 for inhibiting HCC growth and metastasis. We screened 1697 chemicals and found ethylglyoxal bisthiosemicarbazon (ETS) has effective anti-HCC activity probably via targeting LAPTM4B-35. Bel-7402 and HepG2 cell lines that highly express LAPTM4B-35 and a primarily cell line from naturally abortioned human fetal liver were used as the cell models and a control, respectively. Cell survival curve and apoptosis examination in vitro, and HCC xenograft growth and metastases in nude mice were measured to confirm the anti-HCC efficacy in vivo. Western blot, Co-IP, cDNA chips and RNAi were applied for mechanism study. The results showed that ETS can kill HCC cells but not human fetal liver cells *in vitro*, and also attenuate xenograft growth and metastasis of HCC and extend the life span of mice with HCC *in vivo*. When the endogenious over-expression of LAPTM4B-35 was knock-down by RNAi, the killing efficacy of ETS on HepG2 cells was significantly decreased. Also ETS inhibited the phosphorylation of LAPTM4B-35 Tyr_{285}, which involves in activation of PI3K/Akt signaling pathway induced by LAPTM4B-35 over-expression. In addition, all of the molecular alterations in HepG2 cells induced by LAPTM4B-35 over-expression can be reversed by ETS, including significantly decrease of c-Myc, Bcl-2 and phosphorylated Akt, but increase of Bax and phosphorylated p53. Accordingly, apoptosis was induced by ETS, and a number of pro-apoptotic genes were upregulated, while anti-apoptotic genes were downregulated. It is thus suggested that ETS may be a potential promising drug candidate for treatment of HCC by targeting LAPTM4B-35 protein.

In summary, our previous study demonstrated that *LAPTM4B* is a driver gene of HCC, targeting LAPTM4B may provide potential therapy for HCC. Targeting *LAPTM4B* includes bio-targeted therapy and chemical-targeted therapy. The bio-targeted therapy may further explore aimed at inhibiting over-expression of *LAPTM4B* gene via RNAi, miRNA or antisense RNA etc, as well as at blacking the functions of LAPTM4B-35 protein via specific antibody. The chemical-targeted therapy may further explore aimed at attenuating the over-activated signaling pathways in HCC by chemical inhibitors.

Keywords: LAPTM4B, Targeted HCC thrapy, ETS

1. Introduction

Hepatocellular carcinoma (HCC) is one of the most common cancers worldwide with high prevalence, recurrence, and lethality. The curative rate is not satisfactory. Lysosomal protein transmembrane 4 beta (*LAPTM4B*) is a novel driver gene of HCC first cloned and indentified by our group [1,2]. *LAPTM4B* maps to chromosome 8q22.1 and encodes three isoforms of glycoprotein with four transmembrane regions, two extracellular domains (EC1 and EC2), and one small intracellular loop, together with both N-terminal and C-terminal tails, which reside in the cytoplasm. Three isoforms of LAPTM4B protein were designated as LAPTM4B-40, LAPTM4B-35, and LAPTM4B-24 according to their molecular weights [2]. Interestingly, overexpression of LAPTM4B-35 and LAPTM4B-24 show antagonist functions: LAPTM4B-35 promotes oncogenesis and the malignant cellular and molecular phenotypes, but LAPTM4B-24 promotes apoptosis and autophage [2].

LAPTM4B mRNA is overexpressed in 87.3% (48/55) of HCC by Northern blot analysis. The expression levels of the encoded protein LAPTM4B-35 is also over-expressed in 86.2% (T/N≥1.5 in 56/65) of HCC by Western blot analysis [4] and 71.8% (51/71) of HCC by immunohistochemistry [3] and show a significant positive correlation with pathological grade, metastasis, and recurrence and a negative correlation with postoperative survival of HCC patients [3-5]. Moreover, HCC cells with a high expression of LAPTM4B-35 show a strong tendency to motivate drug resistance [6]. The over-expression of this gene promotes tumorigenesis, faster growth, and metastasis of human HCC xenografts in nude mice [5,7] and leads to antiapoptosis, deregulation of proliferation, enhancement of migration and invasion, and multidrug resistance [5]. In addition, the overexpression of LAPTM4B-35 leads to the accumulation of a number of oncoproteins and downregulation of a number of tumor suppressing proteins. Conversely, knockdown of endogenous LAPTM4B-35 via RNAi results in remarkable inhibition of xenograft growth and metastasis of human HCC in nude mice [5,7]. Meanwhile, the RNAi knockdown of LAPTN4B-35 can reverse the cellular and molecular malignant phenotypes noted above [5]. It was also found in a number of solid cancers, including non-small cell lung cancer (NSCLC) that the level of LAPTM4B-35 expression was not only significantly higher than that in normal tissues and associated with histopathologic differentiation, lymph node metastasis, and TNM stage but also associated with microvessel density [8]. Taken together, it is suggested that *LAPTM4B* is a cancer driver gene and LAPTM4B-35 is a key oncoprotein, which are both predicted to be a diagnostic marker and a therapeutic target for cancer.

The extensive effects caused by LAPTM4B-35 overexpression are based on its critical function on cell trafficking and signaling network. Recently, Tan et al. [9] reported that the oncoprotein LAPTM4B not only interacts with EGFR but also regulates EGFR internalization and trafficking, and thus increases the amount and enhances the functions of EGFR on cell surface. Moreover, LAPTM4B can play a kinase-independent role for EGFR in autophagy initiation [10]. We found that the over-expression of LAPTM4B-35 can activate several signaling pathways that are commonly known to be associated with oncogenesis and progression [2]. The activation of PI3K/Akt signaling pathway induced by the overexpression of LAPTM4B-35 has been demonstrated to associate with drug resistance [6]. In this paper, we further present the functions of LAPTM4B-35 on signaling and a chemical that inhibits HCC *in vitro* and *in vivo* by targeting LAPTM4B-35.

2. Functions of LAPTM4B-35 involved in signaling network

Current evidence indicates that the interaction between cancer cells with their microenvironment plays key roles in oncogenesis and progression. Cancer microenvironment is composed of variant signal molecules, including solvable signal molecules (growth factors, cytokines, etc.), insolvable extracellular matrix (ECM), and variant cells nearby. Cancer cells and their microenvironment are reciprocally affected. Cancer cell proliferation, survival, and migrationare all motivated and dependent on not only solvable signal molecules but also ECM. Cancer cells accept positive or negative regulations of signal molecules from solvable factors, ECM, and other cells in their microenvironment through signal transduction pathways, which are organized as a very complicated network. In other words, cancer may be known as a disease of signaling network. Disturbances of signaling pathways and the converging network initiate at the early stage and go through the whole process of cancer development. In addition, the disturbance of signaling pathways results from oncogenic alternation in genetics and epigenetics and contributes to the molecular and cellular malignant phenotypes of cancer cells, which include disregulations of proliferation, survival/apoptosis, differentiation and metabolism, as well as enhancement of migration/invasion and multidrug resistance. Therefore, signaling pathways and the network are of importance from a therapeutic perspective because targeting them may help reverse, delay, or prevent oncogenesis. Notably, since cirrhosis is associated with hepatic regeneration after tissue damages, which are caused by hepatitis infection, toxins (for example, alcohol oraflatoxin) or metabolic influences, and is often the prerequisite of hepato-oncogenesis, it is noticed that the ECM and the ECM-related signaling pathways, that are commonly alternated in cirrhosis and HCC, are of very importance. Our preliminary study has indicated that LAPTM4B-35 is most likely an assembly platform or organizer for a number of signaling molecules which are integrated in the cell membranes or soluble in the cytoplasm. Overexpression of LAPTM4B-35 would therefore be expected to lead to disturbance of a wide range of signaling pathways and their networks. We found LAPTM4B-35 can interact or co-localize with a number of these signal molecules, including membrane-integrated receptors and cytoplasmic signal molecules. These membrane-integrated receptors involve the growth factor receptors of the RTK (receptor tyrosine kinase) family, such as EGFR [9-11] and IGF-1R (Figure 1a), and ECM receptors of the integrin family, such as $\alpha6\beta1$ [11] and $\alpha5\beta1$ (Figures 1d and 2). The cytoplasmic signaling molecules that can interact with LAPTM4B-35 include FAK (Figure 2c) and PI3K p85α (Figure 3a). Given that LAPTM4B-35 is a tetra-transmembrane protein and localizes in plasma membrane and endomembranes (including lysosomes and endosomes). The interaction of LAPTM4B-35 with both RTK under the stimulation of growth factors, and integrin under ECM stimulation would be expected to integrate related signal transduction pathways triggered by growth factors and ECM components at the cell surface. It is well known that based on binding of growth factors (ligand) to their corresponding RTK receptor, Ras and ERK1/2 (MAPK family)downstream is subsequently activated [12]. At the same time, based on binding of ECM components (ligand), such as fibronectin (FN) or laminin (LN), to their corresponding integrin receptor ($\alpha5\beta1$ or $\alpha6\beta1$, respectively), FAK_{397} is phosphorylated and activated, and may subsequently activate downstream Ras/ERK and PI3K/AKT signaling pathways [13,14]. As has been previously recognized, the RTK/Ras/ERK signaling pathway and the ECM/Integrin/FAK signaling pathway converge at Ras and/or FAK. However, we found that over expression of LAPTM4B-35 can not only dramatically activate Ras (Figure 1b) and the downstream ERK1/2 (MAPK) under the stimulation of growth factors (Figures 1c) or FN (Figure 1f), respectively, but also activates FAK. This was originally suggested by knock down experiments. When LAPTM4B-35 is knocked down by RNAi in HCC cells, binding of integrin $\alpha5$ with LAPTM4B-35 is dramatically decreased under stimulation with FN, as shown in Figure 1d. Knockdown of LAPTM4B-35 also coincidently significantly reduces phosphorylation and activation of FAK_{397} (Figure 1e) under stimulation by FN or LN. These experiments further provide evidence for the involvement of LAPTM4B-35 in the ECM/integrin/FAK signaling pathway. In addition, inhibition of FAK by PP2 (FAK inhibitor) can attenuate phosphorylation/activation of ERK1/2 in both LAPTM4B35-up-regulated HCC cells (AE) and in wild-type HCC control cells (Mock) as shown in Figure 1f. AE and Mock cells are both LAPTM4B-35 overexpressed, but to different extents. These results suggest that in LAPTM4B-35 overexpressed HCC cells, activation of ERK results from both the upstream growth factor/Ras and FN/

Integrin/FAK signaling cascades. Taken together, it is reasonable to propose that overexpressed LAPTM4B-35 as a linker at the cell surface (plasma membrane) simultaneously over activates both the growth factor (EGF or IGF-1R)/RTK/Ras/ERK and the ECM (FN or LN)/ Integrin/FAK/ERK signaling pathways by interacting with growth factor receptor (RTK) and ECM receptor (integrin) under the stimulation of growth factor and ECM components (FN, LN), respectively. In other words, the growth factor/RTK/Ras/ERK and ECM/ integrin/FAK/ERK signaling pathways initiallyconverge at the plasma membrane level through overexpression of membrane-integrated LAPTM4B-35 in HCC cells, instead of at Ras and FAK in the cytoplasm in normal hepatocytes whichexpress LAPTM4B-35 and FAK at rather low level. Moreover, simultaneous overactivation of these two signaling pathways caused by LAPTM4B-35 overexpression would result in enhancement of proliferation, survival, migration and invasion of cancer cells.

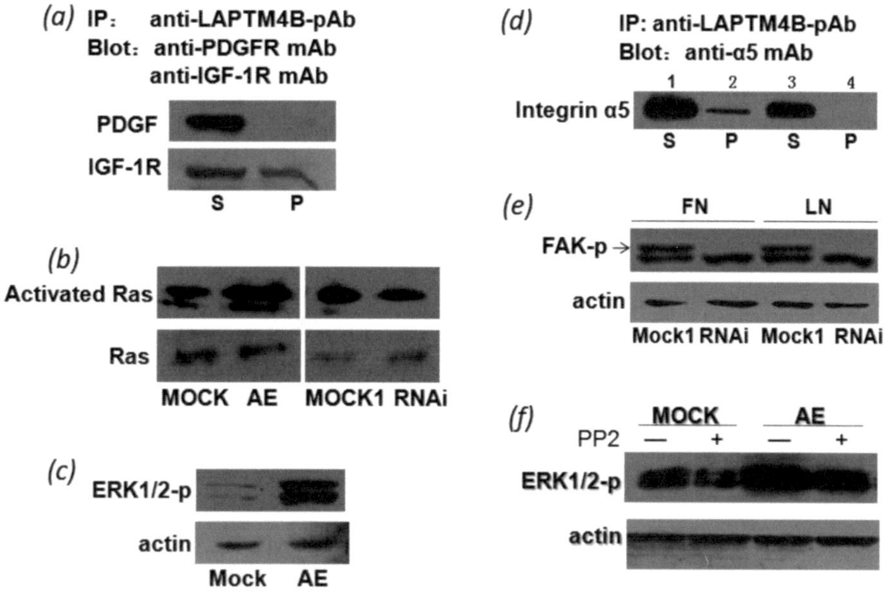

Figure 1. Activation of Ras/ERK and FAK/ERK signaling pathways by LAPTM4B-35 overexpression. *(a)* Co-IP assay indicates the interaction between LAPTM4B-35 and IGF-1R, but not PDGFR. Lysate from BEL-7402 HCC cells was immunoprecipitated by anti-LAPTM4B pAb, and the supernatant (S) and precipitant (P) were then subjected to Western blot with anti-PDGFR-mAb and anti-IGF-1R-mAb. *(b)* GST pull-down experiments with GST-RafRBD fusion protein to show Ras activation under stimulation of 20% fetal calf serum. The left panel indicates that activated Rasis increased inthe LAPTM4B-35 overexpressed BEL-7402 HCC cells (AE) as compared to the control cells (MOCK). The right panelindicates that activated Rasis decreased in the BEL-7402 HCC cells (RNAi)in which theLAPTM4B-35 has been knocked down via transient transfection by LAPTM4B-shRNA as compared with its control cells (MOCK1). It is obvious that activation of Ras in HCC cells is associated with overexpression of LAPTM4B-35. *(c)* Western blot analysis indicates that phosphorylated ERK1 and ERK 2 are increased in LAPTM4B-35 upregulated BEL-7402 HCC cells (AE) as compared with its control (MOCK) under stimulation of 20% fetal calf serum.*(d)* Co-IP assay indicates that the interaction between LAPTM4B-35 and integrin $\alpha5$ and its dependent on the overexpression of LAPTM4B-35. The lysate of BEL-7402 HCC cells was immunoprecipitated with anti-LAPTM4B pAb, the supernatant (S) and precipitant (P) were then separately subjected to Western blot analysis with anti-integrin $\alpha5$-mAb. In the Western blot profiles, Lanes 1 and 2 show the integrin $\alpha5$ from the HCC MOCK1 cells (as a control) in the supernatant and immunoprecipitant, respec-

tively; Lanes 3 and 4 show the integrin α5 from LAPTM4B-35 knocked down (RNAi) HCC cells in the supernatant and immunoprecipitant, respectively. It is obvious, that integrin α5 in Lane 4 from LAPTM4B-immunoprecipitant of RNAi HCC cells Is dramatically reduced (disappear) as compared with Lane 2 from LAPTM4B-immunoprecipitant of wild-type HCC control cells that over express LAPTM4B-35. *(e)* Western blot analysis indicates that the phosphorylation/activation of FAK_{397} is reduced depending on knock down of LAPTM4B-35. The cells are stimulated by ECM component, either fibronectin (FN) or laminin (LN), for 15 min. The lysate of cells was then subjected to Western blot analysis. Anti- phosphorylated FAK_{397} mAb was used for blotting. The Western blot profiles indicate that based on stimulation of FN or LN, the phosphorylated FAK_{397} is reduced in cells which LAPTM4B-35 expression is knocked down as compared with the control cells.*(f)* Western blot analysis indicates that FAK inhibitor (PP2) inhibits the phosphorylation of ERK1/2. After treatment of BEL-7402 HCC cells (AE) by 1 μM PP2, the phosphorylation of ERK1/2 was analyzed via Western blot for the LAPTM4B-35 up-regulated cells and the MOCK cells under the stimulation of laminin substrate. The Western blot profile shows that phosphorylation/activation of ERK1/2 is associated with FAK activity.

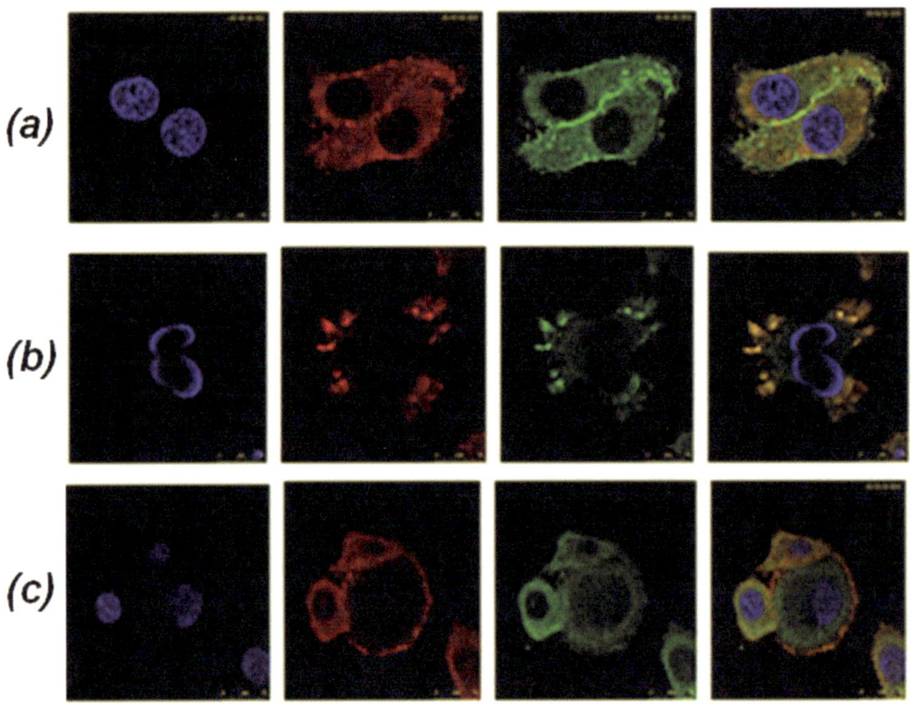

Figure 2. Colocalization between LAPTM4B-35 and integrinα5 or FAK. Cells were attaching and spreading onto fibronectin for 6 h *(a, c)* or 24 h*(b)*. *(a)* and *(b) show* the colocalization of LAPTM4B-35 (red) and integrin α5 (green). *(c)* shows the colocalization of LAPTM4B-35 (red) and FAK(green).

We found that not only membrane-integrated receptors, but also some solvable signaling molecules in cytoplasm can interact with LAPTM4B-35, such as FAK (Figure 2c) and PI3K p85α [6]. It is known that PI3K is a kinase which catalyzes phosphorylation of proteins andlipids. An important phosphorylated product catalyzed byPI3K is membrane-integrated PIP3 which can recruit cytoplasmic PH domain-containing proteins, including Akt and the corresponding kinases (PDK1 and PDK2) to the plasma membrane where Akt is phosphorylated by PDK1 and PDK2. Phosphorylated Akt is commonly known as a marker for PI3K/Akt signaling pathway activation. In view of the fact PI3K consists of two subunits: p110 catalytic subunit and p85α regulatory subunit. The kinase activity of p110 is normally inhibited by binding of p85α. The inhibitory effect of p85αcan be released by binding to an appropriate molecule [15]. We found that LAPTM4B-35 can interact with p85α, but not with p110 (Figure 3a). Moreover, using site-directed mutation experiments we found that binding of LAPTM4B-35 to PI3K p85α is mediated by two motifs. One is the proline-rich motif (PPRP) in the N-terminus of LAPTM4B-35, which may bind to the SH3 domain of PI3K p85αsubunit, and the other is phosphorylated Tyr_{285} in the C-terminus of LAPTM4B-35, which may bind to the SH2 domain of the PI3K p85α subunit (Figure 3b). To demonstrate this a series of HCC cell variants with highly expressed wild type and mutated LAPTM4B-35 were prepared by transfection with variant plasmids containing LAPTM4B-35 with mutation at PPRP or at Try $(Y)_{285}$, or with deleted N-terminus. These plasmids containg a FLAG sequence as a tag are designated as pcDNA3-LAPTM4B-flag (AF) containing wild type LAPTM4B-35, pcDNA3-LAPTM4B-flag (PA) containing P12,13,15A mutated LAPTM4B-35, pcDNA3-LAPTM4B-flag (△N) containing LAPTM4B-35 with a deletion of $N_{10\text{-}19}$ amino acid residues), pcDNA3-LAPTM4B-flag (YF) containing Y285F mutated LAPTM4B-35, or pcDNA3-LAPTM4B-flag (△N+YF). As shown in Figure 3b, the binding of p85α to LAPTM4B-35 in HCC AF cells (up-regulated wild-type LAPTM4B-35) is dramatically increased under the stimulation of fetal calf serum, as compared with Mock cells (the control). In contrast, the binding of p85α to LAPTM4B-35 in the PA, △N, YF, and △N+YF-mutated HCC cell variants are all significantly attenuated under the same condition, as compared with AF cells. Therefore, the overexpression of LAPTM4B-35 in HCC cells would promote the interaction of both PPRP and Tyr-p motifs of LAPTM4B-35 with PI3K p85α and thus release the inhibitory effect of p85α regulatory subunit to the p110 catalytic subunit, and would cause the phosphorylation of the downstream AKT. Accordingly, Western blot analysis (Figure 3c) demonstrated that the phosphorylated Akt (Akt-p) is decreased in the mutated AF(PA) and AF(YF) cells as compared with the wild-type LAPTM4B-35 (AF), indicating that the proline-rich domain in the N-terminal and the Tyr_{285} in the C-terminal tails of LAPTM4B-35 are both required for Akt phosphorylation/activation. We also found that in the serum-starved HCC cells, LAPTM4B-35 and Akt separately distributes (Figure 4a); conversely under the stimulation of fetal calf serum which provides growth factors, co-localization of activated Akt and LAPTM4B-35 appears in the AF cells (Figure 4b); however, there is no co-localization in the PA-mutated cells (Figure 4c), YF-mutated cells (Figure 4d), and also in the cells in which PI3K is inhibited by its inhibitor LY294002 (Figure 4e). It is obvious that the co-localization of LAPTM4B-35 and Akt appears merely in cells wherein wild-type LAPTM4B-35 is up-regulated, but not in the cells transfected by the empty vector (Mock) nor in any of the cells with mutation of PA, ΔN, and YF of LAPTM4B-35. These results further provide evidence that the PI3K-dependent activation of Akt is associated with the up-regulation of LAPTM4B-35 expression via both proline-rich motif in the N-terminus and the Tyr-p in the C-terminus (Figure 5). It is therefore proposed that LAPTM4B-35 activates PI3K/Akt signaling pathway through binding PI3K p85α by a proline-rich domain at the N terminaus and a phosphorylated Tyr_{285} at the C terminus to release the inhibitory effect of p85α on PI3K p110 activity, and consequently result in phosphorylation and activation of Akt.

Moreover, we demponstrated that theTyr_{285} is the one single site for phosphorylation of Tyr residues in the LAPTM4B-35 molecule (Figure 3f). Notably, under stimulation of LN, Tyr_{285} phosphorylation rises quickly and peaks at 10 min. Thereafter phosphorylation decreases steadily out to 40 minutes (Figure 3g -1). It is of importance that LAPTM4B-35 Tyr_{285} phosphorylation can be markedly inhibited by LAPTM4B-EC2-pAb (Figure 3g -2), indicating the EC2 domain is required for Tyr_{285} phosphorylation of LAPTM4B-35. Kazarow (2002) reported that CD151, a member of the tetra-transmembrane protein family, can interact with the integrin α subunit via an QRD motif in the EC2 domain. Similarly, a YRD motif exists in the LAPTM4B-35 EC2 domain. We found that in LAPTM4B-35 $YRD_{233\text{-}235}$INF mutated HCC cells, AKT phosphorylation/activation is significantly inhibited (Figure 3h), suggesting interaction of LAPTM4B-35 EC2 YRD and integrin is involved in PI3K/AKT activation. In addition, LAPTM4B-EC2-pAb and integrin α6-mAb can both inhibit FAK phosphorylation under stimulation by LN (Figure 3i), indicating interaction of LAPTM4B-EC2 with integrin α6 (the specific receptor of LN) is involved in FAK phosphorylation/activation. Moreover, we found that the FAK inhibitor PP2 can simultaneously inhibit phosphorylation of LAPTM4B-35 and interaction of LAPTM4B-35 with PI3K p85α (Figure 3e). These result suggest that FAK is likely the kinase that catalyzes the Tyr phosphorylation of LAPTM4B-35, by which the binding site of LAPTM4B-35 to the PI3K p85α SH2 domain is created, thus releasing inhibition of PI3K p85α to p110 kinase activity, and consequently resulting in activation of downstream AKT (Figure 5).

It is known that FAK, as a functionally complicated signal molecule with Tyr kinase activity and nonkinase scaffolding function, is overexpressed in many cancers (including 60% of HCC) and involves in many aspects of tumor growth, invasion, and metastasis. Given that the phophorylation of FAK Tyr_{397} is critical for trigering its Tyr kinase activity and enhancing its nonkinase scaffolding function, and is induced by binding of integrin with FN or LN. We found that the PI3K/Akt signaling pathway in LAPTM4B-35 overexpressed HCC cells can be activated by stimulation of not only serum but also fibronectin or laminin substrate (Figure 3d); additionally the interaction of LAPTM4B-35 with PI3K p85α is inhibited by FAK inhibitor PP2 (Figure 3e). These results suggest that overexpression and interaction of LAPTM4B-35 and FAK in cancer cells would be expected tocreate an alternative signaling pathway, i.e. ECM/ integrin/FAK/LAPTM4B-35/PI3K/AKT signaling pathway. In which FAK phosphorylation/ activation results from interaction of the LAPTM4B-35 EC2 domain and integrin α6 subunit at the cell surface under the stimulation by LN or FN, and results in phosphorylation of LAPTM4B-35 Tyr_{285} by FAK kinase activity. This model (shown in Figure 5 on the upper right) illustrates a novel putative mechanism by which the PI3K/AKT signaling pathway is over activated through the involvement LAPTM4B-35 in cancer cells. In other words, our preliminary results suggest there might be a novel LAPTM4B-35 dependent pathway which gives rise to overactivation of the PI3K/AKT signaling pathway in HCC cells. In this mechanism, overexpressed LAPTM4B-35 interacts initially with integrin at the cell surface under stimulation of an ECM component (FN or LN) via its EC2 YRD motif. This interaction of LAPTM4B-35 and integrin induces phosphorylation and activation of FAK_{397} through a currently not fully understood mechanism. Activated FAK may catalyze phosphorylation of LAPTM4B-35 Tyr_{285} to create a binding site for PI3K p85α. Consequently, downstream AKT is phosphorylated and activated by PI3K p110, the kinase activity of which comes into play through binding of phosphorylated LAPTM4B-35 Tyr_{285} to PI3K p85α. This proposed molecular mechanism remains to be further studied in detail.

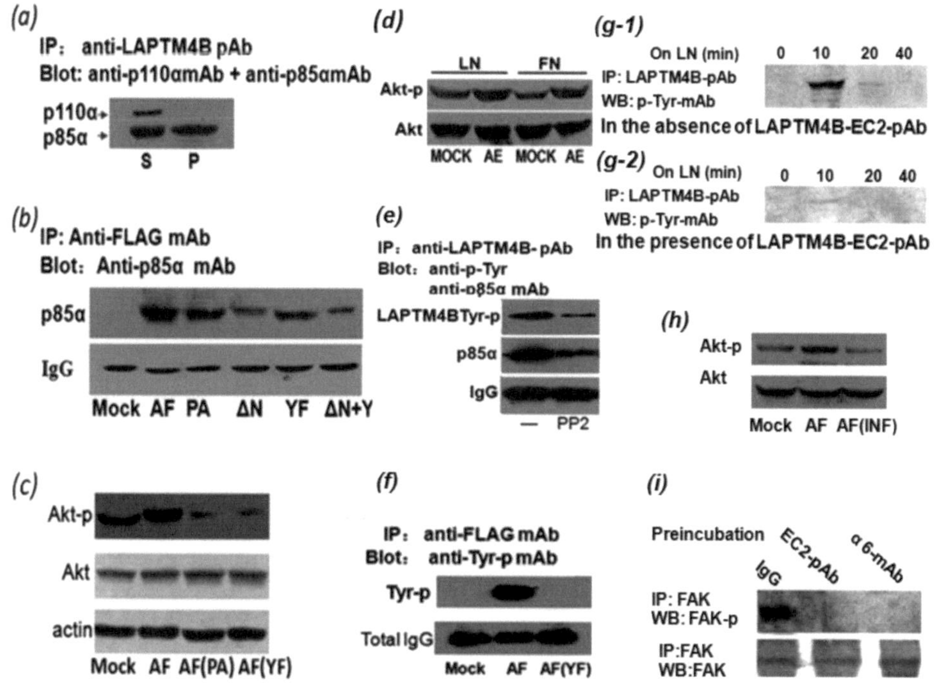

Figure 3. Mechanism for interaction of LAPTM4B-35 with of PI3K p85α and activation of Akt. *(a)* Co-IP analysis demonstrates interaction of LAPTM4B-35 with p85α regulatory subunit, but not PI3K p110 catalytic subunit. Anti-LAPTM4B35-pAb was used to precipitate the binding proteins, and a mixture of anti-PI3K p110-mAb and anti-PI3Kp85α-mAb was applied to blot the binding proteins. *(b)* Co-IP analysis demonstrates that the proline-rich domain in N-terminus and Tyr_{285} in C-terminus of LAPTM4B-35 are involved in the interaction of LAPTM4B-35 with PI3K p85α via a serious of mutants, including PA, ΔN, YF, and ΔN+YF mutants. PA mutant (P): Prolines in the PPRP motif in N-terminus of LAPTM4B-35 were mutated to alanines(P12,13,15A). ΔN mutant: The 10th-19th amino acid residues in the N-terminus of LAPTM4B-35 were deleted. YF mutant: The Tyr_{285} in the C-terminus of LAPTM4B-35 was mutated to phenylalanine (Y285F). ΔN+YF mutant: ΔN mutant plus YF mutant. Anti-FLAG-mAb was used to immunoprecipitate the binding proteins in lysates from variant BEL-7402 HCC cell lines, which were transfected separately by pcDNA3-Mock-flag (Mock), pcDNA3-LAPTM4B-flag (AF), pcDNA3-LAPTM4B-flag (PA), pcDNA3-LAPTM4B-flag (ΔN), pcDNA3-LAPTM4B-flag (YF), or pcDNA3-LAPTM4B-flag (ΔN+YF) plasmids. Then anti-PI3Kp85α-mAb was applied to blot the binding proteins. The interaction of LAPTM4B-35 and PI3K p85α was dramatically enhanced in LAPTM4B-35 up-regulated AF cells as compared with the Mock cells and was significantly attenuated in the variant LAPTM4B-mutated cells as compared with the AF cells. *(c)* Western blot profile demonstrates that Akt-p is decreased in the mutated AF(PA) and AF(YF) cells as compared with wild-type LAPTM4B-35 (AF), indicating that the proline-rich domain in N-terminal and the Tyr_{285} in C-terminal tails of LAPTM4B-35 are necessary for Akt phosphorylation. *(d)* Western blot demonstrates that ECM components, fibronectin (FN) or laminin (LN), can promote phosphorylation/activation of Akt in cells in which LAPTM4B-35 expression is up-regulated, indicating association of phosphorylation/activation of Akt with FN and LN in HCC cells. *(e)* Co-IP analysis demonstrates that FAK inhibitor PP2 can simultaneously inhibit phosphorylation of Tyr_{285} and interaction of p85α with LAPTM4B-35. Anti-LAPTM4B-pAb was used to immunoprecipitate the binding proteins, then anti-phosphorylated Tyr mAb or anti-Akt mAb was used to blot the

binding protein. *(f)* Co-IP and Western blot profile show that LAPTM4B-35 Tyr_{285} is the only phosphorylation site by mutation analysis. HepG2 cells were transfected by AF or AF(YF) mutant. The phosphorylation appeared merely in the wild type HepG2 cells, but not the Tyr $_{285}$ mutated YF cells. *(g)* Co-IP analysis indicates that LAPTM4B-35 Tyr can be phophorylated in a peaky manner under the stimulation of LN. HCC cells were placed on LN-coated vials for variant times, LAPTM4B-EC2-pAb was used to precipitate LAPTM4B protein in the HCC lysates. The immuno-precipitants were subjected to Western blot analysis. The anti-phosphorylated Tyr-mAb was used to blot the phosphorylated LAPTM4B-35. *(g-1)* shows the time course of LAPTM4B-35 phosphorylation with the highest phosphorylation at 10 min. *(g-2)* shows the inhibition of LAPTM4B-35 phosphorylation by LAPTM4B-EC2-pAb. *(h)* Western blot analysis indicates that mutation of YRD motif in EC2 domain of LAPTM4B-35 can inhibit AKT phosphorylation. BEL-7402 HCC cells were transfected by pcDNA3-AF(YRD233-235INF) mutated plasmids (INF) and the wild type pcDNA3-AF (AF) plasmids, respectively. The lysates were analyzed by Western blot with a anti-phosphorylated AKT-mAb. *(i)* Co-IP analysis indicates that both LAPTM4B-EC2-pAb and integrin $\alpha6$ mAb can inhibit FAK phosphorylation. The BEL-7402 HCC cells were pre-incubated with non-immune IgG (as a control), LAPTM4B-EC2-pAb and integrin $\alpha6$ mAb, respectively. The lysates were precipitated by FAK mAb. The immuno-precipitants were then subjected to Western blot analysis, and phosphorylated FAK mAb (the upper panel) or FAK-mAb (the lower panel) was used as the bloting antibody.

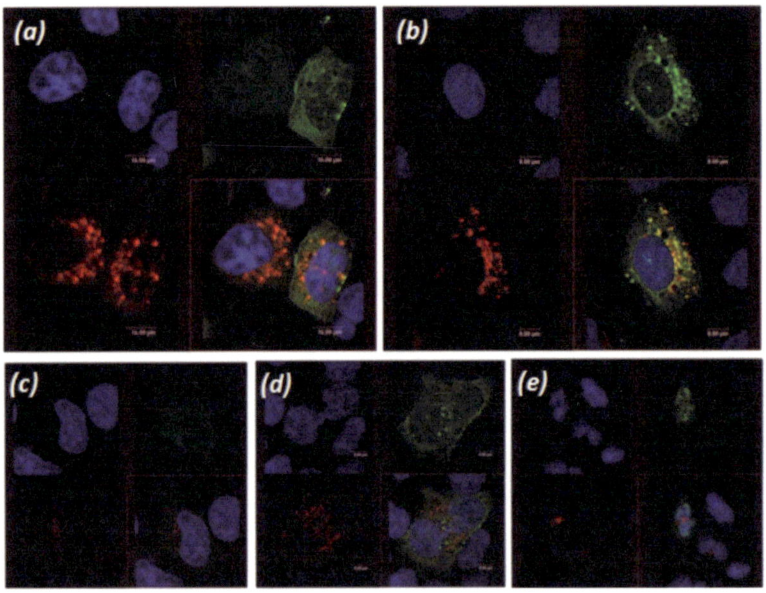

Figure 4. Co-localization of activated Akt and overexpressed LAPTM4B-35 under the stimulation of serum in BEL-7402 HCC cells. *(a)* Nonactivated Akt (green) and LAPTM4B-35 (red) are separately distributed in the cells cotransfected with pEGFP-PH-Akt plasmids and pcDNA3-LAPTM4B-flag plasmids (AF) after serum-starvation for 16 h. *(b)* Colocalization (yellow) of activated Akt (green) and overexpressed LAPTM4B-35 (red) understimulation of serum in HCC cells, which is stimulated by 20% fetal calf serum for 15 min after serum-starvation for 16 h. (c) No colocalization appeared in PA mutant HCC cells under the same conditions as described in *(b)*. (d) No colocalization appeared in YF mutant HCC cells under the same conditions as described in *(b)*. (e) No colocalization appeared in the presence of PI3K inhibitor (LY294002) in AF HCC (wild-type) cells under the same conditions as described in *(b)*.

In summary, cancer-targeted therapy currently focuses primarily on targeting key signaling molecules in one or more signaling pathways which are overactivated in a given cancer. Tetra-transmembrane LAPTM4B-35 is believed to function as an assembly platform or organizer for a number of signaling molecules, which may either be integrated in the cell membranes or

http://dx.doi.org/10.5772/61345

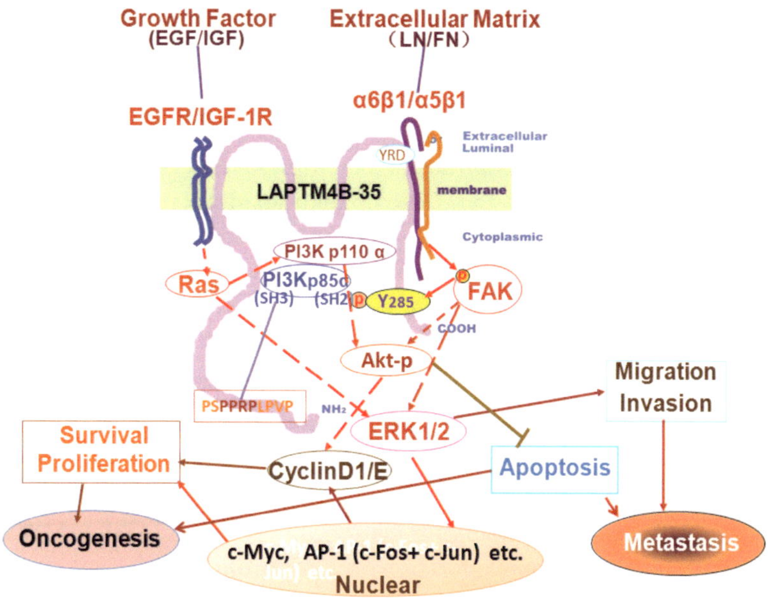

Figure 5. Signaling pathways activated by the overexpression of LAPTM4B-35 in HCC cells.

soluble in the cytoplasm. The LAPTM4B-35 overexpression, which occurs in more than 80% of HCC tissues, and the interactions with membrane-integrated receptors and cytoplasmic signal molecules are expected to act as an amplified assembly platform for upstream signal molecules of several signaling pathways, and leads to over activation of related signaling pathways (Figure 5), such as growth factor/ RTK/Ras/ERK, growth factor/RTK/Ras/PI3K/Akt, ECM/integrin/FAK/ERK, ECM/integrin/FAK/PI3K/Akt, and so on. Since these signaling pathways and their networks are closely associated with malignant molecular and cellular phenotypes, including cell proliferation/differentiation and survival/apoptosis as well as migration/invasion, it is believed that over activation of these signaling pathways is linked with hepatic carcinogenesis and progression [12-15]. Collectively, our data strongly suggest that LAPTM4B-35 would be an ideal target for HCC treatment, and that LAPTM4B-targeted therapy is a promising potential therapeutic strategy for HCC which will act in down regulation of the expression of LAPTM4B-35, or act by obstructing the interaction of LAPTM4B-35 with growth factors, integrins, FAK, PI3K p85α and other LAPTM4B-35 binding signal molecules.

3. Small chemicals targeting LAPTM4B-35

The molecular targets for cancer therapy have expanded from angiogenesis to oncogenic signaling pathways. The target indication has shifted from advanced stage to early or intermediate stages of cancer. Agents targeting EGFR, FGFR, PI3K/Akt/mTOR, TGF-β, c-Met, MEK, IGF signaling, FAK and histone deacetylase have been actively explored [17,20].

Based on the basic characteristics: (1) *LAPTM4B* is a driver oncogene (2) this gene and theencoding LAPTM4B-35 protein are over expressed in more than 85% of HCC and (3) theoverexpression of LAPTM4B-35 can activate multiplesignaling pathways, we propose that *LAPTM4B* gene and the LAPTM4B-35 protein might bean ideal target for HCC treatment. We identified the chemicals that target LAPTM4B-35 for inhibiting HCC growth and metastasis. A total of 1697 synthetic small chemicals from Li and Liu (Pharmaceutical Institute, Chinese Academy of Medical Sciences) were screened. Among these chemicals, ethylglyoxal bis-thiosemicarbazone (ETS) was found to have effective activity for the inhibition of growth and metastasis of human HCC cells *in vitro* and *in vivo* probably via targeting LAPTM4B-35 [18].

Three HCC cell lines (Bel-74402, HepG2, and HLE) from human HCC and a cell line from naturally aborted human fetal were used as the cell models and a control, respectively. Cell survival curve and apoptosis analysis *in vitro* and HCC xenograft growth and metastasis in nude mice were evaluated to confirm the inhibitory efficacy *in vivo*. Western blot, Co-IP, cDNA chips, and RNAi were applied for exploration on mechanism.

We found that ETS can inhibit cell growth of variant HCC cell lines in a dose-dependent manner shown by cell growth curve *in vitro* (Figure 6a, 6b, and 6d). The IC50 of ETS inhibition varies for variant HCC cell lines, such as HepG2 (0.9 μmol/L), Bel-7402 (0.7 μmol/L), HLE (1.1 μmol/L), and H22 (1.6 μmol/L). Convesely, ETS cannot affect the survival of human fetal liver cells even if the concentration of ETS is increasing to as high as 200 times of that used for HCC cells. Notably, both Bel-7402 and HepG2 cells express LAPTM4B-35 at very high level and are most sensitive to ETS; HLE cells express LAPTM4B-35 at relatively low level [19] and are less sensitive to ETS. However, the fetal liver cells that express LAPTM4B-35 at a low level are not sensitive to ETS. Accordinly, when the endogenous overexpression of LAPTM4B-35 was knocked down by RNAi through shRNA transfection, the inhibitory effect of ETS on HepG2 cells was significantly decreased (Figure 6d). Figure 6c demonstrates the killing efficacy of ETS to HepG2 cell as shown by fluorescently double stained with Calcein-AM (1 μmol/L) and EthD-1 (2 μmol/L). Cells emitting green fluorescence were alive cells merely stained by Calcein-AM. Cells emitting red fluorescence were dead cells or apoptotic cells merely stained by EthD-1. Collectively, It is suggested that the inhibitory/killing efficacy of ETS on HCC cells depends on the high expression of LAPTM4B-35. At the same time, the effect of ETS on HepG2 cells was more effective than cisplatin (IC50: 7.5 μmol/L), doxorubicin (IC50: 7.6 μmol/L), mitomycin (IC50: 5.8 μmol/L), and 5-fluorouracil (IC50: >200 μmol/L) *in vitro* (Figure 6b). Moreover, the killing efficacy of ETS was confirmed from two aspects. First, after ETS treatment at a concentration of 1.25 μM for 72 h, HepG2 cells were cultured in a ETS-free medium at 37°C for as long as 12 days. As a result, when compared with 6×10^3 cells seeded in a well at the beginning, only a few colonies appeared after the12 days ETS-free culture, indicating that the vast majority of HepG2 cells were killed by ETS. Second, the significant killing efficacy of ETS on HepG2 cells was further confirmed by Calcein-AM/EthD-1 fluorescence double staining in a time-dependent manner (Figure 7b). The time-dependent growth inhibition was also shown by growth curves of HepG2 cells *in vitro* (Figure 7a) and HCC xenograft *in vivo* (Figure 8a).

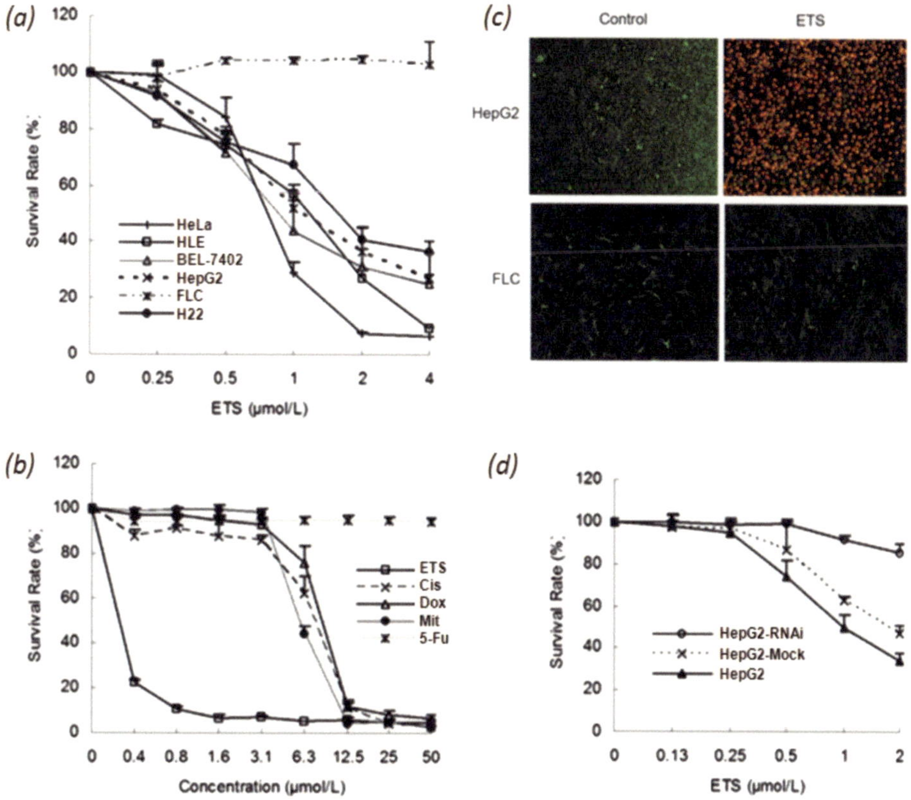

Figure 6. Inhibitory and killing efficiency of ETS on HCC cells. *(a)* Cancer cells of variant lines were incubated in the absence or presence of ETS at indicated concentrations for 48 h. *(b)* HepG2 cells were incubated in the absence or presence of variant drugs at indicated concentrations for 48 h. *(c)* The cells were fluorescently double-stained with Calcein-AM (1 μmol/L) and EthD-1 (2 μmol/L) at 37℃ for 30 min and then surveyed under fluorescence microscope. Cells emitting green fluorescence were alive cells which were merely stained by Calcein-AM. Cells emitting red fluorescence were dead cells or apoptotic cells which merely stained by EthD-1. Upper panel: HepG2 HCC cells were treated by ETS at a concentration of 2 μmol/L for 48 h. The vast majority of HepG2 cells were killed by ETS. Lower panel: human fetal liver cells were treated by ETS at a concentration of 25 μmol/L for 48 h. None of fetal liver cells were killed by ETS. *(d)* HepG2 cell line was transfected by LAPTM4B-shRNA or Mock. The transfected HepG2 cells by LAPTM4B-shRNA (RNAi) or LAPTM4B-Mock plasmids and the parent HepG2 cells were treated by ETS at indicated concentrations for 48 h. The LAPTM4B-35 silenced HepG2 cells showed less sensitive to ETS.The cell survival rate (%) of growth curves was calculated according to ratio of viable cells number determined by acid phosphatase assay (APA) before and after treatment.

ETS also shows significant effect on the inhibition of HCC growth and metastasis *in vivo*. Human HCC BEL-7402 cells were subcutaneously inoculated, and then ETS was administered either by intratumor injection or intraperitoneal injection. Both ways can inhibit the HCC xenograft growth. The effect of ETS on attenuation of growth and metastasis of human HCC xenograft in nude mice is shown in Table 1, as well as Figure 8(a) and 8(b). At the same time, the mice treated by ETS were less lost their body weight than that treated by mitomycin and

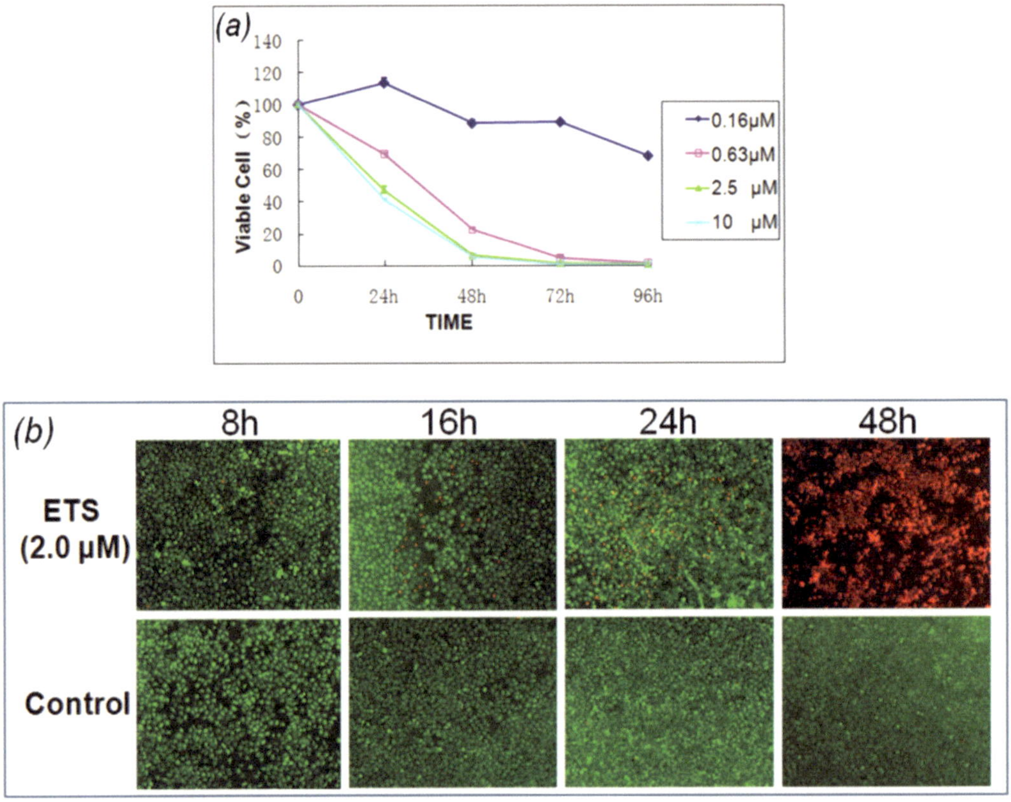

Figure 7. The time- and dose-dependent inhibition and killing of ETS on HepG2 cells. *(a)* HepG2 cells were treated with ETS at variant concentrations or for variant hours. The number of viable cells was determined by ASA. This figure shows that the effect of ETS on inhibiting HCC cell growth is dose and time dependent. *(b)* HepG2 cells were treated as Figure 6(c). Upper panel: with ETS (2 μM) for indicated incubation time. Lower panel: without ETS for comparable incubation time as a control. This figure shows that the effect of ETS on killing HCC cells is time-dependent.

cisplatin. As a matter of fact, the acute toxicity test indicated that ETS had little poison on mice. There is no death of mice in the 1000mg/kg, 464mg/kg, and control groups. Of the 10 mice per group, all died in the 4640mg/kg group, and 4 mice died in the 2150mg/kg group. The LD_{50} of ETS was 2329.9 mg/kg, with a 95% dependable limit of 1846.7-2939.0 mg/kg.

In addition, a murine HCC H22 cell line was applied to study the effect of ETS on the life span of mice with ascetic HCC. A dose-dependent prolongation of life span was observed as shown in Figure 8(c).

To illustrate the mechanism for killing HCC cells of ETS, apoptosis was studied at cellular, molecular, and gene levels. Flow cytometry showed that ETS (2μmol/L) can induce apoptosis of HepG2 cells in a time-dependent manner, i.e., 10.1% (8 h), 15.8% (16 h), 29.1% (24 h), 63.0% (36 h), and ~100% (48 h). The apoptotic cell rate includes all apoptotic cells at early and late apoptotic phases. Western blot analysis showed that along with the prolonged time of ETS treatment, the antiapoptotic Bcl-2 is decreasing and proapoptotic Bax is increasing (Figure

Group	No. of mice	Tumor size (X ± S), cm³	Inhibitory rate (%)	Tumor growth rate	Metastasis of lymph node (number) (X ± S)
PBS control	8	1.96 ± 0.133	0	100%	3.3 ± 0.89
Solvent control	8	2.073 ± 0.118	0	100%	3.5 ± 1.07
ETS (5 mg/kg)	8	1.276 ± 0.104*	38.4%	58.5%	2.8 ± 0.71
ETS (15 mg/kg)	8	0.794 ± 0.090*	61.7%	52.6%	1.8 ± 0.71
ETS (45 mg/kg)	8	0.485 ± 0.123**	76.6%	31.7%	0.8 ± 0.71
Mitomycin (2 mg/kg)	8	0.673 ± 0.119**	67.5%	38.9%	0.9 ± 0.83
Cisplatin (2 mg/kg)	8	0.734 ± 0.098**	64.6%	41.9%	1.0 ± 0.76

*$p < 0.05$ vs. controls.

**$p < 0.01$ vs. controls.

Table 1. Inhibitory efficacy of ETS on the xenograph of human HCC in nude mice

9a). Notably, the phosphorylation of p53 protein is also increasing, suggesting that ETS might stabilize p53 protein, the key apoptosis regulator. Western blot analysis also showed that the key effecter molecule of apoptosis pathway, caspase 3, was activated from procaspase into cleaved caspase by ETS in a time-dependent manner (Figure 9c). At the same time, cDNA array analysis showed that a large number of proapoptotic genes were up-regulated and a large number of antiapoptotic genes were down-regulated by ETS treatment (Figure 9d).

Based on LAPTM4B-35 overexpression in HCC can up-regulate a number of oncogenes that promote cell proliferation and/or resist apoptosis, the effects of ETS on the expression of oncoproteins were detected. We found that all the molecular alterations in HepG2 cells induced by LAPTM4B-35 overexpression can be reversed by ETS (Figures 9-11), such as significant decrease of c-Myc (Figure 9b), cyclinD1, and Bcl-2 (Figure 9a) but increase of Bax and phosphorylated p53 (Figure 9a).

It is well known that PI3K/Akt signaling pathway plays a key role in antiapoptosis and cell survival in a large number of cancers and thus is considered as a target for cancer therapy [20]. We have found that the PI3K/Akt/GSK3β signaling pathway is overactivated by LAPTM4B-35 overexpression [5,6]. The effect of ETS on PI3K/Akt signaling was detected.We found that the phosphorylated Akt (Akt-p) is significantly reduced in the ETS-treated HCC cells either in the presence or absence of serum stimulation (Figure 10a). Then the mechanism was explored. Co-IP and Western blot analyses showed that ETS significantly decreased the phosphorylation of LAPTM4B-35 Tyr_{285} in C-terminus of LAPTM4B-35 (Figure 10b) and therefore the activation of PI3K/Akt signaling pathway is minimized via reducing interaction of LAPTM4B-35 and PI3K p85α (Figure 12).

In summary, our previous study demonstrated that *LAPTM4B* is a driver gene of HCC, and LAPTM4B-35 targeting may provide potential therapy for HCC. To target LAPTM4B for cancer therapy includes bio-targeted therapy and chemical-targeted therapy. The bio-targeted therapy may further explore aimed at inhibiting the overexpression of *LAPTM4B* gene via RNAi, miRNA, or antisense RNA, etc., as well as at blocking the functions of LAPTM4B-35

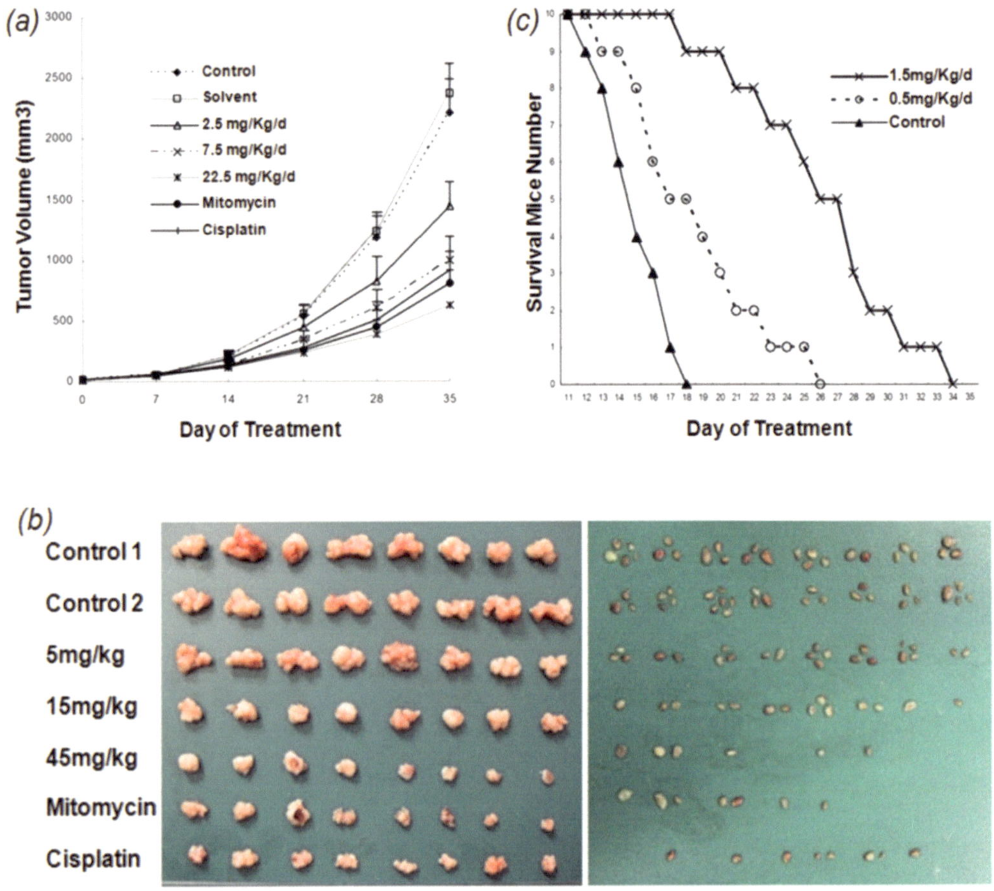

Figure 8. Inhibitory effect of ETS on growth and metastasis of human HCC xenograft in nude mice. Human HCC Bel-7402 cells (1×10^6) were inoculated into each nude mice. ETS (5, 15, or 45 mg/kg), cisplatin (2.0 mg/kg), mitomycin (2.0 mg/kg), PBS (control 1), or solvent (control 2) was administered every other day for each BALB\c-nude mouse in variant groups ($n = 8$), respectively, by intraperitoneal injection from day 9 when the xenograft grew out. Tumor volume was measured twice a week. The inhibitory efficacy on xenograft growth of ETS was observed to be dose-dependent as compared with the control groups of solvent and PBS. Mitomycin and cisplatin were used as the positive controls. *(a)* Tumor growth curves of human HCC xenograft in nude mice with variant treatments. *(b)* Tumor photograph of human HCC xenograft in nude mice with variant treatment for 6 weeks. Left panel: Size of human HCC xenografts in variant groups. Right panel: Number of lymph node metastases in variant groups. *(c)* The survival curves of mice with ascetic HCC in variant groups. Mouse hepatocellular carcinoma H22 cells (1×10^6) were inoculated into peritoneal of each ICR mouse. ETS (0.5 or 1.5 mg/kg) or the solvent was intraperitoneally administered every other day for each ICR mouse in variant groups ($n = 10$). The life span showed a significant prolongation in the ETS groups in a dose-dependent manner.

protein via specific antibody. The chemical-targeted therapy may further explore aimed at attenuating the overactivated signaling pathways by chemical inhibitors and thus inhibiting proliferation and inducing apoptosis. More signaling pathways and more complicated signaling network are supposed to be involved in deregulation induced by LAPTM4B-35 overexpression in cancer. Thus, the mechanism of ETS for targeting LAPTM4B-35 may be more complicated.

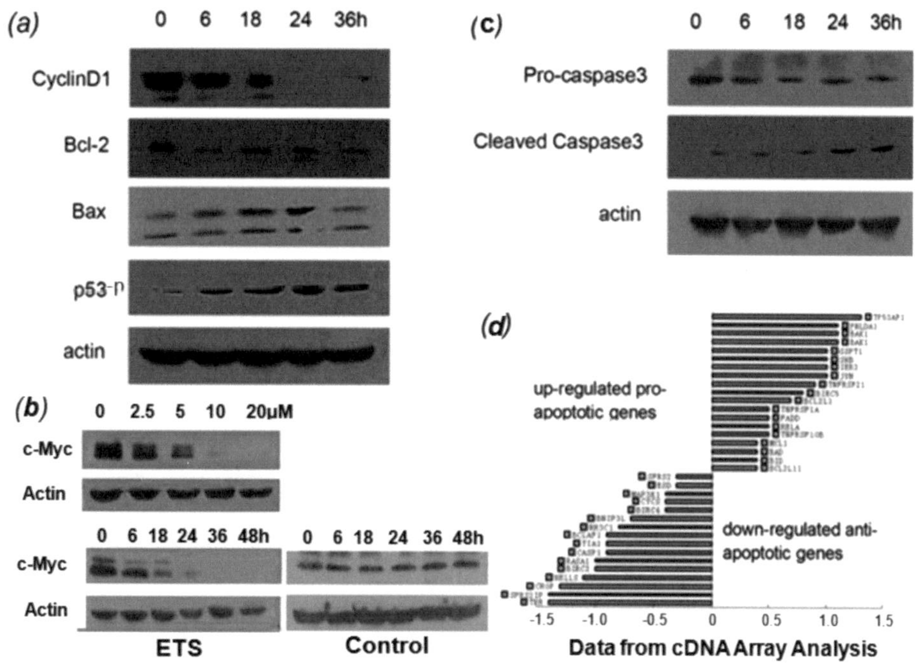

Figure 9. Apoptosis-related molecular alteration induced by ETS. *(a)* Western blot profiles of cyclin D1, Bcl-2, Bax, and phosphorylated p53 proteins from lysates of HepG2 cells incubated in the presence of ETS (2 μM) for indicated times, indicating that proliferation- and apoptosis-related proteins are altered by ETS in a time-dependent manner. *(b)* Western blot profile of cMyc protein from lysates of HepG2 cells incubated in the presence of ETS at indicated concentration for indicated hours, indicating remarkable decrease of c-Myc protein by treatment of ETS in a dose- and time-dependent manner. *(c)* Western blot profile of procaspase 3 and cleaved caspase 3 from lysates of HepG2 cells incubated in the presence of ETS (2 μM) for indicated times, indicating the activation of key effecter molecule in apoptotic pathway by ETS. *(d)* cDNA array analysis shows the up-regulated and down-regulated genes that promote and inhibit apoptosis, respectively, by treatment of ETS.

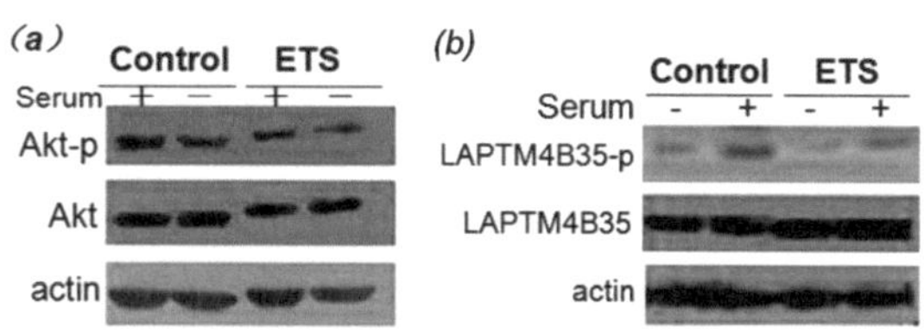

Figure 10. Inhibitory effects of ETS on phosphorylation of Akt and LAPTM4B-35. *(a)* Western blot profile of phosphorylated Akt from lysates of HepG2 cells incubated in the absence and presence of ETS (2 μM), indicating the inhibitory effect of ETS on activation of PI3K/Akt signaling pathway under stimulation with and without serum. *(b)* Co-IP and Western blot profile shows that ETS significantly decreased the phosphorylation of Tyr of LAPTM4B-35 protein. HepG2 cells were first serum-starved for 16 h, then serum and ETS or PBS (control) were added for 15min. The cell lysate was first precipitated by anti-LAPTM4B-N10-pAb, which reacts with LAPTM4B-35. After absorption by protein G/A agarose beads, the precipitant was subjected to Western blot analysis with antiphosphorylated Tyr-mAb. The profile shows that compared with the control, the phosphorylated LAPTM4B-35 is attenuated by ETS treatment in either presence or absence of serum stimulation.

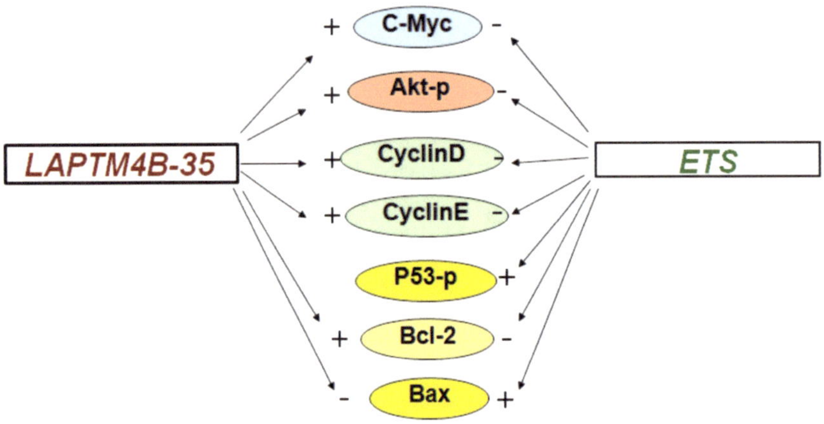

Figure 11. The antagonistic effects of ETS vs LAPTM4B-35 overexpression on expression of oncogenes and tumor suppressor genes in HCC.

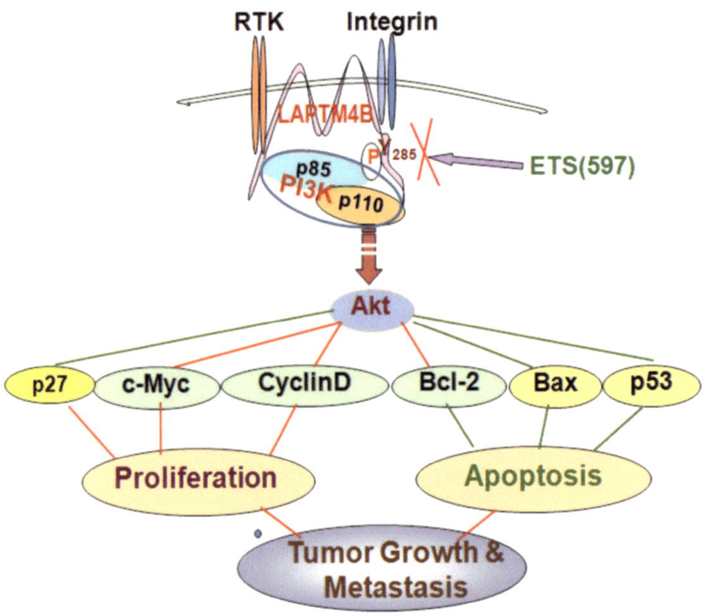

Figure 12. Molecular mechanism of ETS for targeting LAPTM4B-35.

4. Conclusion

Given that *LAPTM4B* is a driver gene of HCC and the encoding LAPTM4B-35 protein is overexpressed in HCC and contributes to the cellular and molecular malignant phenotypes [2], the study on molecular mechanism reveals that the overexpression in HCC of the membrane integrated LAPTM4B-35 functions as an amplified assembly platform or organizer of related signaling molecules that are either integrated in cell membranes or solvable in cytoplasm, and thus activates several signaling pathways, such as growth factor/ RTK/Ras/ERK (MAPK), growth factor/RTK/Ras/PI3K/Akt, ECM/integrin/FAK/ERK (MAPK) or ECM/integrin/FAK/PI3K/Akt, etc. Therefore, it is worth considering the *LAPTM4B* gene and the LAPTM4B-35 protein as novel targets in HCC therapy. A small chemical (ETS) can inhibit HCC cell growth and induce apoptosis *in vitro*, and inhibit growth and metastasis of human HCC xenograft *in vivo*. Notably, ETS can reverse the molecular alterations, that are induced by LAPTM4B-35 overexpression and involved in promotion of proliferation and survival of cancer cells. Moreover, ETS inhibits the phosphorylation of LAPTM4B-35 Tyr_{285}, a key motif forbinding to PI3K p85α regulatory subunit,, and thus inhibits the PI3K/Akt signaling pathway. Taken together, developing strategies for LAPTM4B-35 targeting can be a potential treatment for hepatocellular carcinoma therapy.

Acknowledgements

The authors thank Dr. Liu Gang and Li Li who provided all of the synthetic small chemicals for this study.

Author details

Rou Li Zhou*, Mao Jin Li#, Xuan Hui Wei#, Hua Yang#, Yi Shan, Ly Li and Xin Rong Liu

*Address all correspondence to: rlzhou@bjmu.edu.cn

Department of Cell Biology, School of Basic Medical Sciences, Peking University, Beijing, China

#These authors contributed equally to this article.

References

[1] Shao GZ, Zhou RL, Zhang QY, Zhang Y, Liu JJ,. Rui JA, Wei XH, and Ye DX. Molecular cloning and characterization of LAPTM4B, a novel gene upregulated in hepatocellular carcinoma. *Oncogene* 2003; 22:5060-5069.

[2] Zhou RL, Lau WY. LAPTM4B: a novel diagnostic biomarker and therapeutic target for hepatocellular carcinoma. In: Hepatocellular Carcinoma-Basic Research. Rijeka: InTech; 2012. pp. 1-34.

[3] Yang H, Xiong FX, Lin M, Qi RZ, Liu ZW, Rui, JA, Su J, Zhou RL. LAPTM4B-35 Is a Novel Diagnostic Marker and a Prognostic Factor of Hepatocellular Carcinoma. *J Surgical Oncology* 2010; 101:363-369.

[4] Yang H, Xiong FX, Lin M, Yang Y, Nie X and Zhou RL. LAPTM4B-35 overexpression is a risk factor for tumor recurrence and poor prognosis in hepatocellular carcinoma, *J Cancer Res Clin Oncol.* 2010; 136:275-281.

[5] Yang H, Xiong F, Wei X, Yang Y, McNutt MA, Zhou RL. Overexpression of LAPTM4B-35 promotes growth and metastasis of hepatocellular carcinoma in vitro and in vivo. *Cancer Letters* 2010; 294:236-244.

[6] Li L, Wei XH, Pan YP, Shan Y, Li HC, Yang H, Pang Y, Xiong FX, Shao GZ, Zhou RL. LAPTM4B: A novel cancer-associated gene motivates multi-drug resistance through efflux and activating PI3K/Akt signaling. *Oncogene* 2010; 29(43):.5785-95.

[7] Li L, Shan Y, Yang H, Zhang S, Lin M, Zhu P, Chen XY, Yi J, McNutt MA, Shao GZ and Zhou RL. Upregulation of LAPTM4B-35 promotes malignant transformation and tumorigenesis in L02 human liver cell line. Anat Rec (Hoboken) 2011; 294(7):1135-42.

[8] Tang H, Tian H, Yue W, Li L, Li S, Gao C, Si L, Qi L, Lu M. Overexpression of LAPTM4B is correlated with tumor angiogenesis and poor prognosis in non-small cell lung cancer. Med Oncol. 2014; 31(6): 974.

[9] Tan X, Thapa N, Sun Y, Anderson RA. LAPTM4B is a PtdIns(4,5)P2 effectors that regulates EGFR signaling, lysosomal sorting, and degradation. EMBO J. 2015; 34(4): 475-90.

[10] Tan X, Sun Y, Thapa N, Anderson RA. A kinase-independent role for EGF receptor in autophagy initiation. Cell 2015; 160(1-2):145-60.

[11] Liu XR, Zhou RL, Zhang QY, Zhang Y, Shao GZ, Jin YY, Zhang S, Lin M, Rui JA, Ye DX. Identification and characterization of LAPTM4B encoded by a human hepatocellular carcinoma-associated novel gene. J Peking University (health Sciences) 2003; 35: 340-347.

[12] Min LH, He BK, Hui LJ. Mitogen-activated protein kinases in hepatocellular carcinoma development. Semin Cancer Biol 2011; 21:10-20.

[13] Shang N, Arteaga M, Zaidi A, Stauffer J, Cotler SJ, Zeleznik-Le NJ, Zhang J, Qiu W. FAK is required for c-Met/β-catenin-driven hepatocarcinogenesis. Hepatology 2015;61(1):214-26.

[14] Chen JS, Huang XH, Wang Q, Huang JQ, Zhang LJ, Chen XL, Lei J, Cheng ZX. Sonic hedgehog signaling pathway induces cell migration and invasion through focal adhesion kinase/AKT signaling-mediated activation of matrix metalloproteinase (MMP)-2 and MMP-9 in liver cancer. Carcinogenesis. 2013;34(1):10-19.

[15] Whittaker S, Marais R, Zhu AX. The role of signaling pathways in the development and treatment of hepatocellular carcinoma. Oncogene 2010; 29(36):4989-5005.

[16] Chen JS, Huang XH, Wang Q, Chen XL, Fu XH, Tan HX, Zhang LJ, Li W, Bi J. FAK is involved in invasion and metastasis of hepatocellular carcinoma. Clin Exp Metastasis 2010, 27: 71-82.

[17] Shen YC, Lin ZZ, Hsu CH, Hsu C, Shao YY, Cheng AL. Clinical trials in hepatocellular carcinoma: an update. Liver Cancer 2013; 2(3-4):345-364.

[18] Li MJ, Zhou RL, Shan Y, Li L, Liu G. Anticancer efficacy of ethylglyoxal bisthiosemicarbazon on human hepatocellular carcinoma in vitro and in vivo through targeting a novel cancer-associated gene and its encoding protein. Manuscript in preparation.

[19] Liu XR, Zhou RL, Zhang QY, Zhang Y, Jin YY, Lin M, Rui JA, Ye DX. Structure analysis and expressions of a novel tetratransmembrane protein, lysosomal-associated protein transmembrane 4 beta associated with hepatocellular carcinoma. World J Gastroenterol 2004; 10: 1555-1559.

[20] Buitrago-Molina LE, Vogel A. mTOR as a potential target for the prevention and treatment of hepatocellular carcinoma. Current Cancer Drug Targets 2012; 12:1-17.

Chapter 7

Hepatic Surgery for Colorectal Cancer Metastasis — Possibilities and Prerequisites

Ilze Strumfa, Ervins Vasko, Andrejs Vanags, Zane Simtniece, Peteris Trapencieris and Janis Gardovskis

Additional information is available at the end of the chapter

http://dx.doi.org/10.5772/60971

Abstract

Colorectal cancer is among the most frequent malignant tumours. Liver metastases develop in 70–75% of patients affected by colorectal carcinoma. Nowadays, surgical treatment can significantly improve the 5-year survival ranging 40–58% of the patients undergoing liver surgery. The operation extent ranges from nonanatomic minor resection to major hepatectomy. Recently, liver transplantation has been performed for metastatic colorectal cancer. Laparoscopic approach and robotic surgery can be used by experienced specialists. The prerequisites for successful surgical treatment include exact radiologic diagnostics to determine the number and size of metastases and their association with anatomic structures; individual anatomic peculiarities and remnant liver volume, ranging 20–40% in respect to functional liver status. Magnetic resonance imaging is the most sensitive method that has marked advantages in the diagnostics of lesions smaller than 1 cm and metastases on the background of liver steatosis. Computed tomography is an acceptable alternative that benefits from high spatial resolution and optimal reconstructions to evaluate the anatomy. Additional information can be obtained from tumour markers, including traditional, e.g., carcinoembryonic antigen (CEA) and novel, e.g., microRNAs. To ensure that each colorectal cancer patient receives the best care, the medical society should be well informed about the possibilities in the treatment of liver metastases of colorectal cancer regarding the methods, indications and limits.

Keywords: Colorectal cancer, liver metastasis, liver resection, magnetic resonance imaging

1. Introduction

Colorectal cancer (CRC) represents one of the leading malignant tumours both by incidence and death rate [1, 2]. Metastatic spread to liver occurs in 70–75% of patients, and 20–35% of CRC patients present with synchronous liver metastases [1, 3, 4]. Although the presence of metastatic disease significantly adversely affects the survival, a wide scope of treatment options exists. To ensure that each colorectal cancer patient receives the best care, the medical society should be well informed about the possibilities in the treatment of liver metastases of colorectal cancer regarding the methods, indications and limits.

Surgery is the preferred option for long term survival. The operation extent ranges from major hepatic resection (trisegmentectomy, hepatectomy, extended hepatectomy, and hemihepatectomy) to parenchyma-sparing minor resection such as segmentectomy or wedge resection [4]. Laparoscopic approach and robotic surgery can be considered, especially in advanced centres [5, 6]. In patients with questionable adequacy of the liver remnant and wide intrahepatic tumour spread, portal vein occlusion, forced liver hypertrophy and staged resection can be helpful [7, 8]. Recently, liver transplantation for metastatic colorectal cancer has been performed [9].

Surgery at present assumes significant role in treatment of metastatic liver lesions. However, it demands not only appropriate surgical technique but also correct preoperative diagnosis and reliable plan for postoperative treatment.

Adequately timed and exact imaging is necessary prior to the surgical or nonsurgical treatment to reveal the metastases and assess the feasibility of resection. Magnetic resonance imaging (MRI), computed tomography (CT), ultrasonography (US) and 18F-2fluoro-D-glucose positron emission tomography in association with computed tomography (PET-CT) are used for imaging metastatic lesions in the liver [1]. The radiologic evaluation can be combined with traditional and novel cancer markers [10–12] and biopsy examination. Among serological markers, carcinoembryonic antigen (CEA) has been used traditionally despite the limitations [4] and lack of unified guidelines. MicroRNAs represent a rapidly advancing research field hopefully yielding diagnostic blood tests to diagnose the cancer by location and to identify the presence of residual tumour or early recurrence.

If the surgical treatment is not possible, other options must be considered, including systemic or transarterial chemotherapy; embolisation; ablation by cryotreatment, radiofrequency or microwaves; or radiotherapy and targeted external beam radio therapy [1].

Due to the wide scope of treatment options, the median survival of patients affected by metastatic colorectal cancer has increased significantly [13, 14]. The 5-year and 10-year survival reaches 58% and 36%, correspondingly [15].

In conclusion, liver metastases of colorectal cancer represent a frequent and serious condition. The remarkable medical advances request dynamic systematisation of up-to-dated evidence. The present chapter on the surgical treatment of colorectal cancer metastases is intended to summarise the present knowledge in regard to the approach to patient with liver metastases of colorectal cancer, discussing the diagnostics, treatment and evaluation of response.

2. Epidemiology of colorectal cancer

Colorectal cancer is among the leading malignant tumours both by incidence and by death rate [1]. Globally, in the year 2012, it was the 3rd most frequent cancer in men and the 2nd in women [2]. The incidence and mortality is higher in males (Table 1). The highest incidence rates are found in Australia and New Zealand, Europe and North America contrasting with low incidence in Africa and South Central Asia. As shown in Table 2, the incidence is generally higher in more developed countries [2]. The decrease in colorectal cancer incidence in USA reflects successful screening and removal of colorectal adenomas. The incidence growth, recently observed in Western Asia (Kuwait and Israel) and Eastern Europe (Czech Republic and Slovakia), reflects increased prevalence of risk factors as diet, obesity and smoking.

Gender	Incidence		Mortality	
	ASR	Proportion[1], %	ASR	Proportion[1], %
Males	20.6	10.1	10.0	8.0
Females	14.3	9.2	6.9	9.0

[1] Among all cancers.

ASR, age-standardised ratio per 100,000.

Table 1. Global incidence and mortality attributable to colorectal cancer (2012) by Globocan data [16]

Gender and welfare status	Incidence		Mortality	
	ASR	Cumulative risk, %	ASR	Cumulative risk, %
More developed areas[1]				
Males	36.3	4.3	14.7	1.6
Females	23.6	2.7	9.3	1.0
Less developed areas[2]				
Males	13.7	1.6	7.8	0.8
Females	9.8	1.1	5.6	0.6

[1]Includes Europe, North America, Australia, New Zealand and Japan.

[2]Includes Africa, Asia (except Japan), Latin America, Melanesia, Micronesia and Polynesia.

ASR, age-standardised ratio per 100,000.

Table 2. Incidence and mortality caused by colorectal cancer by regional welfare [2]

Colorectal cancer could be prevented avoiding obesity, alcohol, smoking and excessive consumption of red and processed meat, as well as maintaining physical activity. There are also several screening methods, including guaiac-based or immunochemical test for occult blood in stools, faecal DNA test, virtual colonoscopy by computed tomography imaging, double-contrast barium enema, flexible sigmoidoscopy and colonoscopy [2]. MicroRNA stool test could appear in the nearest future. Despite the possibilities of prevention and screening, metastatic disease is common. Metastatic spread to liver occurs in 70–75% of patients, and 20–35% of CRC patients are diagnosed with synchronous liver metastases [1, 3, 4]. Although the presence of metastatic disease significantly adversely affects the survival, a wide scope of treatment options exist.

3. Radiologic imaging techniques in the diagnostics of liver metastases of colorectal cancer

The radiologic techniques of liver examination comprise computed tomography, magnetic resonance imaging, ultrasound evaluation and fluorodeoxyglucose positron emission tomography [17]. CT and MRI represent the cornerstone in the diagnostics of liver metastases of colorectal cancer [1, 18]. US has the benefits of wide accessibility and lack of irradiation. However, it is considered a historical method in developed countries as USA [18] due to lower sensitivity and specificity. These parameters can be improved by contrast-enhanced US [19]. Positron emission tomography (PET) has certain indications.

MRI is characterised by the highest specificity and sensitivity, especially regarding metastases smaller than 1 cm in diameter [1, 20]. The imaging technology is based on different physical status of water and fat protons [18]. To identify liver metastases, MRI routinely includes T1, T2 and diffusion-weighted sequences before and after administration of gadolinium-containing contrast agent. The CRC metastases are hypointense on T1 but hyperintense on T2 and diffusion-weighted imaging sequences. The contrasting reveals metastasis as a hypovascular focus with an irregular rim of enhancement [18].

In the identification of liver metastases, MRI is characterised by the highest sensitivity that reaches 76.0–85.7% if enhancement by extracellular contrast agents and dynamic acquisition is used. The sensitivity can be further improved by diffusion-weighted imaging. Diffusion-weighted imaging is based on the assessment of Brownian motion of water molecules and water diffusion within a voxel (a tridimensional pixel). As cell membranes limit the diffusion, greater cellularity results in diffusion restriction [21]. Thus, the metastasis creates an obstacle in water molecule diffusion and is revealed by diffusion-weighted imaging at higher sensitivity and specificity than routine MRI [17, 22, 23]. The hepatobiliary phase MRI represents another improvement in the diagnostics of liver metastases by contrast agents that are absorbed by hepatocytes and excreted in biliary system, e.g., gadoxetate disodium and gadobenate dimeglumine. These agents differ from the traditional MRI contrast agents by the dual elimination, including both biliary excretion (50%) and renal glomerular filtration, while the traditional agents, as gadopentetic acid, are almost completely excreted via kidneys [1, 18]. The hepatobiliary phase of MRI corresponds to the peak parenchymal enhancement due to contrast uptake in hepatocytes. It is observed 20 min after injection. Metastatic foci lack liver cells and therefore do not absorb hepatobiliary contrast agents. In the diagnostics of colorectal cancer liver metastases, the sensitivity of hepatobiliary phase MRI reaches even 90–97% [1, 24, 25]. In comparison with diffusion-weighted imaging, hepatobiliary phase MRI enhances sensitivity for the detection of colorectal cancer metastasis, e.g., from 78.3–97.5% to 94.4–100.0%. The combination of diffusion-weighted imaging with hepatobiliary phase MRI yields better results than isolated techniques [26].

Gadolinium-containing contrast agents can induce nephrogenic systemic fibrosis in a subfraction of patients (2.9–4%) with severe renal insufficiency [1, 27, 28]. Sufficient enhancement quality can be reached by half-dose gadoxetic acid [29]. However, other research groups have not observed any case of gadoxetate-related nephrogenic systemic fibrosis in a prospective multicentre study [30]. The risk of nephrogenic systemic fibrosis also varies by different contrast agents [1].

In comparison with CT, MRI has advantage in the diagnostics of lesions measuring less than 1 cm and shows better ability to discriminate metastases on the background of spontaneous or treatment-induced (e.g., 5-fluoruracil and irinotecane) liver steatosis [1, 17, 31]. However, CT provides better resolution of anatomic details that are necessary to plan the surgery [18]. Consequently, controversies have been expressed if the liver imaging in colorectal cancer patient should be started with CT or MRI [1, 18].

MRI is contraindicated in patients having incompatible implants, e.g., pacemakers; affected by claustrophobia or impaired glomerular filtration rate, or unable to hold the breath for longer than 20 seconds. CT should be performed in these patients [1, 18].

Multidetector CT can be used for chest, abdominal and pelvic imaging to reveal the total visceral metastatic burden. Contrasting with intravenous iodinated agents is necessary to reveal liver metastases that represent hypodense hypovascular foci with variable heterogeneity, seen in portal venous phase [18]. Rim enhancement can be observed [17]. Due to low tumour vascularity, arterial phase is more important for detection of arterial anatomy than for identification of metastases. In nonenhanced CT, the metastases are hypointense but can be inconspicuous [17, 18]. The possibilities of CT are limited in detection of small lesions and inhassessment of steatotic liver. MRI is helpful in these situations. The benefits of multidetector CT include high spatial and temporal resolution exceeding that of MRI. Thus, CT is useful for planning before surgery. The individual anatomic features can also be detailed by CT [18].

PET-CT reflects the metabolic activity in tumour cells by analysing glucose uptake. It has advantage in detecting extrahepatic metastatic spread [1] or local recurrence and in evaluation of indeterminate liver lesions [17]. In a prospective study of 133 consecutive patients, PET-CT had a major impact on staging of extrahepatic spread in 20% of patients. It resulted in upstaging (from surgically treatable to inoperable) in 6% of patients and downstaging (from indeterminate or suspected inoperable to operable) in another 6% of patients [32]. As extrahepatic spread is more likely in patients who already have liver metastases, PET-CT should be considered a standard evaluation prior to curative liver surgery for metastatic colorectal cancer. PET-CT reduces futile laparotomies by 38% [33]. Combination with diagnostic intravenous contrast-enhanced CT is strongly advised as opposed to noncontrast low-dose CT providing anatomic data only [1, 34]. The sensitivity of PET-CT is impaired after chemotherapy [1, 35].

In the early studies, liver US was considered effective in the follow-up after surgical treatment of colorectal cancer metastases as it disclosed all the resectable cancer metastases as it disclosed all the resectable with thoracic X-ray [36]. However, more recent data evidence that transabdominal US has limited sensitivity in the diagnostics of CRC liver metastases: 50–75% [17]. Despite the serious shortcoming, US still can be used for screening purposes by experienced specialist who is aware of these limitations and will combine US by more sensitive methods of radiologic diagnostics. Intravenous contrast-enhanced US imaging using microbubbles to contrast blood increases the sensitivity of US by 20% [17, 19] and exceeds the sensitivity of CT, especially for small lesions [17]. Contrast-enhanced US affords diagnostic benefit in 13.7% patients with liver mass lesions [19]. The increased sensitivity of contrast-enhanced US in detection of tumours is explained by the vascularisation pattern and the phagocytosis of contrasting microbubbles by Kupffer cells that are present in liver parenchyma but absent in liver tumours. Thus, CRC metastases would be an adequate object for contrast US. The tumours are hypoechoic. The sensitivity and specificity of US and contrast-enhanced US in diagnosing malignant liver tumours is around 58.8% and 50.7% for US versus 68.7–90% and 67–88% for the contrast-enhanced modality. Deep lesions, small metastases and liver steatosis are known limiting factors. Colorectal cancer metastases may occasionally be hyperechogenic and lack hypoechoic structure on contrast-enhanced US embarrassing differential diagnosis with benign lesions, e.g., haemangioma [19].

Hepatic lesions can be missed even by combined radiologic investigation, including US, CT and MRI. The proportion of such lesions can be as high as 30% [19]. Intraoperatively, US can be applied. The sensitivity of intraoperative imaging is again enhanced by contrast US [37].

4. Preoperative radiologic evaluation: the target parameters

To plan the surgical treatment, the number, the size and the location of metastases must be detected [1]. The number of affected segments, the relations between metastases and arteries, veins and bile ducts as well as the size of remnant liver must be ascertained as well [18]. The anatomical variations of bile ducts as well as arterial and portal blood vessels must be established. CT or MRI can be used for these purposes. Although similar efficacy of both methods has been shown regarding vascular anatomic evaluation, CT can yield better contrast [1].

Diagnostic problems can be associated with identification of small lesions, imaging of metastases on the background of liver fibrosis, steatosis or sinusoidal congestion due to preceding chemotherapy (or other reasons) and detailed characteristics of deep metastasis that necessitates careful planning of surgical approach and exact data on the involvement of anatomical structures. Occasionally, differential diagnosis with benign lesions can be complicated. The presence and extent of extrahepatic disease must be estimated [18].

Software-based three-dimensional CT volumetrics is used to calculate the volume of the remnant and total liver volumes excluding nonfunctional spaces as tumours, cysts and ablation cavities. The remnant liver volume is expressed as a proportion of the preoperative total liver volume. The minimal volume of remnant liver has not been established by exact experimental studies therefore the described desirable values differ slightly. The remnant liver volume after the operation is expected to be 25–30% in young patients with normal liver parenchyma and 40% in cirrhotic patients [4, 18]. In a consensus statement, remnant liver volume is recommended to be at least 20% for patients with normal extratumoural liver tissue, 30% for patients having chemotherapy-induced liver injury and 40% in cirrhotic patients [17, 38–40]. As metastatic tumour is spreading systemically and recurs in most patients, higher preserved proportion of liver parenchyma provides more options for repeated future surgery if necessary. The risk factors for postoperative liver dysfunction due to insufficient remnant include older age, liver fibrosis, cirrhosis and preoperative chemotherapy. Except liver cirrhosis, these factors are frequent as many patients with CRC liver metastasis are elderly and have received chemotherapy [4]. To estimate the compromised liver function more exactly, functional tests are helpful. The liver function is reflected by albumin level, hemostasis, bilirubin level, lidocaine conversion test or clearance of indocyanine green [18].

5. Traditional and novel tumour markers in the diagnostics of colorectal cancer

The patients with metastatic colorectal cancer nowadays survive longer, thus they need prolonged follow-up. CT is a sensitive method but some authors have expressed fears that the patient is subjected to radiation exposure [41]. MRI benefits from high sensitivity and lack of ionising radiation, but it is expensive. Blood test for surveillance thus seems to be an attractive, patient-friendly and radiation-free option. Although the follow-up of colorectal cancer patients after resection of the primary tumour is controversial, increased blood level of the carcinoembryonic antigen (CEA) can disclose cancer recurrence and is used traditionally. In a recent study, 25% increase of CEA level in comparison with the previous value detected 23% of recurrences while 46% of recurrences were evident both by radiology and CEA and 31%—only by radiology data. The radiologic imaging in this study comprised US after surgical treatment and CT after thermal ablation as well as in difficult cases. The resectability of the recurrent cancer did not differ in patients who were identified through CEA or by imaging [41]. Thus, CEA alone is not sensitive enough to identify the recurrence but can be helpful in complex diagnostic protocol. In contrast, CEA alone did not identify any additional case of curable recurrence after liver resection for metastatic colorectal cancer in comparison with CT [42].

CEA has several benefits, including cheapness and availability. In addition, prognostic information can be obtained. High perioperative CEA levels indicate worse survival after liver resection for CRC metastases [43].

CEA has been explored in association with other biological markers both for comparison and in order to create wider diagnostic protocol. Regarding circulating tumour cells, the findings along with CEA level added prognostic information in patients with metastatic colorectal cancer undergoing chemotherapy. In a multivariate analysis, circulating tumour cells but not CEA at the baseline predicted the survival, but both parameters predicted survival at 6–12 weeks after the initiation of treatment. There was no correlation between CEA and circulating tumour cells [10]. The levels of circulating tumour cells in colorectal cancer are reported to be lower than in other cancers due to homing within the liver [44]. The complex mechanism of metastasis involving epithelial–mesenchymal and mesenchymal–epithelial transformation as well as blood clearing in the liver and secondary spread from liver metastasis to systemic circulation hypothetically can influence the results and interpretation of circulating tumour cell tests.

Plasma levels of the tissue inhibitor of matrix metalloproteinase 1 (TIMP-1) have also been explored in parallel with CEA in patients undergoing chemotherapy for metastatic colorectal cancer. High plasma TIMP-1 and CEA levels both before and during treatment were related to poor response. Worse survival was predicted by high TIMP-1 level before or during chemotherapy, and by high CEA values before treatment [45]. However, chemotherapy and radiation treatment itself influenced serum levels of these markers, decreasing CEA and increasing TIMP-1 [46]. The treatment-induced switches in the biomarker levels would limit their application in the surveillance.

MicroRNAs (miRNAs) are small noncoding RNAs that post-transcriptionally modulate the expression of the target genes [47, 48]. These endogenous molecules are evolutionarily highly conserved, suggesting an important functional role in cell biology [48]. MiRNAs are located either between protein-coding genes, or in the introns of protein-coding genes. Transcription of miRNAs results in primary miRNAs that undergo processing within the nucleus. The processing yields miRNA precursors that are transported to the cytoplasm and transformed into mature miRNAs. These molecules perform their regulatory function by complementary binding to mRNA [11]. miRNAs regulate such crucial steps in cancer development (Table 3) as cell proliferation, invasion, angiogenesis, epithelial-mesenchymal transformation and the reverse process [47]. The value of miRNAs is the ability to function as large genomic switches.

Target process	Result	MicroRNAs
Angiogenesis	Activation	miR-194; miR-17-92; miR-126; miR-210; miR-424
	Suppression	miR-221; miR-222; miR-497
Invasion	Activation	miR-31; miR-122; miR-200; miR-145; miR-103; miR-107; miR-29a; miR-21; miR-17; miR-19a
	Suppression	miR-122; miR-328; miR-143
Metastasis	Vascular invasion	miR-21
	Loss of cell adhesion	miR-126
	Immune regulation	miR-155; miR-17-92
	Colonisation	miR-328; miR-103; miR-107
Apoptosis	Induction	miR-26b

Table 3. MiRNAs involved in different steps of carcinogenesis

From the practical standpoint, miRNAs at present are explored as diagnostic markers and therapeutic targets [11]. In contrast to mRNA, miRNAs are stable in formalin-fixed, paraplast embedded tissues [48–50]. In the blood and plasma, MiRNA also circulate in persistent form, suitable for testing [51, 52]. The stability might be ensured by development of extracellular microvesicles [52]. The specificity and sensitivity issues still must be finalised, but promising results have already been reported. Thus, 6 serum miRNA-based biomarker signature, including miR-21, let-7g, miR-31, miR-92a, miR-181b and miR-203, had high sensitivity (93%) and specificity (91%) in the diagnosis of colorectal cancer. The sensitivity of such traditional serum markers as CEA and CA19-9 was significantly lower: 23% and 35%, respectively. The tested panel could discriminate stage I and II colorectal cancer from healthy controls [12], thus showing appropriate sensitivity for low tumour burden. Moreover, miR-92a, miR-21 and miR-29a serum levels could discriminate healthy controls from patients affected by colorectal cancer or advanced adenomas, the well-established precursor lesion of colorectal cancer [53, 54]. The levels of miR-17-3p, miR-92 and miR-221 also differed in plasma of colorectal cancer patients and healthy controls [55, 56].

Early relapse of colorectal cancer is associated with increased plasma levels of miR-29c [48, 57]. More intense surveillance or postoperative treatment could be offered to these patients.

Patients with liver metastasis exhibit significantly higher miR-21 level in colorectal cancer tissues. MiR-29a serum level is increased in colorectal cancer patients affected by liver metastasis and is considered a promising novel marker for early detection of liver metastasis [58]. In more recent studies, increased serum levels of miR-141 and miR-21 as well as down-regulation of miR-126 were advised for early diagnosis of liver metastasis of colorectal cancer while let7a up-regulation was associated with extrahepatic metastases [59]. The applicability of this or similar biomarker signature for metastatic cancer remains to be subjected to deeper analysis as at least few controversies can be expected. It has been shown in gastric and hepatocellular carcinoma that serum and tissue levels of miRNAs can change in opposite directions [60–62], possibly because cancer cells can selectively retain certain miRNAs [63]. In colorectal cancer, liver metastasis exhibits higher levels of miR-29c, although miR-29c is significantly down-regulated in primary colorectal cancers giving rise to distant metastasis. The seeming controversy can be explained by epithelial–mesenchymal and mesenchymal–epithelial transition [64]. In addition, surgical treatment can influence the miRNA level; thus, in hepatocellular carcinoma, miR-92a levels are high in tumour tissue, low in plasma before the treatment and high in plasma after the operation [61]. In colorectal cancer with liver metastases, tissue levels of 28 miRNAs were different (Table 4) from nonmetastatic cancers [65]. The tissue miRNA profile hypothetically could also discriminate between colorectal cancer metastases in liver and lymph nodes [66].

MicroRNA	**Change in the target tissue compared to the control**	**Target tissue or body liquid**	**Control tissues or body liquid**
miR-21; let-7g	Increase	Plasma of cancer patients	Plasma of healthy controls
miR-31; miR-181b; miR-92a; miR-203	Decrease	Plasma of cancer patients	Plasma of healthy controls
miR-21	Increase	Colorectal cancer	Normal colonic tissue
miR-143	Decrease	Colorectal cancer	Normal colonic tissue
miR-21; miR-224; miR-96; miR-31; miR-155	Increase	Colorectal cancer	Normal colonic tissue
miR-21	Increase	Liver metastasis of colorectal cancer	Normal colonic tissue

MicroRNA	Change in the target tissue compared to the control	Target tissue or body liquid	Control tissues or body liquid
miR-143	Decrease	Liver metastasis of colorectal cancer	Normal colonic tissue
miR-21	No difference	Liver metastasis of colorectal cancer	Colorectal cancer
miR-143	Decrease	Liver metastasis of colorectal cancer	Colorectal cancer
miR-150; miR-125b-2; miR-1179; miR139-3p	Increase	Colorectal cancer with liver metastasis	Colorectal cancer without distant metastasis
miR-93; miR-548e; miR-19b; miR-96; miR-548c-5p; miR-140-5p; miR-19a; miR-17-5p:9.1; miR-101; miR-579; miR-18b; miR-18a; miR-455-5p; miR-549; miR-219-5p; miR-33b; miR-330-5p; miR-301a	Decrease	Colorectal cancer with liver metastasis	Colorectal cancer without distant metastasis
miR-196a-5p; miR-200b-3p; miR-223-3p	Decrease	Colorectal cancer with liver metastasis	Colorectal cancer without distant metastasis
miR-UL70-3p; miR-154-5p; miR-221-3p; miR-301b; miR-320b; miR-371a-5p; miR-486-5p; miR-572; miR-654-3p; miR-923	Increase	Colorectal cancer with liver metastasis	Colorectal cancer without distant metastasis
miR-29c	Decrease	Colorectal cancer with liver metastasis	Colorectal cancer without distant metastasis
miR-29c	Increase	Liver metastasis of colorectal cancer	Colorectal cancer
miR-21; miR-31; miR-93; miR-103	Increase	Colorectal cancer	Normal tissues
miR-566	Decrease	Colorectal cancer	Normal tissues
miR-21; miR-31; miR-93	Increase	Liver metastasis of colorectal cancer	Normal tissues
miR-21	Increase	Lymph node metastasis	Normal tissues
miR-181a	Increase	Colorectal cancer with liver metastasis	Colorectal cancer without liver metastasis

[1]References: [12, 64–69].

Table 4. MiRNAs in colorectal cancer[1]

Prognostic value has been reported regarding has been reported. In colorectal cancer, shorter disease-free interval was found in patients who exhibited higher miR-21 and higher miR-143

http://dx.doi.org/10.5772/60971

levels in tumour tissues. Notably, in this study, higher miR-21 and lower miR-143 was found in cancer and liver metastases in comparison to normal colonic and liver tissues [67]. The seeming logic discrepancy between the prognostic levels and the differences in normal and neoplastic tissues suggests multiple mechanisms of a single miRNA. These findings are warning about high complexity in the elaboration of diagnostic tests. MiRNAs have also been explored to predict the response to treatment. Thus, increased plasma concentrations of miR-106a, miR-484 and miR-130 are associated with lack of response to oxaliplatin-based treatment [48, 70]. Similar markers would be valuable to identify patients that would benefit from preoperative tumour burden reduction by chemotherapy. The predicted nonresponders could be treated by ablation techniques. As miRNAs function as large genomic switches, they are also attractive potential targets of therapy [11].

6. Biopsy in the differential diagnostics of liver lesions

Biopsy evaluation can yield reliable diagnosis of colorectal cancer. The tubular and cribrous glandular architecture in combination with high cylindrical neoplastic cells frequently is straightforward (Figure 1). Upon necessity, immunohistochemical evaluation can be applied as colorectal cancer is characterised by specific markers. Thus, the cytoplasmic expression of cytokeratin 20 (Figure 2) and nuclear presence of CDX2 protein (Figure 3) is virtually diagnostic of colorectal cancer.

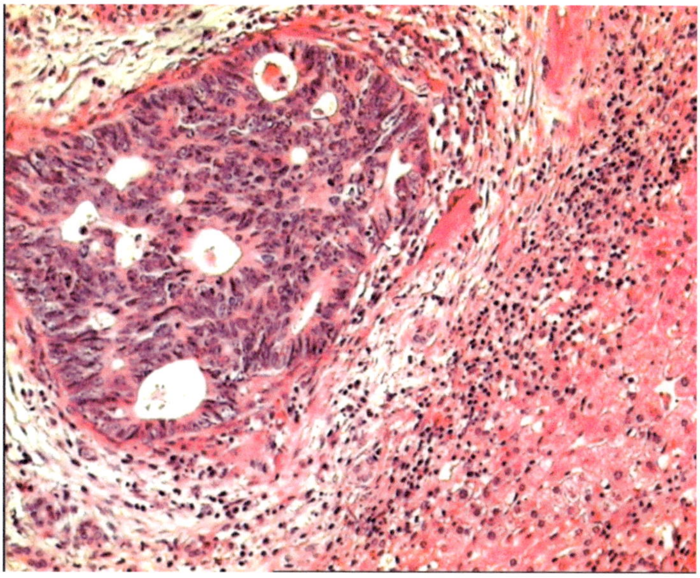

Figure 1. Metastasis of colorectal cancer in liver tissue. Haematoxylin–eosin, original magnification 50×.

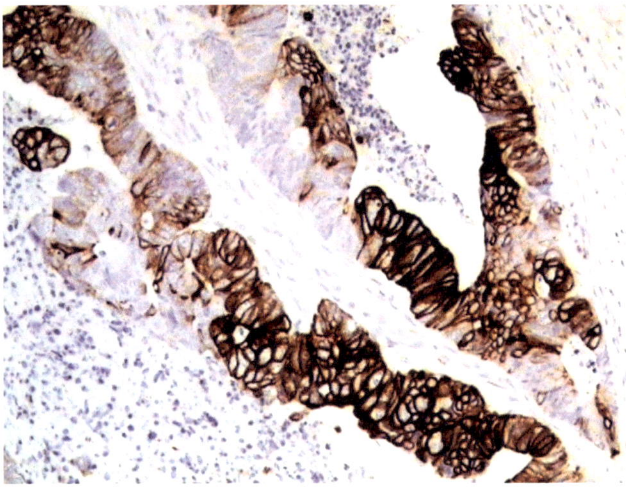

Figure 2. Intense cytoplasmic expression of cytokeratin 20 in colorectal cancer. Note the heterogeneity. Immunoperoxidase, anti-cytokeratin 20, original magnification 50×.

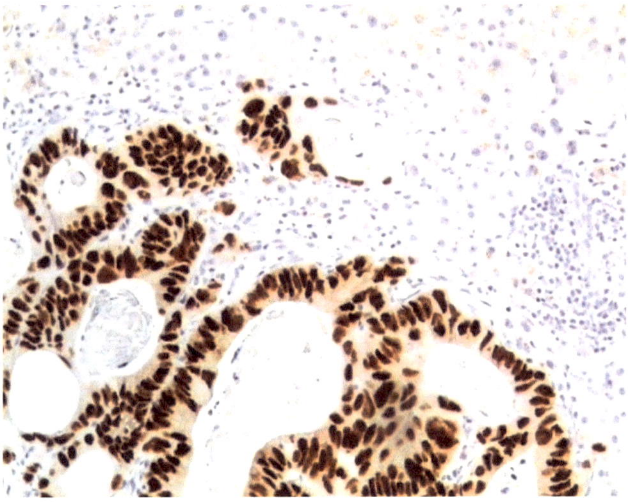

Figure 3. Diffuse intense nuclear expression of CDX2 in colorectal cancer. Immunoperoxidase, anti-CDX2, original magnification 100×.

In contrast to many other metastatic carcinomas, colorectal cancer lacks cytokeratin 7. Metastatic neuroendocrine tumours (Figures 4 and 5) can be excluded by the absence of chromogranin A, synaptophysin and CD56. The combination of several neuroendocrine markers is advisable, especially in a patient with clinically and/or endoscopically identified colorectal tumour, due to differential expression of these markers by gut origin (foregut *versus* midgut *versus* hindgut). The clinical relevance of correct differential diagnosis between metastatic colorectal adenocarcinoma and neuroendocrine tumours is high.

http://dx.doi.org/10.5772/60971

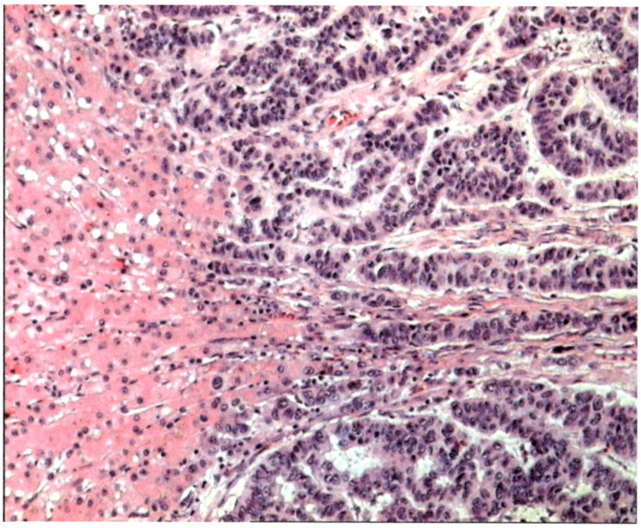

Figure 4. Metastasis of neuroendocrine carcinoma in the liver tissue. Haematoxylin–eosin, original magnification 50×.

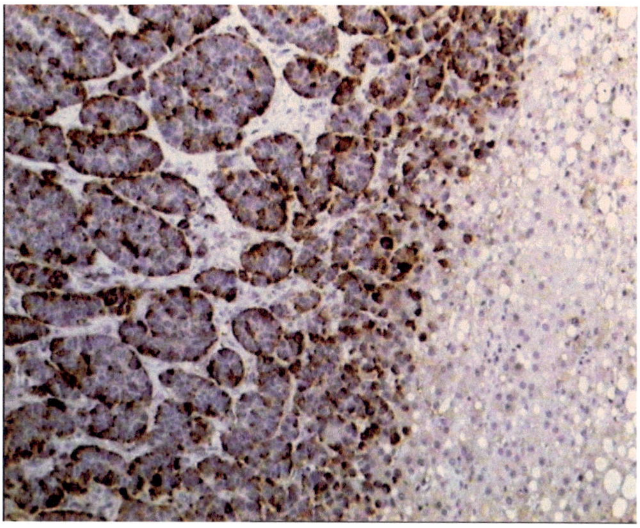

Figure 5. Metastasis of neuroendocrine carcinoma in the liver tissue. Immunoperoxidase, anti-chromogranin A, original magnification 50×.

In contrast to hepatocellular carcinoma, colorectal cancer lacks hepatocyte antigen, glypican and cytoplasmic TTF-1 expression. Alpha-fetoprotein is absent from colorectal cancer tissues, although the differential diagnostic value is lower because of relatively infrequent expression in hepatocellular carcinoma. CD10 can be misleading in the differential diagnosis of hepatocellular and metastatic colorectal cancer. Hepatocellular cancer mostly develops in the background of liver cirrhosis while metastases are rare in cirrhotic liver. However, hepatocellular carcinoma, and especially fibrolamellar variant, can arise in the absence of cirrhosis. In contrast, colorectal cancer metastasis can be surrounded by liver tissue that is damaged by peritumoural or treatment-related cell damage, fibrosis and inflammation [71].

The tissue analysis of cardinal tumour features and cancer microenvironment, production of cytokinesand growth factors in the metastasis, evaluation of circulating neoplastic cells, analysis of tumour hypoxia and angiogenesis atprotein, gene and miRNA levels can also bring prognostic and predictive information [72–77]. Besides the tumour characteristics, hepatic lymphatic anatomy and its involvement by tumour can be evaluated to predict the recurrence [15].

7. Surgical treatment of the liver metastasis of colorectal cancer

The prognosis of metastatic colorectal cancer is serious. The 5-year survival of patients receiving chemotherapy is low. In contrast, hepatic metastasectomy is an accepted procedure with low perioperative mortality (2.3–2.8%) ensuring 5-year survival 28–58% and 10-year survival 22-36% [15, 18, 78, 79]. The median survival of surgically treated patients is 42.5 months [4].

The CRC metastases can be treated surgically if all metastases can be completely resected, at least 2 adjacent liver segments can be spared and sufficient liver function is expected [1].

The liver is composed of segments defined by vascular branching. As described by the International Hepato-Pancreato-Biliary Association, the liver segments are unified in four sections: left lateral and medial, right lateral and medial. Thus, segmentectomy, singular sectionectomy, hemihepatectomy involving two sections and trisectionectomy can be performed [4]. Nonanatomic liver resection shows no differences from anatomic resection regarding morbidity, mortality, recurrence rate or survival. In addition, it has the benefit of parenchymal sparing providing more opportunities for repeated resections that are usually limited by insufficient remnant liver. Nonanatomic resections can be carried out during shorter operation time and are associated with less blood loss [80].

Extrahepatic vascular anatomy must be carefully considered before the operation as only 55% of persons have typical arterial anatomy. Aberrant right hepatic arteries can arise from superior mesenteric artery and from left gastric artery. The trifurcation of portal vein can be observed. Computed tomography is the method of choice for vascular imaging [4].

Liver resection necessitates parenchymal dissection and haemostasis. The liver parenchyma can be divided by finger-fracture or crush-clamp technique, by scissors using scratch or sharp dissection technique, or by ultrasound or radiofrequency knives. Small vessels must be occluded by bipolar coagulation, titan clipping or ligation. Bipolar or ultrasound coagulation devices can be used for dissection and closure of small vessels. Larger vessels must be ligated. Liver resection with staplers involves tissue dissection and automatic vessel clamping [4].

To limit the bleeding, total inflow occlusion can be used but can result in ischemia/reperfusion injury if prolonged. Intermittent occlusion (15 min, alternating with 5 min of perfusion) better preserves liver function. Bleeding from hepatic veins can be decreased by low central venous pressure (less than 4 mm Hg) or total vascular occlusion of the liver with or without in-situ cooling of the liver [4].

Laparoscopic approach sincreasinglyapplied for liver resections, including even hemihepatectomy [4, 81]. The best indications for laparoscopic resection are single metastases, not exceeding 5 cm in diameter, in readily accessible segments 2–6. In contrast, segments 1, 7 and 8 are considered difficult to access except for skilled professionals. Single incision laparoscopic surgery has been used for liver resection but faces technical difficulties in spatial manoeuvres with the instruments. As human ergonomics is limited, robotic surgery has been developed and applied for liver resections facilitating the manipulations with the instruments and improving the overview of operating field at the expense of remote contact with tissues and patient. The lack of tactile feedback compromises the estimation of interaction strength and pressure applied on the tissues. The conversion to open operation necessitates reorganisation of the operation team [82]. Despite these shortcomings, in a recent review, robotic liver resection was found to be a safe procedure [83]. Robotic malfunction is rare (2.4–4.5%). Major hepatectomies have been performed by robotic surgery [82]. However, the greatest advance of robotic surgery can be the possibility to remove small, but hardly accessible lesions by small sectoral, segmental or subsegmental resections instead of extensive routine liver resection [82, 84].

The surgical treatment can be precluded by involvement of portal vein, hepatic artery or common bile duct. The goal of surgery is to resect all malignant tissue. If this would lead to insufficient remnant liver, as in case of multiple bilobar metastases or deep metastases close to hilum or major vessels, the surgery also is contraindicated [18]. To increase the size of liver remnant, two-stage hepatectomy [85] or portal vein embolisation or ligation can be applied. Both procedures take advantage of the regenerative capacity of the liver [4]. Portal vein embolisation increases the resectability rate [86]. The portal vein occlusion can be performed as intraoperative ligation of portal vein branches, transileocolic embolisation or percutaneous transhepatic ipsilateral or contralateral embolisation. The spectrum of applied embolisation materials includes polyvinyl alcohol particles, coils, gelatine sponge, fibrin glue, lipoiodol or butyl cyanoacrylate. In a recent review, authors showed that preoperative portal vein embolisation has a high technical and clinical success rate. Liver cirrhosis impaired the regeneration. However, cirrhosis is rarely encountered in association with metastatic cancers. Cholestasis and preceding chemotherapy had no negative impact [87]. The resectability can also be improved by chemotherapy-induced downstaging [86, 88, 89]. By chemotherapy, resectability can be achieved in up to 40% of patients [90]. If the downstaging is successful and followed by the resection, the 5-year survival reaches 33% that is comparable with the results in patients with initially resectable metastases [86]. Preoperative chemotherapy is not indicated for resectable lesions [89] and should not be excessively extended (9 cycles or more) to avoid marked hepatotoxicity without improving the pathologic response [91]. Among the chemotherapy-related liver damage, steatosis can be induced by 5-fluorouracil, nonalcoholic steatohepatitis by irinotecan and sinusoidal obstruction syndrome by oxaliplatin [92]. For successful downstaging, the type of chemotherapy is more important than the number of cycles. Thus, the inclusion of bevacizumab in the chemotherapy schedule in addition to FOLFOX improves the outcome in terms of achieving resectability [91].

The planning of liver surgery can be challenging in patients presenting with colorectal cancer and synchronous liver metastases. Simultaneous resection of primary tumours and liver metastases can be performed in selected patients. Liver resection can safely be performed as the first operation followed by the large bowel operation [93]. The safety of liver-first approach has been confirmed in a recent review [94].

The risk factors of cancer recurrence include the presence of lymph node or extrahepatic metastases, high CEA (above 200 ng/mL), multiple and large (above 5 cm) metastases, short disease-free survival [18], high tumour grade and positive resection lines [4]. Regarding the resection line, the minimal requirements are under discussion regarding R0 resection with distance between tumour and resection line less than 1 cm. In the recent literature, lack of 1 cm margin is not considered a contraindication for liver resection [80], and generally the requirement for tumour-free tissue border has decreased from 10 to 2 mm or even 0 mm [95–98]. The presence of hilar lymph node metastases is an adverse prognostic factor in comparison to metastases affecting only liver but can be less hazardous in prognostic terms than metastases in lymph nodes adjacent to truncus coeliacus or aorta [4].

After resection, MRI or CT should be used for surveillance. The examinations must be repeated every 3–6 months for 2 years after resection and every 6 months for 3–5 years after the surgery [1]. Perioperative chemotherapy, including adjuvant treatment, increases recurrence-free survival [99].

8. Liver transplantation for colorectal cancer metastases

Liver transplantation is indicated for end-stage chronic liver disease and acute liver failure. In addition, transplantation has certain indications regarding malignant tumours. The classic indications include hepatocellular carcinoma on the background of liver cirrhosis if the patient corresponds to the Milan criteria; fibrolamellar hepatocellular carcinoma, hepatoblastoma and epithelioid haemangioendothelioma. Transplantation is researched in patients having hepatocellular carcinoma with tumour burden exceeding the Milan criteria, hepatocellular carcinoma in noncirrhotic liver, cholangiocellular cancer and liver metastases from neuroendocrine tumours. Hepatocellular carcinoma with extrahepatic spread or portal vein invasion, hepatoblastoma with uncontrolled extrahepatic spread and other malignancies are regarded as contraindications for liver transplantation. Thus, until recently, colorectal cancer metastases to the liver also were considered a contraindication for liver transplantation [100] due to allocation justice in the background of organ shortage and due to the risk of tumour recurrence on the background of immunosuppression.

A revolutionary approach has been undertaken in Norway by Hagness et al. offering liver transplantation to patients with unresectable liver metastases of colorectal cancer. The resulting life quality was good. The 5-year survival was 60%, that exceeds the survival obtained by chemotherapy and is comparable to the survival after liver resection in suitable cases [9].

Interestingly, the recurrence patterns after liver transplantation differ from those after liver resection. The most frequent event is single-site recurrence in the lungs, followed by recurrence in multiple sites. In the present group of patients, no single-site recurrences in liver were observed, although the liver was involved by tumour metastases in patients having recurrence in multiple sites. Regarding the outcome, the pulmonary metastases followed indolent course, but metastases to the transplanted liver were prognostically adverse. The immunosuppressive treatment did not enhance the growth of those pulmonary metastases that were present at the time of transplantation [9]. The m-TOR inhibitors used for immunosuppression can have beneficial influence as they block angiogenesis and proliferation [9, 100].

9. Nonsurgical treatment of liver metastases of colorectal cancer

Although surgical treatment ensures the best 5-year survival, only 15–25% of liver metastases are amenable to resection [98]. If surgical treatment is not possible, radiofrequency ablation, cryotherapy, microwave ablation, stereotactic body radiotherapy, radioembolisation or percutaneous alcohol injection canbe used to decrease the tumour burden [101, 102]. Generally, ablation therapies are not recommended for resectable lesions [103].

The liver metastases can be targeted by radiofrequency ablation although the benefits of it are controversial. Positive estimates have been published [104, 105]. However, later data showed that radiofrequency ablation alone or in combination with surgery resulted in inferior survival in comparison with liver resection. The outcome of radiofrequency ablation was only slightly better than the results of chemotherapy [39]. The resulting 5-year survival was around 24% [106–110]. Still later, 5-year survival of 43% has been reported [98]. After the procedure, either local recurrence or new liver metastases can develop. The risk of local recurrence is higher if the lesion is larger than 3 cm: 21.7% vs. 1.6–3.8% [111–113]. The development of new metastases predominates over local recurrence and can be promoted by liver regeneration and production of cytokines [98, 113]. To avoid complications, proximity to bile ducts but not vessels is of utmost importance as the blood vessels are moderately sensitive to heat and can be protected by vascular clamping and Pringle manoeuvre involving alternation of clamping and perfusion. In contrast, bile ducts are very sensitive to heat-induced damage [113].

Radiofrequency ablation belongs to the group of thermal ablation procedures comprising also laser-induced interstitial thermotherapy. In this method, laser light is directly transmitted to the neoplastic tissue through flexible optic fibres, and the absorption of laser photon energy causes local rise of temperature inducing coagulation necrosis. The results are highly dependent on the completeness of tumour destruction. The 5-year survival after thermal ablation is 44% if the ablation is complete and 20% if it is partial. The frequency of partial ablation ranges from 38% to 52% [114–116]. The size of neoplastic mass is the main predictive factor for the completeness of the ablation, with better results achieved in metastases smaller than 3 cm [116, 117].

Cryoablation involves tissue destruction by low temperature, i.e., intended freezing of the target in order to induce local necrosis. Although percutaneous, laparoscopic or open surgical approach generally is possible, cryotreatment of liver tumours is mostly performed via open surgical access. Occasionally, laparoscopic approach is used [118]. The temperature is decreased by liquid nitrogen or argon gas that is delivered to the target by special probe under US guidance. The freezing is rapid, so the formed ice crystals destroy the cells, including tumour cells. Ice crystals also propagate in the microvessels. The procedure includes alternating cycles of freezing and thawing. Multiple masses are treated consecutively rather than simultaneously. Necrosis develops within the next 2 days and is well-demarcated in the third to fourth day after the procedure. Large masses (>5 cm) are not amenable to complete treatment. Another limitation includes tumours close to large blood vessels [119]. Cryoablation ensures 5-year survival in 17% of patients [109, 120–122].

In microwave ablation, tissue destruction is induced by microwaves. The electrode is inserted in the tumour mass under US or CT guidance using percutaneous, laparoscopic or open surgical access. An alternating high-frequency (900–2450 Hz) electromagnetic field induces vibration of water molecules representing dipoles. The energy created by the induced movement of water molecules is released as heat that results in coagulative necrosis [3]. The method can ensure wider and quicker tissue destruction than radiofrequency ablation. It is not limited by the temperature 100°C, does not rely on the conduction of electricity and is less limited by impedance of the destroyed tissues or scars [123]. The 5-year survival after microwave ablation was 16% in the older reports [109, 124, 125]. Recently, intraoperative microwave ablation ensured 4-year survival of 35.2% [123] and 3-year survival of 36% [126].

External beam radiation treatment for liver metastases has limited effect due to high sensitivity of hepatocytes towards ionising radiation. Thus, therapeutic radiation doses would induce serious liver damage but small doses lack efficacy. The treatment of liver metastases by external beam radiation is associated with high rate of local recurrence and side effects, both contributing to low survival. Three-dimensional conformal radiotherapy is more targeted. In stereotactic body radiation treatment, a robotic arm is used to target the lesion in synchronisation with the respiratory movements. This allows delivering higher radiation dose to the lesion while retaining appropriate safety profile with only tolerable complications. After stereotactic body radiation treatment, the 1-year survival of complex, pretreated patients with the frequent presence of extrahepatic metastases was 45.5% [110]. The 2-year survival is reported to be 45% [127].

Hepatic arterial infusion can be applied due to the fact that metastases larger than 3 mm receive 95% of blood supply from the hepatic artery. This technique yields higher concentration (up to 16 times higher) of the medication within the metastasis in association with lower systemic toxicity due to concentrated supply and first-pass effect with maximum absorption in the liver. Skilled team and qualitative radiologic imaging are the prerequisites [102]. There are several technically related approaches that also involve direct supply of the therapeutic agent to the target via hepatic artery, such as placement of hepatic arterial infusion pumps, selective internal radiation therapy, drug-eluting bead embolisation and irinotecan-containing drug-eluting particles [128].

Although successful surgery can yield long term survival, recurrence develops either in liver or in other distant sites in 60–70% of patients [15]. Therefore, adjuvant systemic chemotherapy, hepatic arterial infusion chemotherapy and molecular targeted therapy represent important adjuncts to surgical treatment. Systemic chemotherapy results in significantly better survival [129, 130] but can cause systemic adverse effects along with vascular liver damage and steatosis [131]. Hepatic arterial infusion of specific chemotherapeutic agents has the benefits of directly targeting the metastasis within liver and thus causing less systemic toxicity. However, biliary tract damage can follow [132, 133]. Monoclonal antibodies against VEGF and EGFR are attractive by the targeted mechanism [101, 134]. However, bevacizumab, cetuximab and panitumumab have also caused controversies regarding liver metastases of colorectal cancer [13].

10. Radiologic evaluation before nonsurgical treatment

In general, the metastatic process must be characterised similarly as before the operation. If ablation is planned, the relation between the metastasis and the intrahepatic bile ducts and vessels must be carefully established to avoid heat-induced damage [1]. If the medical centre has the necessary skills to provide hepatic artery infusion with chemotherapeutic agents for neoadjuvant therapy to decrease lesion size and allow resection, for adjuvant for treatment after resection or treatment of unresectable liver disease, hepatic artery must be visualised by CT angiography [18].

11. Radiologic assessment of the treatment outcome

Classically, the tumour response to treatment is measured by decrease of the tumour mass diameter as defined by the Response Evaluation Criteria in Solid Tumours (RECIST). The RECIST criteria, described in 2000 and refined in 2009 [1, 135, 136], necessitate one-dimensional measurements to detect the sum of maximal diameter of five lesions. The relative difference of this parameter before and after treatment is interpreted as follows: progressive disease, increase of at least 20% and at least 5 mm in the sum, or appearance of a new lesion; stable disease, lack of dynamics or changes within the borders between progressive disease and partial response; partial response, decrease for at least 30%; and complete radiologic response, disappearance of all lesions. It must be emphasised that radiologic complete response is not always equivalent to pathologic complete response; therefore, all the responded lesions still must be removed surgically [17]. Several controversies exist regarding RECIST criteria. First, it is suggested that early response for 10% correlates with the outcome better than the border of 30% [17, 137]. Further, not only size but also the composition of the mass lesion matters as it can include not only viable tumour but also necrosis, fibrosis, granulations or haemorrhage. By ablation techniques, the surrounding liver tissue is intentionally damaged and fuses together with the metastatic mass. After intra-arterial treatment by chemotherapy, drug-eluting beads, irinotecan drug-eluting beads or radio embolisation, the response evaluation is confounded by haemorrhage, necrosis resulting in size enlargement, peripheral thin rim of granulation tissue mimicking metastasis, fibrosis, peritumoural ischemia or hepatitis [1]. Therefore, the evaluation of treatment response includes not only the changes in the lesionsize, but also its morphology and functional status [17].

Morphologic radiologic features, including changes in tumour heterogeneity and internal structure, enhancement and margins, can indicate favourable tumour response to treatment [138]. On CT, CRC metastases in the liver have heterogeneous structure and ill-defined margins. Responding lesions obtain homogeneous structure and outlined margins [17]. The morphologic response on CT correlates with pathologic response and with the survival [138].

PET-CT characterises the metabolic activity in the lesions [1], suggesting pathogenetically substantiated accurate estimate of tumour response. However, the sensitivity of PET decreases after chemotherapy [17]. Clinically importantly, PET can identify lack of chemotherapy efficacy just after 1 cycle [139].

Preceding treatment can induce not only tumour shrinkage but also liver parenchymal damage. By CT, steatosis that affects more than 30% of parenchyma can be diagnosed by the liver attenuation index characterising the difference in the attenuation between liver and spleen. By MRI, the analysis of water and fat proton signals is possible, leading to more accurate estimates of steatosis than by CT and US [1, 140]. Sinusoid obstructive syndrome can be caused by oxaliplatin-based chemotherapy. It is characterised by sinusoidal injury that may lead to fibrosis or veno-occlusive disease. The radiologic findings are nonspecific [1].

12. Complete radiologic response

Complete radiologic response can be obtained in 5–38% of patients. The frequency of complete radiologic response depends on the efficacy of preoperative treatment and on the quality and completeness of radiologic investigation. Metastasis can become difficult to observe on CT if the size decreases and/or the surrounding liver tissue develops steatosis. MRI can be used to identify the residual lesions. The MRI-documented disappearance of the metastasis is suggestive of true complete histologic response.

The correlation between radiologic and pathologic complete response ranges 20–100% in different studies. Thus, at present, all sites of disease should be resected surgically. A fraction of lesions (up to 24% of patients with complete response on CT) can be grossly identified during the operation. Full mobilisation of liver and palpation, followed by intraoperative conventional and contrast-enhanced US, are the subsequent options rising the yield to 45% of patients. Contrast-enhanced US identifies additional 10–15% of nodules, compared with palpation and conventional ultrasonography technique. The intraoperative yield is lower in patients who have had preoperative MRI, suggesting that MRI is the method of choice to identify true small residual metastases that are missed by less sensitive CT [17].

If the radiologically regressed metastases are not resected, they tend to recur. The frequency of durable clinical response, usually defined as disease-free period for 1 year, correlates with the frequency of complete pathologic response. The recurrence mostly develops in 10–20 months. The median time to recurrence is 11 months. The recurrence occurs more frequently in patients who have unresected radiologically disappeared metastases in comparison to those who underwent the surgery, although a more effective adjuvant treatment can diminish these differences. Hepatic arterial infusion treatment lowers the incidence of intrahepatic recurrence and increases the frequency of durable response similarly as increasing the rate of complete pathologic response [17].

13. Survival

The median survival of patients affected by metastatic colorectal cancer has increased significantly, e.g., from 27.3 months in 1994 to 39.4 months in 2007 [13]. Analogous increase in the survival is reported also by other authors [14]. The 5-year and 10-year survival can reach even 58% and 36%, correspondingly [15]. Lower 5-year survival after surgical treatment has been reported earlier, e.g., 25–40% [78, 110, 141–144], contrasting with the 5-year survival of 15% in patients with unresectable metastases [33, 145, 146]. The 10-year survival of 25–26% has been described [123, 147, 148]. Better survival is observed in case of delayed metastases [14].

14. Conclusions

1. In conclusion, liver metastases of colorectal cancer must be treated surgically whenever possible as surgery ensures the best survival.

2. Contraindications for surgery include wide tumour spread within the liver or to extrahepatic organs, expected insufficient liver remnant and poor general status. Neoadjuvant treatment should be attempted to downstage the tumour.

3. If the metastatic lesions are not amenable to surgery,ablation or radiation modalities can be applied in association with chemotherapy.

4. High-quality radiologic investigation is necessary to reveal the metastases of colorectal cancer. Magnetic resonance imaging is considered the most sensitive technique that has remarkable advantages revealing subcentimeter metastases and lesions within steatotic liver. Computed tomography benefits from high discrimination and can be used to replace magnetic resonance.

Acknowledgements

The present work has been carried out within the frames of scientific project no. 2013/0004/1DP/1.1.1.2.0./13/APIA/VIAA/020, supported by the European Social Fund (ESF).

Author details

Ilze Strumfa[1], Ervins Vasko[1], Andrejs Vanags[2], Zane Simtniece[1], Peteris Trapencieris[3] and Janis Gardovskis[2]

*Address all correspondence to: Ilze.Strumfa@rsu.lv

1 Department of Pathology, Riga Stradins University, Riga, Latvia

2 Department of Surgery, Riga Stradins University, Riga, Latvia

3 Department of Organic Chemistry, Latvian Institute of Organic Synthesis, Riga, Latvia

References

[1] Fowler KJ, Linehan DC, Menias CO. Colorectal liver metastases: state of the art imaging. Ann Surg Oncol. 2013;20:1185–1193. DOI: 10.1245/s10434-012-2730-7.

[2] Torre LA, Bray F, Siegel RL, Ferlay J, Lortet-Tieulent J, Jemal A. Global cancer statistics, 2012. CA Cancer J Clin. 2015;65:87–108. DOI: 10.3322/caac.21262

[3] Bala MM, Riemsma RP, Wolff R, Kleijnen J. Microwave coagulation for liver metastases. Cochrane Database Syst Rev. 2013;10:CD010163. DOI: 10.1002/14651858.CD010163.pub2

[4] Heinrich S, Lang H. Liver metastases from colorectal cancer: technique of liver resection. J Surg Oncol. 2013;107:579–584. DOI: 10.1002/jso.23138

[5] Carr AD, Ali MR, Khatri VP. Robotic hepatobiliary surgery: update on the current status. Minerva Chir. 2013;68:479–487.

[6] Tan-Tam C, Chung SW. Minireview on laparoscopic hepatobiliary and pancreatic surgery. World J Gastrointest Endosc. 2014;6:60–67. DOI: 10.4253/wjge.v6.i3.60

[7] Lim C, Farges O. Portal vein occlusion before major hepatectomy in patients with colorectal liver metastases: rationale, indications, technical aspects, complications and outcome. J Visc Surg. 2012;149:e86–e96. DOI: 10.1016/j.jviscsurg.2012.03.003

[8] Frankel TL, D'Angelica MI. Hepatic resection for colorectal metastases. J Surg Oncol. 2014;109:2–7. DOI: 10.1002/jso.23371

[9] Hagness M, Foss A, Egge TS, Dueland S. Patterns of recurrence after liver transplantation for nonresectable liver metastases from colorectal cancer. Ann Surg Oncol. 2014;21:1323–1329. DOI: 10.1245/s10434-013-3449-9

[10] Aggarwal C, Meropol NJ, Punt CJ, Iannotti N, Saidman BH, Sabbath KD, Gabrail NY, Picus J, Morse MA, Mitchell E, Miller MC, Cohen SJ. Relationship among circulating

tumor cells, CEA and overall survival in patients with metastatic colorectal cancer. Ann Oncol. 2013;24:420–428. DOI: 10.1093/annonc/mds336

[11] Muhammad S, Kaur K, Huang R, Zhang Q, Kaur P, Yazdani HO, Bilal MU, Zheng J, Zheng L, Wang XS. MicroRNAs in colorectal cancer: role in metastasis and clinical perspectives. World J Gastroenterol. 2014;20:17011–17019. DOI: 10.3748/wjg.v20.i45.17011

[12] Wang J, Huang SK, Zhao M, Yang M, Zhong JL, Gu YY, Peng H, Che YQ, Huang CZ. Identification of a circulating microRNA signature for colorectal cancer detection. PLoS One. 2014;9:e87451. DOI: 10.1371/journal.pone.0087451

[13] Michl M, Holtzem B, Koch J, Moosmann N, Holch J, Hiddemann W, Heinemann V. [Metastatic colorectal cancer--analysis of treatment modalities and survival now and then]. Dtsch Med Wochenschr. 2014;139:2068–2072. DOI: 10.1055/s-0034-1387283

[14] Landreau P, Drouillard A, Launoy G, Ortega-Deballon P, Jooste V, Lepage C, Faivre J, Facy O, Bouvier AM. Incidence and survival in late liver metastases of colorectal cancer. J Gastroenterol Hepatol. 2015;30:82–85. DOI: 10.1111/jgh.12685

[15] Lupinacci RM, Paye F, Coelho FF, Kruger JA, Herman P. Lymphatic drainage of the liver and its implications in the management of colorectal cancer liver metastases. Updates Surg. 2014;66:239–245. DOI: 10.1007/s13304-014-0265-0

[16] Globocan 2012: estimated cancer incidence, mortality and prevalence worldwide in 2012 [Internet]. 2015. Available from: http://globocan.iarc.fr/Default.aspx [Accessed: 2015-03-01]

[17] Adams RB, Aloia TA, Loyer E, Pawlik TM, Taouli B, Vauthey JN. Selection for hepatic resection of colorectal liver metastases: expert consensus statement. HPB (Oxford). 2013;15:91–103. DOI: 10.1111/j.1477-2574.2012.00557.x

[18] Frankel TL, Gian RK, Jarnagin WR. Preoperative imaging for hepatic resection of colorectal cancer metastasis. J Gastrointest Oncol. 2012;3:11–18. DOI: 10.3978/j.issn.2078-6891.2012.002

[19] Chami L, Lassau N, Malka D, Ducreux M, Bidault S, Roche A, Elias D. Benefits of contrast-enhanced sonography for the detection of liver lesions: comparison with histologic findings. AJR Am J Roentgenol. 2008;190:683–690. DOI: 10.2214/ajr.07.2295

[20] Niekel MC, Bipat S, Stoker J. Diagnostic imaging of colorectal liver metastases with CT, MR imaging, FDG PET, and/or FDG PET/CT: a meta-analysis of prospective studies including patients who have not previously undergone treatment. Radiology. 2010;257:674–684. DOI: 10.1148/radiol.10100729

[21] Guimaraes MD, Hochhegger B, Benveniste MF, Odisio BC, Gross JL, Zurstrassen CE, Tyng CC, Bitencourt AG, Marchiori E. Improving CT-guided transthoracic biopsy of mediastinal lesions by diffusion-weighted magnetic resonance imaging. Clinics (Sao Paulo). 2014;69:787–791. DOI: 10.6061/clinics/2014(11)13

[22] Bruegel M, Gaa J, Waldt S, Woertler K, Holzapfel K, Kiefer B, Rummeny EJ. Diagnosis of hepatic metastasis: comparison of respiration-triggered diffusion-weighted echo-planar MRI and five t2-weighted turbo spin-echo sequences. AJR Am J Roentgenol. 2008;191:1421–1429. DOI: 10.2214/ajr.07.3279

[23] Parikh T, Drew SJ, Lee VS, Wong S, Hecht EM, Babb JS, Taouli B. Focal liver lesion detection and characterization with diffusion-weighted MR imaging: comparison with standard breath-hold T2-weighted imaging. Radiology. 2008;246:812–822. DOI: 10.1148/radiol.2463070432

[24] Muhi A, Ichikawa T, Motosugi U, Sou H, Nakajima H, Sano K, Sano M, Kato S, Kitamura T, Fatima Z, Fukushima K, Iino H, Mori Y, Fujii H, Araki T. Diagnosis of colorectal hepatic metastases: comparison of contrast-enhanced CT, contrast-enhanced US, superparamagnetic iron oxide-enhanced MRI, and gadoxetic acid-enhanced MRI. J Magn Reson Imaging. 2011;34:326–335. DOI: 10.1002/jmri.22613

[25] Holzapfel K, Eiber MJ, Fingerle AA, Bruegel M, Rummeny EJ, Gaa J. Detection, classification, and characterization of focal liver lesions: value of diffusion-weighted MR imaging, gadoxetic acid-enhanced MR imaging and the combination of both methods. Abdom Imaging. 2012;37:74–82. DOI: 10.1007/s00261-011-9758-1

[26] Koh DM, Collins DJ, Wallace T, Chau I, Riddell AM. Combining diffusion-weighted MRI with Gd-EOB-DTPA-enhanced MRI improves the detection of colorectal liver metastases. Br J Radiol. 2012;85:980–989. DOI: 10.1259/bjr/91771639

[27] Marckmann P, Skov L, Rossen K, Dupont A, Damholt MB, Heaf JG, Thomsen HS. Nephrogenic systemic fibrosis: suspected causative role of gadodiamide used for contrast-enhanced magnetic resonance imaging. J Am Soc Nephrol. 2006;17:2359–2362. DOI: 10.1681/asn.2006060601

[28] Shabana WM, Cohan RH, Ellis JH, Hussain HK, Francis IR, Su LD, Mukherji SK, Swartz RD. Nephrogenic systemic fibrosis: a report of 29 cases. AJR Am J Roentgenol. 2008;190:736–741. DOI: 10.2214/ajr.07.3115

[29] Song KD, Kim SH, Lee J, Kang KA, Kim J, Yoo H. Half-dose gadoxetic acid-enhanced liver magnetic resonance imaging in patients at risk for nephrogenic systemic fibrosis. Eur J Radiol. 2015;84:378–383. DOI: 10.1016/j.ejrad.2014.12.010

[30] Lauenstein T, Ramirez-Garrido F, Kim YH, Rha SE, Ricke J, Phongkitkarun S, Boettcher J, Gupta RT, Korpraphong P, Tanomkiat W, Furtner J, Liu PS, Henry M, Endrikat J. Nephrogenic systemic fibrosis risk after liver magnetic resonance imaging with gadoxetate disodium in patients with moderate to severe renal impairment: results of a prospective, open-label, multicenter study. Invest Radiol. 2015. DOI: 10.1097/rli.0000000000000145

[31] Kulemann V, Schima W, Tamandl D, Kaczirek K, Gruenberger T, Wrba F, Weber M, Ba-Ssalamah A. Preoperative detection of colorectal liver metastases in fatty liver: MDCT or MRI? Eur J Radiol. 2011;79:e1–e6. DOI: 10.1016/j.ejrad.2010.03.004

[32] Lake ES, Wadhwani S, Subar D, Kauser A, Harris C, Chang D, Lapsia S. The influence of FDG PET-CT on the detection of extrahepatic disease in patients being considered for resection of colorectal liver metastasis. Ann R Coll Surg Engl. 2014;96:211–215. DOI: 10.1308/003588414x13814021679195

[33] Wiering B, Adang EM, van der Sijp JR, Roumen RM, de Jong KP, Comans EF, Pruim J, Dekker HM, Ruers TJ, Krabbe PF, Oyen WJ. Added value of positron emission tomography imaging in the surgical treatment of colorectal liver metastases. Nucl Med Commun. 2010;31:938–944. DOI: 10.1097/MNM.0b013e32833fa9ba

[34] Badiee S, Franc BL, Webb EM, Chu B, Hawkins RA, Coakley F, Singer L. Role of IV iodinated contrast material in 18F-FDG PET/CT of liver metastases. AJR Am J Roentgenol. 2008;191:1436–1439. DOI: 10.2214/ajr.07.3750

[35] Glazer ES, Beaty K, Abdalla EK, Vauthey JN, Curley SA. Effectiveness of positron emission tomography for predicting chemotherapy response in colorectal cancer liver metastases. Arch Surg. 2010;145:340–345; discussion 45. DOI: 10.1001/archsurg.2010.41

[36] Mann CD, Metcalfe MS, Neal CP, Rees Y, Dennison AR, Berry DP. Role of ultrasonography in the detection of resectable recurrence after hepatectomy for colorectal liver metastases. Br J Surg. 2007;94:1403–1407. DOI: 10.1002/bjs.5855

[37] Torzilli G, Botea F, Donadon M, Cimino M, Procopio F, Pedicini V, Poretti D, Montorsi M. Criteria for the selective use of contrast-enhanced intra-operative ultrasound during surgery for colorectal liver metastases. HPB (Oxford). 2014;16:994–1001. DOI: 10.1111/hpb.12272

[38] Abdalla EK, Hicks ME, Vauthey JN. Portal vein embolization: rationale, technique and future prospects. Br J Surg. 2001;88:165–175. DOI: 10.1046/j.1365-2168.2001.01658.x

[39] Abdalla EK, Vauthey JN, Ellis LM, Ellis V, Pollock R, Broglio KR, Hess K, Curley SA. Recurrence and outcomes following hepatic resection, radiofrequency ablation, and combined resection/ablation for colorectal liver metastases. Ann Surg. 2004;239:818–825; discussion 25–27.

[40] Vauthey JN, Pawlik TM, Abdalla EK, Arens JF, Nemr RA, Wei SH, Kennamer DL, Ellis LM, Curley SA. Is extended hepatectomy for hepatobiliary malignancy justified? Ann Surg. 2004;239:722–730; discussion 30–32.

[41] Verberne CJ, Wiggers T, Vermeulen KM, de Jong KP. Detection of recurrences during follow-up after liver surgery for colorectal metastases: both carcinoembryonic antigen (CEA) and imaging are important. Ann Surg Oncol. 2013;20:457–463. DOI: 10.1245/s10434-012-2629-3

[42] Metcalfe M, Mann C, Mullin E, Maddern G. Detecting curable disease following hepatectomy for colorectal metastases. ANZ J Surg. 2005;75:524–527. DOI: 10.1111/j.1445-2197.2005.03421.x

[43] Oussoultzoglou E, Rosso E, Fuchshuber P, Stefanescu V, Diop B, Giraudo G, Pessaux P, Bachellier P, Jaeck D. Perioperative carcinoembryonic antigen measurements to predict curability after liver resection for colorectal metastases: a prospective study. Arch Surg. 2008;143:1150–1158; discussion 58–59. DOI: 10.1001/archsurg.143.12.1150

[44] Deneve E, Riethdorf S, Ramos J, Nocca D, Coffy A, Daures JP, Maudelonde T, Fabre JM, Pantel K, Alix-Panabieres C. Capture of viable circulating tumor cells in the liver of colorectal cancer patients. Clin Chem. 2013;59:1384–1392. DOI: 10.1373/clinchem.2013.202846

[45] Aldulaymi B, Bystrom P, Berglund A, Christensen IJ, Brunner N, Nielsen HJ, Glimelius B. High plasma TIMP-1 and serum CEA levels during combination chemotherapy for metastatic colorectal cancer are significantly associated with poor outcome. Oncology. 2010;79:144–149. DOI: 10.1159/000320686

[46] Aldulaymi B, Christensen IJ, Soletormos G, Jess P, Nielsen SE, Laurberg S, Brunner N, Nielsen HJ. Chemoradiation-induced changes in serum CEA and plasma TIMP-1 in patients with locally advanced rectal cancer. Anticancer Res. 2010;30:4755–4759.

[47] Ha TY. MicroRNAs in human diseases: from cancer to cardiovascular disease. Immune Netw. 2011;11:135–154. DOI: 10.4110/in.2011.11.3.135

[48] Fesler A, Jiang J, Zhai H, Ju J. Circulating microRNA testing for the early diagnosis and follow-up of colorectal cancer patients. Mol Diagn Ther. 2014;18:303–308. DOI: 10.1007/s40291-014-0089-0

[49] Li J, Smyth P, Flavin R, Cahill S, Denning K, Aherne S, Guenther SM, O'Leary JJ, Sheils O. Comparison of miRNA expression patterns using total RNA extracted from matched samples of formalin-fixed paraffin-embedded (FFPE) cells and snap frozen cells. BMC Biotechnol. 2007;7:36. DOI: 10.1186/1472-6750-7-36

[50] Xi Y, Nakajima G, Gavin E, Morris CG, Kudo K, Hayashi K, Ju J. Systematic analysis of microRNA expression of RNA extracted from fresh frozen and formalin-fixed paraffin-embedded samples. RNA. 2007;13:1668–1674. DOI: 10.1261/rna.642907

[51] Mitchell PS, Parkin RK, Kroh EM, Fritz BR, Wyman SK, Pogosova-Agadjanyan EL, Peterson A, Noteboom J, O'Briant KC, Allen A, Lin DW, Urban N, Drescher CW, Knudsen BS, Stirewalt DL, Gentleman R, Vessella RL, Nelson PS, Martin DB, Tewari M. Circulating microRNAs as stable blood-based markers for cancer detection. Proc Natl Acad Sci U S A. 2008;105:10513–10518. DOI: 10.1073/pnas.0804549105

[52] Chaffer CL, Weinberg RA. A perspective on cancer cell metastasis. Science. 2011;331:1559–1564. DOI: 10.1126/science.1203543

[53] Huang Z, Huang D, Ni S, Peng Z, Sheng W, Du X. Plasma microRNAs are promising novel biomarkers for early detection of colorectal cancer. Int J Cancer. 2010;127:118–126. DOI: 10.1002/ijc.25007

[54] Liu GH, Zhou ZG, Chen R, Wang MJ, Zhou B, Li Y, Sun XF. Serum miR-21 and miR-92a as biomarkers in the diagnosis and prognosis of colorectal cancer. Tumour Biol. 2013;34:2175–2181. DOI: 10.1007/s13277-013-0753-8

[55] Ng EK, Chong WW, Jin H, Lam EK, Shin VY, Yu J, Poon TC, Ng SS, Sung JJ. Differential expression of microRNAs in plasma of patients with colorectal cancer: a potential marker for colorectal cancer screening. Gut. 2009;58:1375–1381. DOI: 10.1136/gut.2008.167817

[56] Pu XX, Huang GL, Guo HQ, Guo CC, Li H, Ye S, Ling S, Jiang L, Tian Y, Lin TY. Circulating miR-221 directly amplified from plasma is a potential diagnostic and prognostic marker of colorectal cancer and is correlated with p53 expression. J Gastroenterol Hepatol. 2010;25:1674–1680. DOI: 10.1111/j.1440-1746.2010.06417.x

[57] Yang IP, Tsai HL, Huang CW, Huang MY, Hou MF, Juo SH, Wang JY. The functional significance of microRNA-29c in patients with colorectal cancer: a potential circulating biomarker for predicting early relapse. PLoS One. 2013;8:e66842. DOI: 10.1371/journal.pone.0066842

[58] Wang LG, Gu J. Serum microRNA-29a is a promising novel marker for early detection of colorectal liver metastasis. Cancer Epidemiol. 2012;36:e61–e67. DOI: 10.1016/j.canep.2011.05.002

[59] Yin J, Bai Z, Song J, Yang Y, Wang J, Han W, Zhang J, Meng H, Ma X, Yang Y, Wang T, Li W, Zhang Z. Differential expression of serum miR-126, miR-141 and miR-21 as novel biomarkers for early detection of liver metastasis in colorectal cancer. Chin J Cancer Res. 2014;26:95–103. DOI: 10.3978/j.issn.1000-9604.2014.02.07

[60] Wang K, Zhang S, Marzolf B, Troisch P, Brightman A, Hu Z, Hood LE, Galas DJ. Circulating microRNAs, potential biomarkers for drug-induced liver injury. Proc Natl Acad Sci U S A. 2009;106:4402–4407. DOI: 10.1073/pnas.0813371106

[61] Shigoka M, Tsuchida A, Matsudo T, Nagakawa Y, Saito H, Suzuki Y, Aoki T, Murakami Y, Toyoda H, Kumada T, Bartenschlager R, Kato N, Ikeda M, Takashina T, Tanaka M, Suzuki R, Oikawa K, Takanashi M, Kuroda M. Deregulation of miR-92a expression is implicated in hepatocellular carcinoma development. Pathol Int. 2010;60:351–357. DOI: 10.1111/j.1440-1827.2010.02526.x

[62] Liu H, Zhu L, Liu B, Yang L, Meng X, Zhang W, Ma Y, Xiao H. Genome-wide microRNA profiles identify miR-378 as a serum biomarker for early detection of gastric cancer. Cancer Lett. 2012;316:196–203. DOI: 10.1016/j.canlet.2011.10.034

[63] Pigati L, Yaddanapudi SC, Iyengar R, Kim DJ, Hearn SA, Danforth D, Hastings ML, Duelli DM. Selective release of microRNA species from normal and malignant mammary epithelial cells. PLoS One. 2010;5:e13515. DOI: 10.1371/journal.pone.0013515

[64] Zhang JX, Mai SJ, Huang XX, Wang FW, Liao YJ, Lin MC, Kung HF, Zeng YX, Xie D. MiR-29c mediates epithelial-to-mesenchymal transition in human colorectal carcinoma metastasis via PTP4A and GNA13 regulation of beta-catenin signaling. Ann Oncol. 2014;25:2196–2204. DOI: 10.1093/annonc/mdu439

[65] Lin M, Chen W, Huang J, Gao H, Ye Y, Song Z, Shen X. MicroRNA expression profiles in human colorectal cancers with liver metastases. Oncol Rep. 2011;25:739–747. DOI: 10.3892/or.2010.1112

[66] Drusco A, Nuovo GJ, Zanesi N, Di Leva G, Pichiorri F, Volinia S, Fernandez C, Antenucci A, Costinean S, Bottoni A, Rosito IA, Liu CG, Burch A, Acunzo M, Pekarsky Y, Alder H, Ciardi A, Croce CM. MicroRNA profiles discriminate among colon cancer metastasis. PLoS One. 2014;9:e96670. DOI: 10.1371/journal.pone.0096670

[67] Kulda V, Pesta M, Topolcan O, Liska V, Treska V, Sutnar A, Rupert K, Ludvikova M, Babuska V, Holubec L, Jr., Cerny R. Relevance of miR-21 and miR-143 expression in tissue samples of colorectal carcinoma and its liver metastases. Cancer Genet Cytogenet. 2010;200:154–160. DOI: 10.1016/j.cancergencyto.2010.04.015

[68] Ji D, Chen Z, Li M, Zhan T, Yao Y, Zhang Z, Xi J, Yan L, Gu J. MicroRNA-181a promotes tumor growth and liver metastasis in colorectal cancer by targeting the tumor suppressor WIF-1. Mol Cancer. 2014;13:86. DOI: 10.1186/1476-4598-13-86

[69] Zhou J, Zhang M, Huang Y, Feng L, Chen H, Hu Y, Chen H, Zhang K, Zheng L, Zheng S. MicroRNA-320b promotes colorectal cancer proliferation and invasion by competing with its homologous microRNA-320a. Cancer Lett. 2015;356:669–675. DOI: 10.1016/j.canlet.2014.10.014

[70] Kjersem JB, Ikdahl T, Lingjaerde OC, Guren T, Tveit KM, Kure EH. Plasma microRNAs predicting clinical outcome in metastatic colorectal cancer patients receiving first-line oxaliplatin-based treatment. Mol Oncol. 2014;8:59–67. DOI: 10.1016/j.molonc.2013.09.001

[71] Strumfa I, Vilmanis J, Vanags A, Vasko E, Sulte D, Simtniece Z, Abolins A, Gardovskis J. Primary and metastatic tumours of the liver: expanding scope of morphological and immunohistochemical details in the biopsy. In: Tagaya N, editor. Liver Biopsy—Indications, Procedures, Results. Croatia: InTech; 2012. p. 115–159. DOI: 10.5772/52838

[72] Groot Koerkamp B, Rahbari NN, Buchler MW, Koch M, Weitz J. Circulating tumor cells and prognosis of patients with resectable colorectal liver metastases or widespread metastatic colorectal cancer: a meta-analysis. Ann Surg Oncol. 2013;20:2156–2165. DOI: 10.1245/s10434-013-2907-8

[73] Lim C, Eveno C, Pocard M. Microenvironment and colorectal liver metastases angiogenesis: surgical implications. Bull Cancer. 2013;100:343–350. DOI: 10.1684/bdc.2013.1725

[74] Xu B, Shen F, Cao J, Jia L. Angiogenesis in liver metastasis of colo-rectal carcinoma. Front Biosci (Landmark Ed). 2013;18:1435–1443.

[75] Kim KY, Kim NK, Cha IH, Ahn JB, Choi JS, Choi GH, Lim JS, Lee KY, Baik SH, Min BS, Hur H, Roh JK, Shin SJ. Novel methods for clinical risk stratification in patients with colorectal liver metastases. Cancer Res Treat. 2014. DOI: 10.4143/crt.2014.066

[76] Sun C, Zargham R, Shao Q, Gui X, Marcus V, Lazaris A, Salman A, Metrakos P, Qu X, Gao Z. Association of CD98, integrin beta1, integrin beta3 and Fak with the progression and liver metastases of colorectal cancer. Pathol Res Pract. 2014;210:668–674. DOI: 10.1016/j.prp.2014.06.016

[77] Toiyama Y, Hur K, Tanaka K, Inoue Y, Kusunoki M, Boland CR, Goel A. Serum miR-200c is a novel prognostic and metastasis-predictive biomarker in patients with colorectal cancer. Ann Surg. 2014;259:735–743. DOI: 10.1097/SLA.0b013e3182a6909d

[78] Nordlinger B, Guiguet M, Vaillant JC, Balladur P, Boudjema K, Bachellier P, Jaeck D. Surgical resection of colorectal carcinoma metastases to the liver. A prognostic scoring system to improve case selection, based on 1568 patients. Association Francaise de Chirurgie. Cancer. 1996;77:1254–1262.

[79] Fong Y, Fortner J, Sun RL, Brennan MF, Blumgart LH. Clinical score for predicting recurrence after hepatic resection for metastatic colorectal cancer: analysis of 1001 consecutive cases. Ann Surg. 1999;230:309–318; discussion 18–21.

[80] Lalmahomed ZS, Ayez N, van der Pool AE, Verheij J, JN IJ, Verhoef C. Anatomical versus nonanatomical resection of colorectal liver metastases: is there a difference in surgical and oncological outcome? World J Surg. 2011;35:656–661. DOI: 10.1007/s00268-010-0890-9

[81] Cheung TT, Poon RT, Yuen WK, Chok KS, Tsang SH, Yau T, Chan SC, Lo CM. Outcome of laparoscopic versus open hepatectomy for colorectal liver metastases. ANZ J Surg. 2013;83:847–852. DOI: 10.1111/j.1445-2197.2012.06270.x

[82] Leung U, Fong Y. Robotic liver surgery. Hepatobiliary Surg Nutr. 2014;3:288–294. DOI: 10.3978/j.issn.2304-3881.2014.09.02

[83] Ho CM, Wakabayashi G, Nitta H, Ito N, Hasegawa Y, Takahara T. Systematic review of robotic liver resection. Surg Endosc. 2013;27:732–739. DOI: 10.1007/s00464-012-2547-2

[84] Troisi RI, Patriti A, Montalti R, Casciola L. Robot assistance in liver surgery: a real advantage over a fully laparoscopic approach? Results of a comparative bi-institutional analysis. Int J Med Robot. 2013;9:160–166. DOI: 10.1002/rcs.1495

[85] Lam VW, Laurence JM, Johnston E, Hollands MJ, Pleass HC, Richardson AJ. A systematic review of two-stage hepatectomy in patients with initially unresectable colorectal liver metastases. HPB (Oxford). 2013;15:483–491. DOI: 10.1111/j.1477-2574.2012.00607.x

[86] Wicherts DA, de Haas RJ, Andreani P, Sotirov D, Salloum C, Castaing D, Adam R, Azoulay D. Impact of portal vein embolization on long-term survival of patients with primarily unresectable colorectal liver metastases. Br J Surg. 2010;97:240–250. DOI: 10.1002/bjs.6756

[87] van Lienden KP, van den Esschert JW, de Graaf W, Bipat S, Lameris JS, van Gulik TM, van Delden OM. Portal vein embolization before liver resection: a systematic review. Cardiovasc Intervent Radiol. 2013;36:25–34. DOI: 10.1007/s00270-012-0440-y

[88] Lam VW, Spiro C, Laurence JM, Johnston E, Hollands MJ, Pleass HC, Richardson AJ. A systematic review of clinical response and survival outcomes of downsizing systemic chemotherapy and rescue liver surgery in patients with initially unresectable colorectal liver metastases. Ann Surg Oncol. 2012;19:1292–1301. DOI: 10.1245/s10434-011-2061-0

[89] Lehmann K, Rickenbacher A, Weber A, Pestalozzi BC, Clavien PA. Chemotherapy before liver resection of colorectal metastases: friend or foe? Ann Surg. 2012;255:237–247. DOI: 10.1097/SLA.0b013e3182356236

[90] Wong R, Cunningham D, Barbachano Y, Saffery C, Valle J, Hickish T, Mudan S, Brown G, Khan A, Wotherspoon A, Strimpakos AS, Thomas J, Compton S, Chua YJ, Chau I. A multicentre study of capecitabine, oxaliplatin plus bevacizumab as perioperative treatment of patients with poor-risk colorectal liver-only metastases not selected for upfront resection. Ann Oncol. 2011;22:2042–2048. DOI: 10.1093/annonc/mdq714

[91] Kishi Y, Zorzi D, Contreras CM, Maru DM, Kopetz S, Ribero D, Motta M, Ravarino N, Risio M, Curley SA, Abdalla EK, Capussotti L, Vauthey JN. Extended preoperative chemotherapy does not improve pathologic response and increases postoperative liver insufficiency after hepatic resection for colorectal liver metastases. Ann Surg Oncol. 2010;17:2870–2876. DOI: 10.1245/s10434-010-1166-1

[92] Zorzi D, Laurent A, Pawlik TM, Lauwers GY, Vauthey JN, Abdalla EK. Chemotherapy-associated hepatotoxicity and surgery for colorectal liver metastases. Br J Surg. 2007;94:274–286. DOI: 10.1002/bjs.5719

[93] Brouquet A, Mortenson MM, Vauthey JN, Rodriguez-Bigas MA, Overman MJ, Chang GJ, Kopetz S, Garrett C, Curley SA, Abdalla EK. Surgical strategies for synchronous colorectal liver metastases in 156 consecutive patients: classic, combined or reverse strategy? J Am Coll Surg. 2010;210:934–941. DOI: 10.1016/j.jamcollsurg.2010.02.039

[94] Lam VW, Laurence JM, Pang T, Johnston E, Hollands MJ, Pleass HC, Richardson AJ. A systematic review of a liver-first approach in patients with colorectal cancer and

synchronous colorectal liver metastases. HPB (Oxford). 2014;16:101–108. DOI: 10.1111/hpb.12083

[95] Cady B, Stone MD, McDermott WV, Jr., Jenkins RL, Bothe A, Jr., Lavin PT, Lovett EJ, Steele GD, Jr. Technical and biological factors in disease-free survival after hepatic resection for colorectal cancer metastases. Arch Surg. 1992;127:561–568; discussion 68–69.

[96] Kokudo N, Miki Y, Sugai S, Yanagisawa A, Kato Y, Sakamoto Y, Yamamoto J, Yamaguchi T, Muto T, Makuuchi M. Genetic and histological assessment of surgical margins in resected liver metastases from colorectal carcinoma: minimum surgical margins for successful resection. Arch Surg. 2002;137:833–840.

[97] de Haas RJ, Wicherts DA, Flores E, Azoulay D, Castaing D, Adam R. R1 resection by necessity for colorectal liver metastases: is it still a contraindication to surgery? Ann Surg. 2008;248:626–637. DOI: 10.1097/SLA.0b013e31818a07f1

[98] Evrard S, Rivoire M, Arnaud J, Lermite E, Bellera C, Fonck M, Becouarn Y, Lalet C, Puildo M, Mathoulin-Pelissier S. Unresectable colorectal cancer liver metastases treated by intraoperative radiofrequency ablation with or without resection. Br J Surg. 2012;99:558–565. DOI: 10.1002/bjs.8724

[99] Wieser M, Sauerland S, Arnold D, Schmiegel W, Reinacher-Schick A. Peri-operative chemotherapy for the treatment of resectable liver metastases from colorectal cancer: a systematic review and meta-analysis of randomized trials. BMC Cancer. 2010;10:309. DOI: 10.1186/1471-2407-10-309

[100] Hackl C, Schlitt HJ, Kirchner GI, Knoppke B, Loss M. Liver transplantation for malignancy: current treatment strategies and future perspectives. World J Gastroenterol. 2014;20:5331–5344. DOI: 10.3748/wjg.v20.i18.5331

[101] Macedo FI, Makarawo T. Colorectal hepatic metastasis: evolving therapies. World J Hepatol. 2014;6:453–463. DOI: 10.4254/wjh.v6.i7.453

[102] Vogl TJ, Zangos S, Eichler K, Yakoub D, Nabil M. Colorectal liver metastases: regional chemotherapy via transarterial chemoembolization (TACE) and hepatic chemoperfusion: an update. Eur Radiol. 2007;17:1025–1034. DOI: 10.1007/s00330-006-0372-5

[103] Abdalla EK, Bauer TW, Chun YS, D'Angelica M, Kooby DA, Jarnagin WR. Locoregional surgical and interventional therapies for advanced colorectal cancer liver metastases: expert consensus statements. HPB (Oxford). 2013;15:119–130. DOI: 10.1111/j.1477-2574.2012.00597.x

[104] Curley SA, Izzo F, Delrio P, Ellis LM, Granchi J, Vallone P, Fiore F, Pignata S, Daniele B, Cremona F. Radiofrequency ablation of unresectable primary and metastatic hepatic malignancies: results in 123 patients. Ann Surg. 1999;230:1–8.

[105] Elias D, Goharin A, El Otmany A, Taieb J, Duvillard P, Lasser P, de Baere T. Usefulness of intraoperative radiofrequency thermoablation of liver tumours associated or

not with hepatectomy. Eur J Surg Oncol. 2000;26:763–769. DOI: 10.1053/ejso.2000.1000

[106] Gillams AR, Lees WR. Radiofrequency ablation of colorectal liver metastases. Abdom Imaging. 2005;30:419–426. DOI: 10.1007/s00261-004-0256-6

[107] Siperstein AE, Berber E, Ballem N, Parikh RT. Survival after radiofrequency ablation of colorectal liver metastases: 10-year experience. Ann Surg. 2007;246:559–565; discussion 65–67. DOI: 10.1097/SLA.0b013e318155a7b6

[108] Veltri A, Sacchetto P, Tosetti I, Pagano E, Fava C, Gandini G. Radiofrequency ablation of colorectal liver metastases: small size favorably predicts technique effectiveness and survival. Cardiovasc Intervent Radiol. 2008;31:948–956. DOI: 10.1007/s00270-008-9362-0

[109] Pathak S, Jones R, Tang JM, Parmar C, Fenwick S, Malik H, Poston G. Ablative therapies for colorectal liver metastases: a systematic review. Colorectal Dis. 2011;13:e252–265. DOI: 10.1111/j.1463-1318.2011.02695.x

[110] Choron RL, Kwiatt ME, LaCouture TA, Hunter K, Kubicek G, Spitz FR. Stereotactic body radiation therapy (SBRT) for liver metastasis: early experience with the cyberknife robotic radio-surgery system. Am J Clin Cancer Res. 2014;2:21–32.

[111] Mulier S, Ni Y, Jamart J, Ruers T, Marchal G, Michel L. Local recurrence after hepatic radiofrequency coagulation: multivariate meta-analysis and review of contributing factors. Ann Surg. 2005;242:158–171.

[112] Abitabile P, Hartl U, Lange J, Maurer CA. Radiofrequency ablation permits an effective treatment for colorectal liver metastasis. Eur J Surg Oncol. 2007;33:67–71. DOI: 10.1016/j.ejso.2006.10.040

[113] Leblanc F, Fonck M, Brunet R, Becouarn Y, Mathoulin-Pelissier S, Evrard S. Comparison of hepatic recurrences after resection or intraoperative radiofrequency ablation indicated by size and topographical characteristics of the metastases. Eur J Surg Oncol. 2008;34:185–190. DOI: 10.1016/j.ejso.2007.09.028

[114] Hori T, Nagata K, Hasuike S, Onaga M, Motoda M, Moriuchi A, Iwakiri H, Uto H, Kato J, Ido A, Hayashi K, Tsubouchi H. Risk factors for the local recurrence of hepatocellular carcinoma after a single session of percutaneous radiofrequency ablation. J Gastroenterol. 2003;38:977–981. DOI: 10.1007/s00535-003-1181-0

[115] Poon RT, Ng KK, Lam CM, Ai V, Yuen J, Fan ST. Effectiveness of radiofrequency ablation for hepatocellular carcinomas larger than 3 cm in diameter. Arch Surg. 2004;139:281–287. DOI: 10.1001/archsurg.139.3.281

[116] Wiggermann P, Puls R, Vasilj A, Sieron D, Schreyer AG, Jung EM, Wawrzynek W, Stroszczynski C. Thermal ablation of unresectable liver tumors: factors associated with partial ablation and the impact on long-term survival. Med Sci Monit. 2012;18:CR88–CR92.

[117] Ayav A, Germain A, Marchal F, Tierris I, Laurent V, Bazin C, Yuan Y, Robert L, Brunaud L, Bresler L. Radiofrequency ablation of unresectable liver tumors: factors associated with incomplete ablation or local recurrence. Am J Surg. 2010;200:435–439. DOI: 10.1016/j.amjsurg.2009.11.009

[118] Mala T. Cryoablation of liver tumours—a review of mechanisms, techniques and clinical outcome. Minim Invasive Ther Allied Technol. 2006;15:9–17. DOI: 10.1080/13645700500468268

[119] Bala MM, Riemsma RP, Wolff R, Kleijnen J. Cryotherapy for liver metastases. Cochrane Database Syst Rev. 2013;6:CD009058. DOI: 10.1002/14651858.CD009058.pub2

[120] Seifert JK, Morris DL. Prognostic factors after cryotherapy for hepatic metastases from colorectal cancer. Ann Surg. 1998;228:201–208.

[121] Yan TD, Padang R, Morris DL. Longterm results and prognostic indicators after cryotherapy and hepatic arterial chemotherapy with or without resection for colorectal liver metastases in 224 patients: longterm survival can be achieved in patients with multiple bilateral liver metastases. J Am Coll Surg. 2006;202:100–111. DOI: 10.1016/j.jamcollsurg.2005.08.026

[122] Niu R, Yan TD, Zhu JC, Black D, Chu F, Morris DL. Recurrence and survival outcomes after hepatic resection with or without cryotherapy for liver metastases from colorectal carcinoma. Ann Surg Oncol. 2007;14:2078–2087. DOI: 10.1245/s10434-007-9400-1

[123] Eng OS, Tsang AT, Moore D, Chen C, Narayanan S, Gannon CJ, August DA, Carpizo DR, Melstrom LG. Outcomes of microwave ablation for colorectal cancer liver metastases: a single center experience. J Surg Oncol. 2015;111:410–413. DOI: 10.1002/jso.23849

[124] Shibata T, Niinobu T, Ogata N, Takami M. Microwave coagulation therapy for multiple hepatic metastases from colorectal carcinoma. Cancer. 2000;89:276–284.

[125] Tanaka K, Shimada H, Nagano Y, Endo I, Sekido H, Togo S. Outcome after hepatic resection versus combined resection and microwave ablation for multiple bilobar colorectal metastases to the liver. Surgery. 2006;139:263–273. DOI: 10.1016/j.surg.2005.07.036

[126] Stattner S, Jones RP, Yip VS, Buchanan K, Poston GJ, Malik HZ, Fenwick SW. Microwave ablation with or without resection for colorectal liver metastases. Eur J Surg Oncol. 2013;39:844–849. DOI: 10.1016/j.ejso.2013.04.005

[127] Chang DT, Swaminath A, Kozak M, Weintraub J, Koong AC, Kim J, Dinniwell R, Brierley J, Kavanagh BD, Dawson LA, Schefter TE. Stereotactic body radiotherapy for colorectal liver metastases: a pooled analysis. Cancer. 2011;117:4060–4069. DOI: 10.1002/cncr.25997

[128] Liu DM, Thakor A, Baerlocher M, Alshammari MT, Lim H, Kos S, Kennedy AS, Wasan H. A review of conventional and drug-eluting chemoembolization in the treat-

ment of colorectal liver metastases: principles and proof. Future Oncol. 2015:1–8. DOI: 10.2217/fon.15.3

[129] Hasegawa K, Takahashi M, Ohba M, Kaneko J, Aoki T, Sakamoto Y, Sugawara Y, Kokudo N. Perioperative chemotherapy and liver resection for hepatic metastases of colorectal cancer. J Hepatobiliary Pancreat Sci. 2012;19:503–508. DOI: 10.1007/s00534-012-0509-7

[130] Wang CC, Li J. An update on chemotherapy of colorectal liver metastases. World J Gastroenterol. 2012;18:25–33. DOI: 10.3748/wjg.v18.i1.25

[131] Sugihara K, Uetake H. Therapeutic strategies for hepatic metastasis of colorectal cancer: overview. J Hepatobiliary Pancreat Sci. 2012;19:523–527. DOI: 10.1007/s00534-012-0524-8

[132] Sadahiro S, Suzuki T, Tanaka A, Okada K, Kamata H, Koisumi J. Clinical significance of and future perspectives for hepatic arterial infusion chemotherapy in patients with liver metastases from colorectal cancer. Surg Today. 2013;43:1088–1094. DOI: 10.1007/s00595-012-0416-1

[133] Richardson AJ, Laurence JM, Lam VW. Transarterial chemoembolization with irinotecan beads in the treatment of colorectal liver metastases: systematic review. J Vasc Interv Radiol. 2013;24:1209–1217. DOI: 10.1016/j.jvir.2013.05.055

[134] Tsujii M. Search for novel target molecules for the effective treatment or prevention of colorectal cancer. Digestion. 2012;85:99–102. DOI: 10.1159/000334678

[135] Therasse P, Arbuck SG, Eisenhauer EA, Wanders J, Kaplan RS, Rubinstein L, Verweij J, Van Glabbeke M, van Oosterom AT, Christian MC, Gwyther SG. New guidelines to evaluate the response to treatment in solid tumors. European Organization for Research and Treatment of Cancer, National Cancer Institute of the United States, National Cancer Institute of Canada. J Natl Cancer Inst. 2000;92:205–216.

[136] Eisenhauer EA, Therasse P, Bogaerts J, Schwartz LH, Sargent D, Ford R, Dancey J, Arbuck S, Gwyther S, Mooney M, Rubinstein L, Shankar L, Dodd L, Kaplan R, Lacombe D, Verweij J. New response evaluation criteria in solid tumours: revised RECIST guideline (version 1.1). Eur J Cancer. 2009;45:228–247. DOI: 10.1016/j.ejca.2008.10.026

[137] Suzuki C, Blomqvist L, Sundin A, Jacobsson H, Bystrom P, Berglund A, Nygren P, Glimelius B. The initial change in tumor size predicts response and survival in patients with metastatic colorectal cancer treated with combination chemotherapy. Ann Oncol. 2012;23:948–954. DOI: 10.1093/annonc/mdr350

[138] Chun YS, Vauthey JN, Boonsirikamchai P, Maru DM, Kopetz S, Palavecino M, Curley SA, Abdalla EK, Kaur H, Charnsangavej C, Loyer EM. Association of computed tomography morphologic criteria with pathologic response and survival in patients

treated with bevacizumab for colorectal liver metastases. JAMA. 2009;302:2338–2344. DOI: 10.1001/jama.2009.1755

[139] Hendlisz A, Golfinopoulos V, Garcia C, Covas A, Emonts P, Ameye L, Paesmans M, Deleporte A, Machiels G, Toussaint E, Vanderlinden B, Awada A, Piccart M, Flamen P. Serial FDG-PET/CT for early outcome prediction in patients with metastatic colorectal cancer undergoing chemotherapy. Ann Oncol. 2012;23:1687–1693. DOI: 10.1093/annonc/mdr554

[140] van Werven JR, Marsman HA, Nederveen AJ, Smits NJ, ten Kate FJ, van Gulik TM, Stoker J. Assessment of hepatic steatosis in patients undergoing liver resection: comparison of US, CT, T1-weighted dual-echo MR imaging, and point-resolved 1H MR spectroscopy. Radiology. 2010;256:159–168. DOI: 10.1148/radiol.10091790

[141] Scheele J, Stangl R, Altendorf-Hofmann A. Hepatic metastases from colorectal carcinoma: impact of surgical resection on the natural history. Br J Surg. 1990;77:1241–1246.

[142] Fong Y, Cohen AM, Fortner JG, Enker WE, Turnbull AD, Coit DG, Marrero AM, Prasad M, Blumgart LH, Brennan MF. Liver resection for colorectal metastases. J Clin Oncol. 1997;15:938–946.

[143] Adam R, Avisar E, Ariche A, Giachetti S, Azoulay D, Castaing D, Kunstlinger F, Levi F, Bismuth F. Five-year survival following hepatic resection after neoadjuvant therapy for nonresectable colorectal. Ann Surg Oncol. 2001;8:347–353.

[144] Simmonds PC, Primrose JN, Colquitt JL, Garden OJ, Poston GJ, Rees M. Surgical resection of hepatic metastases from colorectal cancer: a systematic review of published studies. Br J Cancer. 2006;94:982–999. DOI: 10.1038/sj.bjc.6603033

[145] Lorenz M, Muller HH. Randomized, multicenter trial of fluorouracil plus leucovorin administered either via hepatic arterial or intravenous infusion versus fluorodeoxyuridine administered via hepatic arterial infusion in patients with nonresectable liver metastases from colorectal carcinoma. J Clin Oncol. 2000;18:243–254.

[146] Saltz LB, Cox JV, Blanke C, Rosen LS, Fehrenbacher L, Moore MJ, Maroun JA, Ackland SP, Locker PK, Pirotta N, Elfring GL, Miller LL. Irinotecan plus fluorouracil and leucovorin for metastatic colorectal cancer. Irinotecan Study Group. N Engl J Med. 2000;343:905–914. DOI: 10.1056/nejm200009283431302

[147] Choti MA, Sitzmann JV, Tiburi MF, Sumetchotimetha W, Rangsin R, Schulick RD, Lillemoe KD, Yeo CJ, Cameron JL. Trends in long-term survival following liver resection for hepatic colorectal metastases. Ann Surg. 2002;235:759–766.

[148] Tomlinson JS, Jarnagin WR, DeMatteo RP, Fong Y, Kornprat P, Gonen M, Kemeny N, Brennan MF, Blumgart LH, D'Angelica M. Actual 10-year survival after resection of colorectal liver metastases defines cure. J Clin Oncol. 2007;25:4575–4580. DOI: 10.1200/jco.2007.11.0833.

Chapter 8

Surgical Indications, Timing, and Strategy in Non-colorectal Liver Metastases

Alessandro Uzzau, Serena Bertozzi,
Ambrogio P Londero, Stefano Bacchetti,
Enrico Maria Pasqual and Andrea Risaliti

Additional information is available at the end of the chapter

http://dx.doi.org/10.5772/61079

Abstract

Taking into consideration all primary solid tumors, the liver represents the most common site involved in distant metastasization, also due to its important blood reception from the majority of digestive organs. Despite the abundant literature and guidelines about colorectal liver metastases, there is still great debate about the treatment strategy in the case of non-colorectal ones. Therefore, in this chapter, we reviewed the treatment strategy and surgical indications for the most frequent non-colorectal liver metastases. In the case of neuroendocrine hepatic secondaries, the literature suggests that surgery should be always considered for patients with resectable hepatic disease, as this treatment results more likely to offer the best long-term outcome. For what concerns liver metastases from gastric cancer, surgical approach should always be undertaken if indications are appropriate, after a multidisciplinary discussion to plan an adequate multidisciplinary adjuvant treatment, a proper patient selection, and the exclusion of additional secondary tumors or extrahepatic metastases. Taking into consideration liver secondaries from breast cancer and their chemosensitivity, in the absence of brain and lung lesions, it can be considered a space for liver surgery, especially in the case of single lesions or a maximum of two lesions with dimensions within 3 cm. However, as the number of cancer survivors is progressively increasing and, with it, the number of patients affected by non-colorectal liver metastases, further randomized controlled trials are required in order to better define the benefit of hepatic surgery in these kinds of patients.

Keywords: Non-colorectal liver metastases, Non-colorectal hepatic metastases, Metastatic neuroendocrine tumors, Metastatic breast cancer

1. Introduction

Cancer metastasization is a highly selective, sequential, interdependent, nonrandom process which causes transient or permanent changes in different genes at the DNA and/or mRNA, creating a complex phenotype which favors the survival of a population of tumor cells within an organ environment, distant from the primary tumor [1, 2]. This kind of complex process usually requires many years in order to complete the great series of cumulative DNA changes which consent neoplastic cells to metastasize. As the primary tumor growth may be very slow and the metastasization process does not directly depend on primary tumor size, we can observe two kinds of metastases based on the timing of their diagnosis: synchronous metastases are defined as secondary lesions diagnosed within the first year after primary tumor diagnosis, although this time, interval may vary in the literature between six months and one year, while metachronous metastases are usually diagnosed after one year from the primary tumor diagnosis.

Taking into consideration all primary tumors, the liver represents the most common site of the distant metastases. This particular affinity for distant metastases may have different explanations. First, it may be attributable to the site specificity patterns of neoplastic cells from various primary cancers, which found the liver as the adequate soil where to seed their circulating neoplastic cells [3, 4]. Furthermore, the liver receives 30% of the whole cardiac output, second only to the kidney for the quantity of blood which every day will perfuse its parenchyma, and is consequently more susceptible to neoplastic cell attachment. Moreover, anatomical or mechanical considerations, such as the efferent venous blood stream or the loco-regional lymphatic drainage, may be strongly responsible for this preference in the metastasization site [5]. In fact, most intra-abdominal cancers, and in particular those which originated in the digestive tract, result in having a great affinity for liver metastasization.

In spite of the great progresses of surgical techniques against the primary tumors, as well as the improvement of adjuvant therapies, metastatic disease continues to be the greatest challenge for the medical and the surgical oncologists. In fact, metastases are well recognized as being the major cause of death among neoplastic patients, and the prognosis of patients affected by unresectable liver metastases is very poor. However, although once metastatic malignancies were commonly considered as a terminal neoplastic stage, nowadays, many different therapeutical options have been introduced in order to provide a safe and efficient treatment for these kinds of patients and improve both their quantity and quality of life [6–9].

Despite the abundant literature about colorectal liver metastases and the existence of a great number of guidelines about this argument, there is still great debate about the treatment strategy in the case of non-colorectal ones and controversies especially about the management of rare liver secondaries. On the other hand, a recent review about non-colorectal non-neuroendocrine liver metastases demonstrated surgery to be a benefit for these kinds of metastatic patients, especially for those affected by primary testicular, ovarian, and renal cell cancers but also for women with isolated breast cancer metastases to the liver [10].

Obviously, patients affected by rare hepatic metastases should be conveyed into bigger and more experienced centers, which could be able to more appropriately treat this kind of disease. However, metastatic patients are always more numerous – thanks to the improvement of chemotherapy and the introduction of targeted biological drugs – and deserve as many chances of treatment as possible in order to continue their long battle against cancer. In this chapter, we will then discuss indications and timing of surgery in cases of the most frequent non-colorectal liver metastases.

2. Liver Metastases from Neuroendocrine Tumors

Neuroendocrine tumors (NETs) include a heterogeneous group of neoplasms with different origins and biological behaviors [11–13]. They are commonly distinguished into two classes based on their primary origin: pancreatic neuroendocrine tumors (also known as islet cell tumors) and gastrointestinal neuroendocrine tumors (also known as carcinoids) [14–16].

The widely promulgated benignity of these neoplasms has been more times brought into question, due to the high prevalence of distant metastases and recurrences, and the current literature recognizes nowadays their malignant potential [12, 17–24]. In particular, the recent classifications of the 7th American Joint Committee on Cancer/Union Internationale Contre le Cancer (AJCC/UICC) 2009 and of the European Neuroendocrine Tumor Society (ENETS) 2006, associated with the WHO classification 2010, classified NETs into well-differentiated neuroendocrine tumors (low and intermediate grade based on the Ki67 labeling index, also named NET-G1 or carcinoid and NET-G2, respectively) and into the group of neuroendocrine carcinomas (high grade, poorly differentiated, also named NEC) [21].

Despite their rarity, liver metastases from NETs are not an infrequent finding, because they are usually characterized by a very slow growth pattern and diagnosed in advanced stages [9, 15, 25–29]. In particular, NETs present with liver metastases in even the 50–75% of cases [30–32]. In an analysis of Modlin and colleagues on 13,715 patients, synchronous distant metastases were already evident in 12.9% of patients with gastrointestinal NETs, whose 5-year overall survival rate resulted 67.2% [13].

The occurrence of hepatic secondaries is one of the most important prognostic factor for survival [9, 21, 33, 34]. In fact, although for patients with unresectable liver disease, biotherapy with somatostatin analogues, peptide-mediated radioreceptor therapy, transarterial chemoembolization, selective intra-arterial radiotherapy, or new molecular target-directed therapy can be employed [16, 35, 36], these therapies are considered as palliative.

The role of liver surgery for patients with liver metastases from gastrointestinal NETs remains to be an argument of great debate. In particular, the very small number of patients affected by NETs explains the lack of randomized control trials in order to better define the role of surgery in these rare cases. Moreover, the usually inert growth of NETs and their long-term natural history make even more difficult to assess the real effectiveness of hepatic surgical approach on their overall survival. Furthermore, it is well known that in most patients, neuroendocrine liver metastases recur after hepatic resection in up to 70–94% of cases at 5 years [21, 24, 25, 33, 37–39], the liver is the most common site of progression of disease (69%) [35], and data on repeat liver directed surgery for recurrent disease have been extremely limited and controversial [36]. In particular, in a study of Saxena and colleagues, most patients with hepatic metastases from NETs experienced treatment failure after liver resection. In particular, 57 patients (79%) developed disease progression at a median time of 23 months, and the liver represented the most common site of progression of disease (69%) [23]. In another multi-institutional study on 339 patients, Mayo and colleagues demonstrated that the majority of liver metastases from NETs came from carcinoid (53%) and, at 5 years after surgery, their recurrence rate was 94% [38]. Therefore, the true curative role of liver-directed surgery results is still very questionable.

A recent meta-analysis performed on five studies, considering 374 patients affected by NETs liver metastases treated in a conservative manner and 161 treated with liver surgery, demonstrated a significant increased survival in the group of patients treated with surgical hepatic resections HR 0.45 (CI.95 0.34–0.60) in comparison to conservative treatments and to embolization HR 0.34 (CI.95 0.21–0.55) [40]. All considered studies showed an increased survival in the groups treated with complete surgical resection of liver metastases, but none of the included studies were randomized so that the clinical evidence was low [21, 41, 42].

A systematic review considering 29 studies (between 1980 and 2009) found 5 years OS of 70.5% (range 31–100%) and a 5-year progression-free survival of 29% (range 6–66%) [43]. Histological grade, extrahepatic disease, and macroscopically incomplete resection of liver metastases were associated with poor prognosis. In another multi-institutional study evaluating 339 patients, Mayo et al. demonstrated at multivariate analysis that synchronous disease, nonfunctional NET hormonal status, and extrahepatic disease were the most important predictive factors of worse survival [36]. Concerning other prognostic parameters for primary NETs and liver metastases, Katz et al. demonstrated that the robust presence of tumor-infiltrating lymphocytes is a significant predictor of outcome [44]. Other recent articles confirmed surgical therapy to be the most efficient approach against solitary hepatic metastases [7, 8, 14, 22, 23, 33, 34, 40, 45, 46], with a potential curative resection of liver secondaries can be undertaken in 13.7 to 24.5% of patients with metastatic NETs [47–49], and a significant reduction of carcinoid symptoms [43], but the majority of studies focused exclusively on resection rather than combined-modality approaches with ablation or chemotherapy.

Taking into consideration our institutional cases of liver metastases from NETs, including 52% of synchronous metastases and 48% of metachronous ones, the overall survival of patients who underwent hepatic resections and OLT resulted, respectively, in 44.9% (95% CI 26.0–77.7%) and 50% (95% CI 12.5–100.0%) at 5 years [45]. The median number of resected hepatic metastases was 3. Surgical radicalness (R0) was reached in 84% of cases. Recurrences happened in 60% of patients, among which, 66.7% were intrahepatic and 33.3% extrahepatic. Postoperative complications affected 12% of patients but required reintervention in a single case.

In our opinion, surgery should be always considered for patients with resectable hepatic disease, as this treatment results more likely to offer the best long-term outcome. All patients should be considered for curative surgical treatment, but also palliative resection of liver metastases can be suggested. The advantage that can be potentially achieved with surgery is that of removing all gross diseases. In the future, new clinical and biological prognostic factors could be of help for the better identification of those patients who might benefit from hepatic surgical therapy.

3. Liver Metastases from Gastric Cancer

Gastric cancer is the fourth most common cancer worldwide [50] and the second cause of cancer-related death worldwide [50]. Despite the significant reduction of gastric cancer incidence in the last 20 years, we observed an increase of advanced stages at diagnosis [51]. In Western Europe and Anglo-Saxon world, the incidence of hepatic metastases from gastric cancer during the course of the disease results about 30%-50%, including both synchronous and metachronous metastases [52, 53]. In particular, at the time of diagnosis, 35% of patients present with evidence of distant metastases, and 4% to 14% have metastatic disease to the liver [54–74], whereas metachronous metastases after curative gastrectomy are detected in up to 25–30% of patients, 80% of which appear within the first 2 postoperative years.

Surgical treatment of hepatic metastases from gastric cancers remains to be an argument of great debate [72, 75–78]. In fact, although many studies observed no survival difference among patients submitted or not to liver surgery, in selected cases, an aggressive treatment can achieve unexpected results [65–68, 70, 73, 74, 79–85]. Moreover, surgical approach is not always possible, due to multiple hepatic metastases or the presence of extrahepatic secondaries [52, 53], and only 0.4 to 1% of metastatic gastric cancer patients result in being eligible for radical surgery [54, 56, 57, 86].

Resection of liver metastases from gastric cancer was initially indicated in patients with synchronous metastases who have no peritoneal dissemination or other distant metastases and in those with metachronous metastases without any other recurrent lesion [68] and only if a complete resection of the metastases can be achieved without compromising postoperative liver function [70]. Thereafter, Roh and colleagues supported surgery indication only in cases of metastases in one lobe of the liver without peritoneal dissemination, hilar node metastases, or distant metastases [64]. Recently, in accordance with these findings, the Japanese Gastric Cancer Association revisited its treatment guidelines, which in the case of stage IV gastric cancer recommend only chemotherapy, radiation, palliative surgery, and best supportive care [87], in favor of surgery with curative intent for potentially resectable M1 disease, including patients with resectable hepatic metastasis, positive cytological examination of peritoneal washes, or swollen nodes in the para-aortic region [88].

Unfortunately, if we review the current literature, hepatectomy was indicated in only 0.4% to 1% of gastric cancer patients with liver metastases, because most hepatic metastases from gastric adenocarcinoma are multiple, bilateral, and combined with peritoneal or lymph node metastases, which directly invade adjacent organs, so that finally very few patients result as good candidates for liver surgery [89]. Moreover, surgical indications for liver metastases of gastric origin must be carefully determined because of the biological, clinical, and pathological aggressiveness of the disease [90, 91]. However, even if the percentage of patients who may benefit from resection is probably small, the majority of authors agree that the local treatment of hepatic metastases, compared to palliation or systemic treatment, significantly improved overall survival among these patients [56]. In particular, overall 5-year survival rate of gastric cancer metastatic to the liver ranges between 0 and 10% [58, 59, 92], whereas it rises up to 20% after curative hepatectomy in the literature [64–68, 73, 93]. Furthermore, taking into consideration the only article about hepatic metastasis local re-treatment after recurrence, the authors found a survival advantage in local treatment repetition [94].

In the current literature, many factors resulted in influencing the survival rate of gastric cancer patients with hepatic metastases. In particular, the prognosis seems to be significantly worsened by greater extent of hepatic involvement (H3) or macroscopic peritoneal dissemination (P1) detected at surgical exploration, by greater number (>1) and size of hepatic metastases in H1-2 and P0 patients [61, 62, 95, 96], by greater tumor size (T4), nodal involvement (N+ independently by the extension of the metastatic spread) or higher grading (G3) [63, 80, 97], and the timing of liver metastases diagnosis if metachronous to the primary tumor diagnosis [68, 70, 91]. Therefore, these factors should be considered as possible confounding factors in the future studies. In addition, considering all these prognostic factors, some authors suggested the necessity to clearly identify the patients which could benefit from surgical treatment, in order to offer a chance to cure the patients who have good prognostic factors and to avoid overtreatment in case of absence of these factors [56].

Taking into account local procedures for hepatic metastases, no consensus about standardized therapeutic regimen for metastatic gastric cancer has been achieved yet, so that a variety of alternative, multidisciplinary therapies have been recommended by clinical practice guidelines, including radiofrequency ablation (RFA) [86], transarterial chemoembolization (TACE) [98], microwave coagulation therapy (MCT) [95], adjuvant chemotherapy, molecular targeted therapy, or palliative supportive care [99–101]. In particular, RFA, MCT, and TACE could additionally be used in the case of an isolated metastasis in either half of the liver, in the absence of extrahepatic disease [102, 103]. For example, in some series of patients treated by RFA, survival rates resulted similar to those reported in the best surgical series [61, 104, 105].

In summary, if indications are appropriate, surgical approach in the case of hepatic metastases from gastric cancer should always be undertaken, after a multidisciplinary discussion, a proper patient selection, and the exclusion of additional secondary tumors or extrahepatic metastases. Neoadjuvant chemotherapy, as well as other multidisciplinary, adjuvant treatment modalities, may have a synergic role if combined with surgery. And in particular, local interventional procedures, such as RFA, MCT, or TACE, may be useful in selected patients.

4. Liver Metastases from Breast Cancer

Breast cancer is the most prevalent cancer among the female population worldwide, with a peak of incidence after menopause. Despite the gradual reduction of locally advanced breast cancers and the consensual increase of early breast cancer – thanks to the introduction of an organized mammographic screening [106, 107] and the evident therapeutic improvement – stage IV breast cancer continues to represent a fatal disease and its incidence does not seem to reduce with the passing of years. The first explanation may be that distant metastasis in the hematogenous way does not depend on tumor size nor on lymph node involvement, which is usually an expression of metastasization in the lymphatic way. Secondly, groups of patients who more frequently present distant metastasis from breast cancer do not usually represent a screening target, such as young premenopausal women.

Typical breast cancer metastasization sites are, in order of frequency, the bones, liver, lungs, and brain. In our institutional casistic, distant metastasis prevalence among breast cancer patients resulted about 10%, which in about the 20% cases are synchronous with the primary cancer diagnosis, whereas the remaining 80% of women developed metachronous metastasis.

In the context of the incidence of distant metastases, hepatic ones vary from 5 to 34% [108–111], with values rising up to over 60% in autopsy series [112]. The prognosis is poor in this area being the median survival of 1–20 months from the diagnosis of liver metastases [108, 109, 113, 114]. Long survivals seem to be related to a positive endocrine treatment response, performed in the subgroup of patients with positive estrogen receptor pattern, with median survivals around 14 months compared to 4 months in the other cases [114]. Overall, with current chemotherapy regimens, survivals ranging from 1 to 25 months are obtained. However, after discontinuation of chemotherapy, only 40% of cases are responsive to the same regimen.

Studies on the outcome of local treatment currently do not offer univocal results, probably because of possible selection bias of cases operated and/or treated with other modalities such as thermal ablation, destruction with yttrium, or chemoembolization. On average, in the cases undergoing liver resection, the median survival is of 27–63 months. In almost all studies, however, there is a subgroup of patients with very encouraging survival responses, and many efforts have been directed toward the identification of the related prognostic factors. At the moment, it seems that the receptor status of the primary tumor, the value of Ki-67, the number of liver lesions removed, resection margin, and menopausal status may play a positive role on prognosis [115]. However, the proportion of patients that presents the favorable characteristics is small, not exceeding 3% of patients [116].

Over the past 20 years, the survival of patients with stage IV has been gradually improving as a function of new chemotherapy regimens, local control with radiation therapy, and other forms of intervention. As previously stated, the metastatic breast cancer involves with a high frequency the bones, lungs, liver, and brain. Individually or predominantly considered within the concept of "oligometastatic state," each of these sites leads to different outcomes with median survival of 43 months for nodal involvement, 33 months for metastatic bones, 22 months for the lung, and 12 months for liver. For multiple sites of metastases or brain metastases, survival values collapse, respectively, to 9 and 3 months [117]. Given the prognostic value represented by each metastatic site, the meticulous choice of the liver resection candidate is obvious. In fact, in the studies that show the reference global population, the rate of resection is absolutely modest, around 0.3%, but with a high resection rate, 81%, being the non-resected cases due to intraoperatively carcinomatosis diagnosis [118–120].

In the most recent and representative case studies series, resection of breast cancer liver metastases shows that the appearance of metastases follows the discovery of the primary tumor of an average of 40 months (23–77), the indication for resection concerns cases with single lesion or a maximum of two lesions, with dimensions within 3 cm in most cases, and that in most cases, major resections were performed (more than 3 liver segments) with values of radical resection (negative margin resection) of more than 80% [118–125]. The average survival values reported by these series range from 32 to 74 months and the 5-year follow-up survival rates are of 34–80%. Interestingly, the rates of postoperative mortality are of 0% and morbidity of 0–44% that make absolutely acceptable the surgical treatment in these cases thus selected. Prognostic factors evaluated in multivariate methods ultimately lead to the conclusion that the only real risk factor is represented by the positive resection margin.

Considering these results and taking into account the chemosensitivity of breast cancer emerges the consideration that even in cases of more consistent hepatic invasion, in the absence of brain and lung lesions, it can be considered a space for liver surgery [126]. It is evident from many series that survival is influenced by the state of the free margin, although not always the gap between R0 and R1 leads to a robust statistical difference [122]. Therefore, considering the possibility of a chemotherapy response and the greater possibility of surgical treatment also linked to the impact of new intraoperative technologies (e.g., radio frequency and microwave), it seems natural to expect in the immediate future an expansion of the surgical indications for breast cancer liver metastasis.

As a paradigm of these considerations, we take as example the case of a woman who after two breast surgeries for two metachronous cancers underwent chemotherapy for the appearance of liver metastases, with partial response, followed by rupture of one of the lesions and therefore emergency surgery for hemoperitoneum. Subsequently, after about six months, she developed a second hemoperitoneum treated again by surgical hemostasis. Afterward, she was transferred to our center and it was then made with palliative intent a major liver resection, left hepatectomy en bloc with part of the stomach and removal of two peritoneal implants. In the same intervention, the other two lesions on the right liver lobe were not treated. These two lesions were later treated by radiofrequency ablation combined with transcatheter arterial chemoembolization. Surprisingly the patient is alive and disease-free 43 months after the last procedure.

5. Conclusive Summary

Thanks to the improvement in the diagnostic and therapeutic pathways, the number of cancer survivors is progressively increasing, as well as the number of metastatic patients. Taking into consideration all primary solid tumors, the liver represents the most frequent site involved by distant metastasization, also due to its anatomical position and its important blood reception from the majority of digestive organs.

Despite the abundant literature and guidelines about colorectal liver metastases, there is still great debate about the treatment strategy in the case of non-colorectal ones. Anyway, many experiences have been published in the last decades about surgical treatment of the most frequent non-colorectal liver metastases. In particular, we reviewed surgical strategies in the case of hepatic secondaries from neuroendocrine tumors, gastric cancer, and breast cancer. And in every case, the literature suggests a role for hepatic surgery for patients with resectable hepatic disease.

However, the number of considered patients is often very limited as well as the statistical strength of the current literature. Therefore, further randomized controlled trials are required in order to better define the benefit of hepatic surgery in these kinds of patients.

http://dx.doi.org/10.5772/61079

Author details

Alessandro Uzzau[1]*, Serena Bertozzi[1,2], Ambrogio P Londero[3], Stefano Bacchetti[1], Enrico Maria Pasqual[1], Andrea Risaliti[1]

*Address all correspondence to: alessandro.uzzau@uniud.it

1 Clinic of Surgery, DISM, DSMB, University of Udine, Italy

2 IRCCS CRO, Aviano (PN), Italy

3 Unit of Obstetrics and Gynecology, S. Polo Hospital, Monfalcone (GO), Italy

References

[1] Fidler IJ. Critical factors in the biology of human cancer metastasis: twenty-eighth G.H.A. Clowes memorial award lecture. Cancer Res. 1990;**50**:6130–6138.

[2] Fidler IJ, Radinsky R. Genetic control of cancer metastasis. J Natl Cancer Inst. 1990; **82**:166–168.

[3] Langley RR, Fidler IJ. The seed and soil hypothesis revisited–the role of tumor-stroma interactions in metastasis to different organs. Int J Cancer. 2011;**128**:2527–2535. .

[4] Fidler IJ, Kim SJ, Langley RR. The role of the organ microenvironment in the biology and therapy of cancer metastasis. J Cell Biochem. 2007;**101**:927–936. .

[5] Sugarbaker E. Patterns of metastasis in human malignancies. Cancer Biol Rev. 1981; **2**:235–278.

[6] Frilling A, Li J, Malamutmann E, Schmid KW, Bockisch A, Broelsch CE. Treatment of liver metastases from neuroendocrine tumours in relation to the extent of hepatic disease. Br J Surg. 2009;**96**:175–184. .

[7] Landry CS, Scoggins CR, McMasters KM, Martin RCG 2nd. Management of hepatic metastasis of gastrointestinal carcinoid tumors. J Surg Oncol. 2008;**97**:253–258. .

[8] Musunuru S, Chen H, Rajpal S, Stephani N, McDermott JC, Holen K, et al. Metastatic neuroendocrine hepatic tumors: resection improves survival. Arch Surg. 2006; **141**:1000–1004; discussion 1005. .

[9] Hellman P, Lundström T, Ohrvall U, Eriksson B, Skogseid B, Oberg K, et al. Effect of surgery on the outcome of midgut carcinoid disease with lymph node and liver metastases. World J Surg. 2002;**26**:991–997. .

[10] Fitzgerald TL, Brinkley J, Banks S, Vohra N, Englert ZP, Zervos EE. The benefits of liver resection for non-colorectal, non-neuroendocrine liver metastases: a systematic review. Langenbecks Arch Surg. 2014;**399**:989–1000. .

[11] Schimmack S, Svejda B, Lawrence B, Kidd M, Modlin IM. The diversity and commonalities of gastroenteropancreatic neuroendocrine tumors. Langenbecks Arch Surg. 2011;**396**:273–298. .

[12] Lawrence B, Gustafsson BI, Chan A, Svejda B, Kidd M, Modlin IM. The epidemiology of gastroenteropancreatic neuroendocrine tumors. Endocrinol Metab Clin N Am. 2011; **40**:1–18, vii. .

[13] Modlin IM, Lye KD, Kidd M. A 5-decade analysis of 13,715 carcinoid tumors. Cancer. 2003;**97**:934–959. .

[14] Oberg K, Castellano D. Current knowledge on diagnosis and staging of neuroendocrine tumors. Cancer Metastasis Rev. 2011;**30 Suppl 1**:3–7. .

[15] Auernhammer CJ, Göke B. Therapeutic strategies for advanced neuroendocrine carcinomas of jejunum/ileum and pancreatic origin. Gut. 2011;**60**:1009–1021. .

[16] Eriksson B. New drugs in neuroendocrine tumors: rising of new therapeutic philosophies? Curr Opin Oncol. 2010;**22**:381–386. .

[17] Turaga KK, Kvols LK. Recent progress in the understanding, diagnosis, and treatment of gastroenteropancreatic neuroendocrine tumors. CA: A Cancer J Clin. 2011; **61**:113–132. .

[18] Klimstra DS, Modlin IR, Coppola D, Lloyd RV, Suster S. The pathologic classification of neuroendocrine tumors: a review of nomenclature, grading, and staging systems. Pancreas. 2010;**39**:707–712. .

[19] Soga J. The term "carcinoid" is a misnomer: the evidence based on local invasion. J Exp Clin Cancer Res. 2009;**28**:15. .

[20] Rorstad O. Prognostic indicators for carcinoid neuroendocrine tumors of the gastrointestinal tract. J Surg Oncol. 2005;**89**:151–160. .

[21] Chamberlain RS, Canes D, Brown KT, Saltz L, Jarnagin W, Fong Y, et al. Hepatic neuroendocrine metastases: does intervention alter outcomes? J Am Coll Surg. 2000; **190**:432–445.

[22] Bonaccorsi-Riani E, Apestegui C, Jouret-Mourin A, Sempoux C, Goffette P, Ciccarelli O, et al. Liver transplantation and neuroendocrine tumors: lessons from a single centre experience and from the literature review. Transpl Int. 2010;**23**:668–678. .

[23] Saxena A, Chua TC, Sarkar A, Chu F, Liauw W, Zhao J, et al. Progression and survival results after radical hepatic metastasectomy of indolent advanced neuroendocrine neoplasms (NENs) supports an aggressive surgical approach. Surgery. 2011;**149**:209–220. .

[24] Nave H, Mössinger E, Feist H, Lang H, Raab H. Surgery as primary treatment in patients with liver metastases from carcinoid tumors: a retrospective, unicentric study over 13 years. Surgery. 2001;**129**:170–175.

[25] Cho C, Wust P, Hildebrandt B, Issels RD, Sehouli J, Kerner T, et al. Regional hyperthermia of the abdomen in conjunction with chemotherapy for peritoneal carcinomatosis: evaluation of two annular-phased-array applicators. Int J Hyperthermia. 2008;**24**:399–408. .

[26] Nikou GC, Lygidakis NJ, Toubanakis C, Pavlatos S, Tseleni-Balafouta S, Giannatou E, et al. Current diagnosis and treatment of gastrointestinal carcinoids in a series of 101 patients: the significance of serum chromogranin-A, somatostatin receptor scintigraphy and somatostatin analogues. Hepato-Gastroenterology. 2005;**52**:731–741.

[27] Mazzaferro V, Pulvirenti A, Coppa J. Neuroendocrine tumors metastatic to the liver: how to select patients or liver transplantation? J Hepatol. 2007;**47**:460–466. .

[28] Norton JA. Endocrine tumours of the gastrointestinal tract. Surgical treatment of neuroendocrine metastases. Best Pract Res Clin Gastroenterol. 2005;**19**:577–583. .

[29] Janson ET, Holmberg L, Stridsberg M, Eriksson B, Theodorsson E, Wilander E, et al. Carcinoid tumors: analysis of prognostic factors and survival in 301 patients from a referral center. Ann Oncol. 1997;**8**:685–690.

[30] Nykjaer KM, Grønbaek H, Nielsen DT, Christiansen P, Astrup LB. Description of patients with midgut carcinoid tumours: clinical database from a Danish centre. In Vivo. 2007;**21**:679–684.

[31] Modlin IM, Oberg K, Chung DC, Jensen RT, de Herder WW, Thakker RV, et al. Gastroenteropancreatic neuroendocrine tumours. Lancet Oncol. 2008;**9**:61–72. .

[32] Gomez D, Malik HZ, Al-Mukthar A, Menon KV, Toogood GJ, Lodge JPA, et al. Hepatic resection for metastatic gastrointestinal and pancreatic neuroendocrine tumours: outcome and prognostic predictors. HPB (Oxford). 2007;**9**:345–351. .

[33] Sarmiento JM, Heywood G, Rubin J, Ilstrup DM, Nagorney DM, Que FG. Surgical treatment of neuroendocrine metastases to the liver: a plea for resection to increase survival. J Am Coll Surg. 2003;**197**:29–37. .

[34] Norton ID, Jones DB. Endoscopic ultrasound: diagnostic and therapeutic applications. Intern Med J. 2003;**33**:26–32.

[35] Strosberg JR, Cheema A, Kvols LK. A review of systemic and liver-directed therapies for metastatic neuroendocrine tumors of the gastroenteropancreatic tract. Cancer Control. 2011;**18**:127–137.

[36] Srirajaskanthan R, Toumpanakis C, Meyer T, Caplin ME. Review article: future therapies for management of metastatic gastroenteropancreatic neuroendocrine tumours. Aliment Pharmacol Ther. 2009;**29**:1143–1154. .

[37] Jaeck D, Oussoultzoglou E, Bachellier P, Lemarque P, Weber JC, Nakano H, et al. Hepatic metastases of gastroenteropancreatic neuroendocrine tumors: safe hepatic surgery. World J Surg. 2001;**25**:689–692.

[38] Mayo SC, de Jong MC, Pulitano C, Clary BM, Reddy SK, Gamblin TC, et al. Surgical management of hepatic neuroendocrine tumor metastasis: results from an international multi-institutional analysis. Ann Surg Oncol. 2010;**17**:3129–3136. .

[39] Yao KA, Talamonti MS, Nemcek A, Angelos P, Chrisman H, Skarda J, et al. Indications and results of liver resection and hepatic chemoembolization for metastatic gastrointestinal neuroendocrine tumors. Surgery. 2001;**130**:677–82; discussion 682–5. .

[40] Bacchetti S, Bertozzi S, Londero AP, Uzzau A, Pasqual EM. Surgical treatment and survival in patients with liver metastases from neuroendocrine tumors: a meta-analysis of observational studies. Int J Hepatol. 2013;**2013**:235040. .

[41] Osborne DA, Zervos EE, Strosberg J, Strosberg J, Boe BA, Malafa M, et al. Improved outcome with cytoreduction versus embolization for symptomatic hepatic metastases of carcinoid and neuroendocrine tumors. Ann Surg Oncol. 2006;**13**:572–581. .

[42] Que FG, Nagorney DM, Batts KP, Linz LJ, Kvols LK. Hepatic resection for metastatic neuroendocrine carcinomas. Am J Surg. 1995;**169**:36–42; discussion 42–3.

[43] Saxena A, Chua TC, Perera M, Chu F, Morris DL. Surgical resection of hepatic metastases from neuroendocrine neoplasms: a systematic review. Surg Oncol. 2012; **21**:e131–e141. .

[44] Katz SC, Donkor C, Glasgow K, Pillarisetty VG, Gönen M, Espat NJ, et al. T cell infiltrate and outcome following resection of intermediate-grade primary neuroendocrine tumours and liver metastases. HPB (Oxford). 2010;**12**:674–683. .

[45] Bacchetti S, Pasqual EM, Bertozzi S, Londero AP, Risaliti A. Curative versus palliative surgical resection of liver metastases in patients with neuroendocrine tumors: a meta-analysis of observational studies. Gland Surg. 2014;**3**:243–251. .

[46] Sutton R, Doran HE, Williams EMI, Vora J, Vinjamuri S, Evans J, et al. Surgery for midgut carcinoid. Endocr Relat Cancer. 2003;**10**:469–481.

[47] Glazer ES, Tseng JF, Al-Refaie W, Solorzano CC, Liu P, Willborn KA, et al. Long-term survival after surgical management of neuroendocrine hepatic metastases. HPB (Oxford). 2010;**12**:427–433. .

[48] Frilling A, Rogiers X, Malagó M, Liedke OM, Kaun M, Broelsch CE. Treatment of liver metastases in patients with neuroendocrine tumors. Langenbecks Arch Surg. 1998; **383**:62–70.

[49] Coppa J, Pulvirenti A, Schiavo M, Romito R, Collini P, Di Bartolomeo M, et al. Resection versus transplantation for liver metastases from neuroendocrine tumors. Transpl Proc. 2001;**33**:1537–1539.

[50] Jemal A, Bray F, Center MM, Ferlay J, Ward E, Forman D. Global cancer statistics. CA Cancer J Clin. 2011;**61**:69–90. .

[51] Fayçal J, Bessaguet C, Nousbaum JB, Cauvin JM, Cholet F, Bideau K, et al. Epidemiology and long term survival of gastric carcinoma in the French district of Finistere between 1984 and 1995. Gastroenterol Clin Biol. 2005;**29**:23–32.

[52] Dicken BJ, Bigam DL, Cass C, Mackey JR, Joy AA, Hamilton SM. Gastric adenocarcinoma: review and considerations for future directions. Ann Surg. 2005; **241**:27–39.

[53] D'Angelica M, Gonen M, Brennan MF, Turnbull AD, Bains M, Karpeh MS. Patterns of initial recurrence in completely resected gastric adenocarcinoma. Ann Surg. 2004; **240**:808–816.

[54] Qiu JL, Deng MG, Li W, Zou RH, Li BK, Zheng Y, et al. Hepatic resection for synchronous hepatic metastasis from gastric cancer. Eur J Surg Oncol. 2013;**39**:694–700. .

[55] Wang D, Zhang GB, Yan L, Wei XE, Zhang YZ, Li WB. CT and enhanced CT in diagnosis of gastrointestinal neuroendocrine carcinomas. Abdom Imaging. 2012; **37**:738–745. .

[56] Romano F, Garancini M, Uggeri F, Degrate L, Nespoli L, Gianotti L, et al. Surgical treatment of liver metastases of gastric cancer: state of the art. World J Surg Oncol. 2012;**10**:157. .

[57] Takemura N, Saiura A, Koga R, Arita J, Yoshioka R, Ono Y, et al. Long-term outcomes after surgical resection for gastric cancer liver metastasis: an analysis of 64 macroscopically complete resections. Langenbecks Arch Surg. 2012;**397**:951–957. .

[58] Shin A, Kim J, Park S. Gastric cancer epidemiology in Korea. J Gastric Cancer. 2011; **11**:135–140. .

[59] Schlansky B, Sonnenberg A. Epidemiology of noncardia gastric adenocarcinoma in the United States. Am J Gastroenterol. 2011;**106**:1978–1985. .

[60] Makino H, Kunisaki C, Izumisawa Y, Tokuhisa M, Oshima T, Nagano Y, et al. Indication for hepatic resection in the treatment of liver metastasis from gastric cancer. Anticancer Res. 2010;**30**:2367–2376.

[61] Cheon SH, Rha SY, Jeung HC, Im CK, Kim SH, Kim HR, et al. Survival benefit of combined curative resection of the stomach (D2 resection) and liver in gastric cancer patients with liver metastases. Ann Oncol. 2008;**19**:1146–1153. .

[62] Sakamoto Y, Sano T, Shimada K, Esaki M, Saka M, Fukagawa T, et al. Favorable indications for hepatectomy in patients with liver metastasis from gastric cancer. J Surg Oncol. 2007;**95**:534–539. .

[63] Koga R, Yamamoto J, Ohyama S, Saiura A, Seki M, Seto Y, et al. Liver resection for metastatic gastric cancer: experience with 42 patients including eight long-term survivors. Jpn J Clin Oncol. 2007;**37**:836–842. .

[64] Roh HR, Suh KS, Lee HJ, Yang HK, Choe KJ, Lee KU. Outcome of hepatic resection for metastatic gastric cancer. Am Surg. 2005;**71**:95–99.

[65] Sakamoto Y, Ohyama S, Yamamoto J, Yamada K, Seki M, Ohta Ki, et al. Surgical resection of liver metastases of gastric cancer: an analysis of a 17-year experience with 22 patients. Surgery. 2003;**133**:507–511. .

[66] Shirabe K, Shimada M, Matsumata T, Higashi H, Yakeishi Y, Wakiyama S, et al. Analysis of the prognostic factors for liver metastasis of gastric cancer after hepatic resection: a multi-institutional study of the indications for resection. Hepatogastroenterology. 2003;**50**:1560–1563.

[67] Saiura A, Umekita N, Inoue S, Maeshiro T, Miyamoto S, Matsui Y, et al. Clinicopathological features and outcome of hepatic resection for liver metastasis from gastric cancer. Hepatogastroenterology. 2002;**49**:1062–1065.

[68] Okano K, Maeba T, Ishimura K, Karasawa Y, Goda F, Wakabayashi H, et al. Hepatic resection for metastatic tumors from gastric cancer. Ann Surg. 2002;**235**:86–91.

[69] Zacherl J, Zacherl M, Scheuba C, Steininger R, Wenzl E, Mühlbacher F, et al. Analysis of hepatic resection of metastasis originating from gastric adenocarcinoma. J Gastrointest Surg. 2002;**6**:682–689.

[70] Ambiru S, Miyazaki M, Ito H, Nakagawa K, Shimizu H, Yoshidome H, et al. Benefits and limits of hepatic resection for gastric metastases. Am J Surg. 2001;**181**:279–283.

[71] Imamura H, Matsuyama Y, Shimada R, Kubota M, Nakayama A, Kobayashi A, et al. A study of factors influencing prognosis after resection of hepatic metastases from colorectal and gastric carcinoma. Am J Gastroenterol. 2001;**96**:3178–3184. .

[72] Elias D, Cavalcanti de Albuquerque A, Eggenspieler P, Plaud B, Ducreux M, Spielmann M, et al. Resection of liver metastases from a noncolorectal primary: indications and results based on 147 monocentric patients. J Am Coll Surg. 1998;**187**:487–493.

[73] Miyazaki M, Itoh H, Nakagawa K, Ambiru S, Shimizu H, Togawa A, et al. Hepatic resection of liver metastases from gastric carcinoma. Am J Gastroenterol. 1997; **92**:490–493.

[74] Ochiai T, Sasako M, Mizuno S, Kinoshita T, Takayama T, Kosuge T, et al. Hepatic resection for metastatic tumours from gastric cancer: analysis of prognostic factors. Br J Surg. 1994;**81**:1175–1178.

[75] Jagric T, Potrc S, Jagric T. Prediction of liver metastases after gastric cancer resection with the use of learning vector quantization neural networks. Dig Dis Sci. 2010; **55**:3252–3261. .

[76] Harrison LE, Brennan MF, Newman E, Fortner JG, Picardo A, Blumgart LH, et al. Hepatic resection for noncolorectal, nonneuroendocrine metastases: a fifteen-year experience with ninety-six patients. Surgery. 1997;**121**:625–632.

[77] Schwartz SI. Hepatic resection for noncolorectal nonneuroendocrine metastases. World J Surg. 1995;**19**:72–75.

[78] Foster JH. Survival after liver resection for secondary tumors. Am J Surg. 1978; **135**:389–394.

[79] Kerkar SP, Kemp CD, Avital I. Liver resections in metastatic gastric cancer. HPB (Oxford). 2010;**12**:589–596. .

[80] Tiberio GAM, Coniglio A, Marchet A, Marrelli D, Giacopuzzi S, Baiocchi L, et al. Metachronous hepatic metastases from gastric carcinoma: a multicentric survey. Eur J Surg Oncol. 2009;**35**:486–491. .

[81] Hirai I, Kimura W, Fuse A, Isobe H, Hachiya O, Moriya T, et al. Surgical management for metastatic liver tumors. Hepatogastroenterology. 2006;**53**:757–763.

[82] Das BC, Kawarada Y. Long-term survival after treatment of gastric carcinoma with liver metastases. A case report. Hepatogastroenterology. 2003;**50**:2282–2284.

[83] Morise Z, Yamafuji K, Takahashi T, Asami A, Takeshima K, Hayashi N, et al. Successful treatment of recurrent liver metastases from gastric cancer by repeated hepatic resections: report of a case. Surg Today. 2000;**30**:1041–1045.

[84] Saito A, Korenaga D, Sakaguchi Y, Ohno S, Ichiyoshi Y, Sugimachi K. Surgical treatment for gastric carcinomas with concomitant hepatic metastasis. Hepatogastroenterology. 1996;**43**:560–564.

[85] Bines SD, England G, Deziel DJ, Witt TR, Doolas A, Roseman DL. Synchronous, metachronous, and multiple hepatic resections of liver tumors originating from primary gastric tumors. Surgery. 1993;**114**:799–805; discussion 804–805.

[86] Chen J, Tang Z, Dong X, Gao S, Fang H, Wu D, et al. Radiofrequency ablation for liver metastasis from gastric cancer. Eur J Surg Oncol. 2013;**39**:701–706. .

[87] Japanese Gastric Cancer Association. Japanese gastric cancer treatment guidelines 2010 (ver. 3). Gastric Cancer. 2011;**14**:113–123.

[88] Kodera Y, Fujitani K, Fukushima N, Ito S, Muro K, Ohashi N, et al. Surgical resection of hepatic metastasis from gastric cancer: a review and new recommendation in the Japanese gastric cancer treatment guidelines. Gastric Cancer. 2014;**17**:206–212. .

[89] Fujisaki S, Tomita R, Nezu T, Kimizuka K, Park E, Fukuzawa M. Prognostic studies on gastric cancer with concomitant liver metastases. Hepatogastroenterology. 2001; **48**:892–894.

[90] Kakeji Y, Morita M, Maehara Y. Strategies for treating liver metastasis from gastric cancer. Surg Today. 2010;**40**:287–294. .

[91] Schildberg CW, Croner R, Merkel S, Schellerer V, Müller V, Yedibela S, et al. Outcome of operative therapy of hepatic metastatic stomach carcinoma: a retrospective analysis. World J Surg. 2012;**36**:872–878. .

[92] Liu J, Chen L. Current status and progress in gastric cancer with liver metastasis. Chin Med J (Engl). 2011;**124**:445–456.

[93] Fujii K, Fujioka S, Kato K, Machiki Y, Kutsuna Y, Ishikawa A, et al. Resection of liver metastasis from gastric adenocarcinoma. Hepatogastroenterology. 2001;**48**:368–371.

[94] Takemura N, Saiura A, Koga R, Yoshioka R, Yamamoto J, Kokudo N. Repeat hepatectomy for recurrent liver metastasis from gastric carcinoma. World J Surg. 2013; **37**:2664–2670. .

[95] Ueda K, Iwahashi M, Nakamori M, Nakamura M, Naka T, Ishida K, et al. Analysis of the prognostic factors and evaluation of surgical treatment for synchronous liver metastases from gastric cancer. Langenbecks Arch Surg. 2009;**394**:647–653. .

[96] Garancini M, Uggeri F, Degrate L, Nespoli L, Gianotti L, Nespoli A, et al. Surgical treatment of liver metastases of gastric cancer: is local treatment in a systemic disease worthwhile? HPB (Oxford). 2012;**14**:209–215. .

[97] Kumagai K, Tanaka T, Yamagata K, Yokoyama N, Shimizu K. Liver metastasis in gastric cancer with particular reference to lymphatic advancement. Gastric Cancer. 2001;**4**:150–155. .

[98] Vogl TJ, Gruber-Rouh T, Eichler K, Nour-Eldin NEA, Trojan J, Zangos S, et al. Repetitive transarterial chemoembolization (TACE) of liver metastases from gastric cancer: local control and survival results. Eur J Radiol. 2013;**82**:258–263. .

[99] Jeurnink SM, Steyerberg EW, Hof Gvt, van Eijck CHJ, Kuipers EJ, Siersema PD. Gastrojejunostomy versus stent placement in patients with malignant gastric outlet obstruction: a comparison in 95 patients. J Surg Oncol. 2007;**96**:389–396. .

[100] Kim HS, Yi SY, Jun HJ, Lee J, Park JO, Park YS, et al. Clinical outcome of gastric cancer patients with bone marrow metastases. Oncology. 2007;**73**:192–197. .

[101] Kim JG, Ryoo BY, Park YH, Kim BS, Kim TY, Im YH, et al. Prognostic factors for survival of patients with advanced gastric cancer treated with cisplatin-based chemotherapy. Cancer Chemother Pharmacol. 2008;**61**:301–307. .

[102] Ojima H, Ootake S, Yokobori T, Mochida Y, Hosouchi Y, Nishida Y, et al. Treatment of multiple liver metastasis from gastric carcinoma. World J Surg Oncol. 2007;**5**:70. .

[103] Kutlu R, Sarac K, Yilmaz S, Kirimlioglu V, Baysal T, Alkan A, et al. Percutaneous right portal vein embolization with polyvinyl alcohol particles in gastric cancer metastasis: report of a case. Surg Today. 2005;**35**:765–769. .

[104] Hwang SE, Yang DH, Kim CY. Prognostic factors for survival in patients with hepatic recurrence after curative resection of gastric cancer. World J Surg. 2009;**33**:1468–1472. .

[105] Yamakado K, Nakatsuka A, Takaki H, Mori Y, Tonouchi H, Kusunoki M, et al. Prospective study of arterial infusion chemotherapy followed by radiofrequency ablation for the treatment of liver metastasis of gastric cancer. J Vasc Interv Radiol. 2005;**16**:1747–1751. .

[106] Driul L, Bernardi S, Bertozzi S, Schiavon M, Londero AP, Petri R. New surgical trends in breast cancer treatment: conservative interventions and oncoplastic breast surgery. Minerva Ginecol. 2013;**65**:289–296.

[107] Cedolini C, Bertozzi S, Londero AP, Bernardi S, Seriau L, Concina S, et al. Type of breast cancer diagnosis, screening, and survival. Clin Breast Cancer. 2014;**14**:235–240. .

[108] Hoe AL, Royle GT, Taylor I. Breast liver metastases–incidence, diagnosis and outcome. J R Soc Med. 1991;**84**:714–716.

[109] Kamby C, Dirksen H, Vejborg I, Daugaard S, Guldhammer B, Rossing N, et al. Incidence and methodologic aspects of the occurrence of liver metastases in recurrent breast cancer. Cancer. 1987;**59**:1524–1529.

[110] Zinser JW, Hortobagyi GN, Buzdar AU, Smith TL, Fraschini G. Clinical course of breast cancer patients with liver metastases. J Clin Oncol. 1987;**5**:773–782.

[111] Nemoto T, Dao TL. Significance of liver metastasis in women with disseminated breast cancer undergoing endocrine ablative surgery. Cancer. 1966;**19**:421–427.

[112] Viadana E, Bross ID, Pickren JW. An autopsy study of some routes of dissemination of cancer of the breast. Br J Cancer. 1973;**27**:336–340.

[113] Elias D, Lasser PH, Montrucolli D, Bonvallot S, Spielmann M. Hepatectomy for liver metastases from breast cancer. Eur J Surg Oncol. 1995;**21**:510–513.

[114] Wyld L, Gutteridge E, Pinder SE, James JJ, Chan SY, Cheung KL, et al. Prognostic factors for patients with hepatic metastases from breast cancer. Br J Cancer. 2003; **89**:284–290. .

[115] Eichbaum MHR, Kaltwasser M, Bruckner T, de Rossi TM, Schneeweiss A, Sohn C. Prognostic factors for patients with liver metastases from breast cancer. Breast Cancer Res Treat. 2006;**96**:53–62. .

[116] Hortobagyi GN. Can we cure limited metastatic breast cancer? J Clin Oncol. 2002; **20**:620–623.

[117] Largillier R, Ferrero JM, Doyen J, Barriere J, Namer M, Mari V, et al. Prognostic factors in 1,038 women with metastatic breast cancer. Ann Oncol. 2008;**19**:2012–2019. .

[118] Rubino A, Doci R, Foteuh JC, Morenghi E, Fissi S, Giorgetta C, et al. Hepatic metastases from breast cancer. Updates Surg. 2010;**62**:143–148. .

[119] Sakamoto Y, Yamamoto J, Yoshimoto M, Kasumi F, Kosuge T, Kokudo N, et al. Hepatic resection for metastatic breast cancer: prognostic analysis of 34 patients. World J Surg. 2005;**29**:524–527. .

[120] Selzner M, Morse MA, Vredenburgh JJ, Meyers WC, Clavien PA. Liver metastases from breast cancer: long-term survival after curative resection. Surgery. 2000;**127**:383–389.

[121] Vlastos G, Smith DL, Singletary SE, Mirza NQ, Tuttle TM, Popat RJ, et al. Long-term survival after an aggressive surgical approach in patients with breast cancer hepatic metastases. Ann Surg Oncol. 2004;**11**:869–874. .

[122] Elias D, Maisonnette F, Druet-Cabanac M, Ouellet JF, Guinebretiere JM, Spielmann M, et al. An attempt to clarify indications for hepatectomy for liver metastases from breast cancer. Am J Surg. 2003;**185**:158–164.

[123] Lubrano J, Roman H, Tarrab S, Resch B, Marpeau L, Scotté M. Liver resection for breast cancer metastasis: does it improve survival? Surg Today. 2008;**38**:293–299. .

[124] Pocard M, Pouillart P, Asselain B, Salmon R. Hepatic resection in metastatic breast cancer: results and prognostic factors. Eur J Surg Oncol. 2000;**26**:155–159. .

[125] Kollmar O, Moussavian MR, Richter S, Bolli M, Schilling MK. Surgery of liver metastasis in gynecological cancer – indication and results. Onkologie. 2008; **31**:375–379. .

[126] Abbott D, Brouquet A, Meric-Bernstam F, Valero V, Green M, Kuerer H, et al. Resection of liver metastases from breast cancer: timing of surgery and estrogen receptor status define outcome (P135). Ann Surg Oncol. 2011;**18**:S80. .

Chapter 9

Old versus New – Tumor Ablation versus Tumor Nanoablation with Particular Emphasis on Liver Tumors

Zeno Sparchez, Tudor Mocan and Pompilia Radu

Additional information is available at the end of the chapter

http://dx.doi.org/10.5772/61008

Abstract

Loco-regional treatments play a key role in the management of hepatocellular carcinoma (HCC). Image-guided tumor ablation is recommended in patients with early-stage HCC when surgical options are precluded. Radiofrequency ablation is currently established as the standard method for local tumor treatment. Despite major advances in tumor ablation techniques the disease recurs in a high proportion of cases. A major limitation in its overall effectiveness is due to the difficulties of heating large tumors. Small regions of viable tumor may still remain even after apparently good tumor ablation by perfusion-mediated tissue cooling, preventing the whole tumor reaching a sufficient temperature for coagulation and necrosis. Moreover simple heating techniques have trouble discriminating between tumors and surrounding healthy tissues leading to many side effects. In order to overcome these major limitations numerous groups are investigating the use of energy-absorbing agents localized within tumor tissues to facilitate localized heating. A personal answer based on the review of the literature will be offered to the following questions: NIR photothermal therapy, RFA with nanoparticles, or magnetic fluid hyperthermia for the long term management of HCC? How should we deliver nanoparticles: systemically or directly intratumoral? Ablation versus mild hyperthermia: Pros and Cons in the majority of cases, hyperthermia is applied in one of two ways: a) high temperature for short time periods commonly referred to as ablation, or b) lower temperatures for long time periods, often called mild hyperthermia. The former is used to kill cells directly with heat and consequently can be used to thermally ablate tumor. The second method is just above physiological temperature, and these temperatures are more often used to trigger release from thermosensitive drug carriers. Both approaches can be combined with heat-sensitive drug targeting. There are many ways to induce nanoparticle mediated thermal therapy in solid tumors including absorption of infrared light, radiofrequency ablation and magnetically induced heating. These approaches have demonstrated high efficacy in preclinical models of HCC and are already tested in human clinical trials.

Keywords: Nanoparticles, liver tumors, percutaneous ablation

1. Introduction

Hepatocellular carcinoma (HCC) occurs predominantly in patients with chronic liver disease and limited hepatic functional reserve. Therefore, surgical removal of HCC is feasible only in 15–20% of cases and non-surgical modalities play a relatively important role in HCC management. There are several non-surgical methods; however, ablation therapy has become a mainstay in particular for early-stage HCC because of its superb local control capability and high safety profile [1].

Ablation modalities currently available include percutaneous ethanol injection (PEI), radiofrequency ablation (RFA), microwave ablation (MWA), cryoablation, laser ablation (LA), and irreversible electroporation.

PEI was one of the first effective ablative techniques to be widely adopted for the treatment of small HCC. Ethanol causes dehydration and subsequently necrosis [2]. As far as PEIs are concerned, the 5-year survival rates in patients with HCCs measuring less than 3 cm range from 47% to 65% and in a recent study of 685 Japanese patients, the 5-, 10-, and 20-year survival rates—49%, 18%, and 7.2%, respectively, were similar to those observed in patients with cirrhosis who did not have HCC [3]. PEI maintains the advantage of allowing the treatment of tumors near sensitive organs and tissues; however the applicability of PEI in larger HCC has been shown to produce incomplete necrosis mainly due to the heterogeneous consistency of these tumors [4]. Moreover, PEI is of little benefit in infiltrating HCC or in metastases.

Current limitations of PEI can be overcome with RFA. Radiofrequency current induces ionic agitation that in turn results in heating. The superiority of RFA to PEI in prolonging patient survival has been shown in a randomized controlled trial [5]. The 3-year survival rates were 48%–67% following PEI and 63%–81% following RFA. Moreover, Chen et al. performed a randomized control trial between RFA and hepatectomy in patients who had HCC ≤ 5 cm and found the same overall and recurrence-free survival between the two patient groups [6]. A major disadvantage of RFA is mainly the difficulty to target HCC located in "problem" areas of the liver, for instance tumors adjacent to blood vessels, settings in which the diffusion of heat is less advisable [7]. This phenomenon is also known as the heat-sink effect.

In the last two years, MWA has gained acceptance as a favorable alternative and in some cases a preferred choice of ablation alternative. In MWA, the mechanism of heat generation is based on rapid frictional movement of water molecules in high-frequency (900–2500 MHz) electromagnetic field. The tissue's polar molecules are forced to continuously realign with the oscillating electric field, increasing their kinetic energy, and hence the temperature of the tissue [8]. Unlike RFA, microwaves are capable of effectively heating and propagating through many types of tissue, even those with low electrical conductivity, high impedance, or low thermal conductivity. Moreover, they can readily penetrate through the charred or desiccated tissues that tend to build up around all hyperthermic ablation applicators, resulting in limited power delivery for non-microwave energy systems [9].

MWA has several theoretical advantages, including greater penetration of energy into tissues resulting in a larger area of ablation, higher intratumoral temperatures, faster ablation times, less susceptibility to the heat-sink effect, no need for grounding pads, and low sensitivity to local variation in tissue physiological properties [10]. In some studies, MWA has been compared with RFA for the treatment of HCCs of different sizes (< 3 cm and < 5 cm) and despite the theoretical advantages of MWA, no significant differences have been observed in either setting with regard to the completeness of tumor necrosis, disease recurrence, survival, or complication rates [11, 12].

Laser thermal ablation is another technique that has been associated with high rates of complete necrosis (an average of 95%) in HCCs measuring less than 3 cm [13]. Unfortunately, there are only a few centers that use this type of ablation and therefore the amount of data is limited. Moreover, it is based on sophisticated technology, requires much more substantial operator experience, and involves placement of multiple optical fibers within the neoplastic lesion according to a programmed spatial distribution scheme [14]. Although more expensive to set up and support than RF, LAs are a little more predictable.

To date, there are only a few studies comparing LA with RFA in hepatocellular carcinoma. In their randomized controlled prospective study, Ferrary et al. [15] treated 81 cirrhotic patients with 95 biopsy proven ≤ 4 cm HCCs comparing LA with RF ablation. Two matched groups were randomized to US-guided RF or LA under general anesthesia. The authors adopted multiple fiber techniques using 5 W per fiber delivering a maximum of 1800 J per fiber per single illumination. They reported no significant overall differences in survival rates between the two methods with cumulative rates of 91.8%, 59%, and 28.4% at 1, 3, and 5 years, respectively. However, they demonstrated a statistically significant higher survival rate for RF over LA for Child A patients ($p=0.9966$) and nodules ≤ 2.5 cm ($p=0.01181$). In a randomized prospective trial in a single center with three years of follow-up, the authors treated 140 patients with 157 biopsy-proven HCCs to compare LA and RFA (70 patients with 77 nodules and 70 patients with 80 nodules, respectively). Median follow-up in RFA and LA groups was 21 and 22.5 months, respectively. Complete response was observed in 97.2% and in 95.8% of RFA and LA group patients, respectively. Median time to tumor recurrence was 25.6 and 37.8 months in RFA and in LA groups, respectively ($P = 0.129$). Estimated probability of survival at 1, 2, and 3 years was 94%, 88%, and 66% in the RFA group and 94%, 81%, and 59% in the LA group, respectively ($p = 0.693$). No major complications or significant treatment-related morbidity were observed in both groups. The authors concluded that LA was non-inferior to RFA either in obtaining the complete ablation of HCC nodules or in the long-term outcome [16].

Another type of percutaneous tumor ablation is represented by cryoablation (CRYO). Percutaneous CRYO is a promising local ablation technique, which is believed to ablate cancer cells by several mechanisms including intracellular ice formation, solute-solvent shifts that cause cell dehydration and rupture, and small-vessel obliteration with resulting hypoxia. Perhaps, the main advantage of CRYO relative to RFA is its precise intraprocedural monitoring of iceball formation via various imaging techniques [17]. There are a few studies comparing CRYO with other types of tumor ablation techniques; however Wang C et al. report the results of a randomized, controlled multicenter trial comparing percutaneous CRYO and RFA in patients with cirrhosis, Child-Pugh class A or B liver function, and 1-2 HCC nodules measuring ≤ 4 cm. The primary endpoints were local tumor progression at 3 years and safety. As for the former,

CRYO proved to be significantly superior to RFA in patients with larger tumors (i.e., those that were 3.1 to 4 cm in diameter). The two methods were not significantly different in terms of complication rates, which were less than 4% in both groups, or survival (overall and tumor-free) at 1, 3, and 5 years [18]. The superiority of CRYO over RFA in the larger tumors suggests that CRYO has the ability to necrotize larger volumes of tissue, hence increasing the chances of ablating microsatellite lesions that are always possible with lesions of this size.

Irreversible electroporation (IRE) is a new treatment method with certain advantages over the existing ablative techniques that have gained widespread attention. With IRE, cell death is induced with electric energy. Under image guidance electrodes are placed around the tumor and through multiple and short high-voltage electric pulses, the existing cell membrane potential is disturbed. As a consequence, nanoscale defects appear in the lipid bilayer of the cell membrane. Although IRE is believed to destroy all cells within the ablation zone effectively, the non-thermal nature of IRE results in relative preservation of the extracellular matrix. Hence, the structural integrity of vessels and bile ducts remain intact. Moreover, IRE is not affected by the heat-sink effect [19]. All these advantages suggest that IRE may be more suitable for the treatment of HCCs ineligible for surgical resections or thermal ablation because of unfavorable location.

Currently, there are no published clinical trials for the treatment of hepatic tumors using IRE. In a recent review, Scheffer J. et al. included 221 patients with 325 lesions in different organs: 227 hepatic tumors, 70 unresectable pancreatic adenocarcinoma, 17 renal tumors, 8 pulmonary tumors, 1 presacral tumor, and 2 lymph nodes. Most of the patients were treated by IRE owing to tumor proximity to bile ducts, bronchi, renal pelvis, presacral neural plexus or large vessels, making the tumor unsuitable for surgery or thermal ablation. They concluded that IRE is a safe procedure with a promising early efficacy on smaller hepatic tumors near vascular structures and portal triads, with reported ablation success reaching 90%, but rapidly decreasing with increasing tumor size [20].

Tremendous efforts have been made in the last decades to improve the currently available techniques. However, given that there is not a single method available that meets all the requirements of an ideal ablation system, based on what has been discussed above and on data from the vast literature available, we can reasonably draw some conclusions.

Firstly, all differences between the techniques in terms of results are modest. Secondly, one technique may be more difficult than another and more rapid than another. Thirdly, each technique has its own major advantages and disadvantages. Finally, the rate of recurrence is still high after tumor ablation despite the major advances in tumor ablation devices, optic fibers, and improved imaging guidance. A major limitation in its overall effectiveness is due to the difficulties of heating large tumors. Small regions of viable tumor may still remain even after apparently good tumor ablation. Moreover, simple heating techniques have trouble discriminating between tumors and surrounding healthy tissues leading to many side effects. In order to overcome these major limitations, numerous groups are investigating the use of different types of nanoparticles, including carbon nanotubes, gold nanoparticles, and magnetic nanoparticles, placed/ introduced within tumor tissues to facilitate localized heating.

2. Molecular mechanism of nanoparticle-mediated tumor ablation

A better understanding of the molecular mechanism of nanoparticle mediated tumor ablation is of great importance in order to improve the current available ablation techniques and also to increase the synergies between specific drugs and tumor ablation. There are several ways in which nanoparticles (NPs) alone can affect biological processes.

Several studies have shown that NPs can increase the production of reactive oxygen species (ROS). Cancer cells are generally deficient in antioxidative enzymes present in normal cells, making them more vulnerable to an oxidative assault. Iron oxide nanoparticles via direct uptake in cancer cells result in acutely elevated intracellular iron concentrations and subsequent ROS generation by Fenton reaction [21]. Moreover, silver nanoparticles have also been linked to ROS generation via a mechanism affecting calcium homeostasis. Silver ions can act on the same sites as calcium ions that could perturbate calcium influx in and out of the mitochondria. As a consequence, mitochondrial membrane damage results in ROS production, inhibition of ATP synthesis, and initiation of apoptotic signaling pathways [22].

From a biological and molecular point of view, NPs can affect different structures of the cancer cells. For instance, cellular uptake of NPs results in changes to the cytoskeleton and further affects many biological processes including cell spreading and adhesion, cell growth, viability, and ECM production [23]. Moreover, the accumulation of NPs in the cytoplasm may lead to physical interactions with the cytoskeleton, an increase in size and/or number of endosomes leading to the rearrangement of the cytoskeleton components in order to form new trafficking routes [24]. We consider that by altering the intracellular trafficking routes many other fundamental processes, including intracellular signaling pathways, different types of cross-talks with other cells and proliferation may also be affected. Furthermore, NPs can be engineered to accumulate preferentially in the nucleus of cancer cells. One study used gold nanoparticles (AuNPs) coated with polyethylene glycocol, bioconjugated with an arginine-gyicine-aspartic acid peptide and a nuclear localization signal peptide in order to transport the nanoparticles into the cancer cell nucleus. The results showed that nuclear targeting of AuNPs in cancer cells cause cytokinesis arrest, leading to the failure of complete cell division and thereby resulting in apoptosis [25].

In the past, cancer was considered an isolated self-sufficient ball of aberrant cells. However nowadays, tumors are viewed as "organs" composed of multiple and highly interactive cell types. Thus, the tumor is made up of primary cancer cells and of a court of stromal cells including mesenchymal derived cells, inflammatory cells, and vascular cells. Each of these cell types can be found in normal stroma, but in a tumorigenic setting, the cancer has appropriated, modified, and corrupted these cells to do its bidding [26]. NPs can also be used to target the tumor stroma changing the tumor microenvironment from its pro-tumorigenic state to an anti-tumorigenic state. One study demonstrated the ability of nanoparticles to target the tumor endothelium and improve the anti-tumoral efficacy of paclitaxel, both *in vivo* and *in vitro* [27]. Another approach would be to target the macrophage because they are inherently phagocytic and may uptake nanoparticles either within the tumor or in the circulation and subsequently migrate towards to the tumor. Another ability of macrophage is to store iron; hence, iron oxide

NPs have been shown to induce cytotoxic effects on themselves and surrounding cells via ROS-mediated activation of the c-jun N-terminal kinase pathway [28].

Understanding how nanomaterials affect live cell function, controlling such effects, and using them in therapy (for example In tumor ablation), is now the most challenging aspects of nanobiotechnology. An ideal NP would be a multifunctional one, targeting both the tumor cells and tumor microenvironment with low toxicity, which is easy to engineer, and has low costs. However, there is still a long way and a great deal of research has to be performed in order to develop what we consider the ideal nanoparticle.

3. Near-infrared photothermal ablation

Near-infrared (NIR) laser light is ideal for *in vivo* hyperthermia applications because of its low absorption by tissue chromophores such as hemoglobin and water. NIR light demonstrates maximal penetration of tissue, thereby reaching deep inside the tissue. Photothermal ablation (PTA) therapy is a recently developed technique that uses NIR laser light-generated heat to destroy tumor cells. In recent years, PTA has gained a lot of popularity mainly because a specific amount of photoenergy is delivered directly into the tumor without causing systemic effects [29]. However, this therapy approach is limited by the fact that the heating is nonspecific and nonuniform mainly in areas peripheral to large blood vessels where heat can be rapidly dissipated by circulating blood.

The efficacy of PTA can be significantly enhanced by using different types of nanoparticles that are applied to the target tissue to mediate selective photothermal effects. For instance, AuNPs including gold nanorods, gold nanocages, gold nanostars, and gold nanopopcorns with unique optical proprieties have been developed [30].

In order to treat a tumor, AuNPs are systemically administered to the subject and allowed to passively localize in the tumor. The tumor is then exposed to an excitation source such as the NIR laser light. The AuNPs absorb the incident energy and convert it into heat, which raises the temperature of the tissue and ablates the cancerous cells by disrupting the cell membrane [31]. AuNPs have unique optical-electronic proprieties as a result of surface plasmon resonances (SPRs). SPR is a phenomenon in which free electrons oscillate collectively at the interface of metal and surrounding medium in resonance with external electromagnetic fields [30].

Nanoparticles in the tissues produce heat strong enough for thermal ablation in both tumors and surrounding cells. Therefore, it is crucial to increase the intratumoral localization of the nanoparticles on the one hand and to protect the surrounding tissue on the other hand. Selective accumulation of AuNPs in the target tumor tissue can be achieved by surface conjugation of targeting agents, such as antibodies and peptides that can recognize specific cell types. For instance Liu et al. reported that gold nanoshells functionalized with the small peptide A54 can significantly increase the efficiency of cancer cell death in the NIR photothermal treatment due to the specific binding (targeting) between the A54-nanoshells and the liver cancer cells, BEL-7404 and BEL-7402 [32].

AuNP can also be functionalized to load various cargoes such as different types of anticancer drugs. As an example in this setting, You et al. investigated DOX-loaded hollow gold nanospheres (DOX@HAuNSs) and conjugated them with a peptide sequence that targets EPHB4, a tyrosine kinase receptor that is often overexpressed in many tumor cell membranes including HCC. NIR laser irradiation after treatment with targeted DOX@HAuNSs resulted in significantly suppressed tumor growth when compared with the control treatment with nontargeted DOX@HAuNSs or HAuNSs [33]. Moreover, another study conducted by the same authors, evaluated the triggered release of paclitaxel via NIR laser irradiation and its antitumor efficacy by hepatic arterial administration of HAuNS and paclitaxel loaded microspheres into rabbits with liver carcinoma in situ [34]. The results showed statistically significant increases in necrosis and apoptosis percentage in the MS-HAuNS-PTX-plus-NIR treatment group compared with the other two treatment groups.

A different approach in the field of NPs, mediated NIR thermal ablation has been developed in the last two years mainly due to the development of therenostic agents, which combine diagnostic and therapeutic modalities. This approach offers tremendous potential for the management of chronic liver injury or HCC. In a recent article, multifunctional nanoprobe based on Glypican-3 anti-body-mediated HCC-targeting Prussian blue nanoparticles (antiGPR-PBNPs) was developed as a novel theranostic agent for the targeted PTT and MR imaging of HCC treatments [35]. They concluded that antiGPC3-PBNPs could be used as a promising nanoprobe for further treating and early diagnosis of HCC.

A major limitation of nanoparticle-assisted drug delivery is represented by their uptake in the reticuloendothelial system leading to undesirable systemic toxicity and reduced efficacy. Hence many researchers have investigated the use of different cell types for drug delivery. Zhao J et al. in their study used adipose-derived mesenchymal cells (AD-MSCs) to deliver superparamagnetic iron oxide (SPIO)-loaded gold nanoparticles (SPIO@AuNP) into HCC tumors [36]. They demonstrated that AD-MSC is an effective carrier for the specific delivery of theranostic agents to liver injuries or HCC and SPIO@AuNP is a host-compatible cargo that enables both MRI enhancement and laser induced thermal ablation.

Besides the different types of gold nanoparticles described above, carbon nanotubes (CNT) also have the ability to efficiently convert NIR into heat. The role on CNT-mediated thermal therapy for the treatment of a wide variety of cancer types both *in vitro* and *in vivo* have been recently reviewed [37]. It is hard to claim that CNTs are better than GNPs because direct comparisons are hard to make; however, some estimates indicate that CNTs can achieve thermal destruction of tumors at 10-fold-lower doses and a 3-fold-lower power than what is required for gold nanorods [23]. On the other hand GNP can be synthesized with great uniformity and have already been tested in human clinical trials.

It is worth to mentioning that there is a massive amount of research in the field of nanoparticles-mediated PTA therapy. We only provided a few examples that we considered most suitable. Describing all the possible applications of nanoparticles mediated thermal therapy is beyond the purpose of this chapter.

4. Magnetic fluid hyperthermia-iron magnetic nanoparticles

Thermotherapy represents a physical treatment induced by hyperthermia. Nowadays, macroscopic thermotherapy (ablative methods: microwave or radiofrequency, optical laser irradiation via fibers, focused ultrasound) is widely used to destroy focal tumors. The mechanism of tumoral damage is the result of an irreparable destruction of molecular constituents of cells (mainly protein denaturation) that appears after an exposure of a few minutes at temperatures higher than 48°C. Even if it has lower side effects when compared to conventional therapy (chemo/radiotherapy) and although it has proved to be a reliable alternative to surgery, this therapy has several limits: the relative higher rate of incomplete destruction for tumors larger than 3 cm and a higher risk of destruction of the proximate healthy tissue. These deficiencies seem to disappear by using a new thermal method known as magnetic termic hyperthermia [38]. This approach uses an external alternating magnetic field applied to a target tumor where magnetic metallic particles (MNPs) have been infiltrated or injected. MNPs show distinguishing phenomena such as superparamagnetism, high field irreversibility, high saturation field, extra anisotropy contributions, or shifted loops after field cooling [39]. According to Reference [40], the distinguished phenomena noticed in MNPs are the result of the interaction between the intrinsic properties (size, distribution, and finite-size effects) and the interparticle interactions. The MNPs have the ability to absorb the energy of the alternating magnetic field energy and transform it into heat. Two factors are implicated in producing hyperthermia, the size of the magnetic material and the strength of the applied magnetic field. Larger implants (seeds) generate heat by resistance to circumferential eddy currents induced on the surface of the seeds by an alternative magnetic field [41]. Multidomain particles produce heat by hysteresis loss effects. On the contrary, nanoparticle, particularly subdomain particle, suspensions generate heat mainly by Brownian relaxation (heat is the result of friction arising from the total particle oscillations) and Neel relaxation (heat is the result of friction arising from the rotation of the magnetic moment with each field oscillation) [42, 43].

Superparamagnetic particles are particles that have sufficient high thermal motion after the magnetic field is removed, which can be randomly reoriented so as not to leave a residual magnetization [43].

Due to their properties, these particles may have several applications in clinical practice such as hyperthermia (HT), drug delivery and diagnosis (s.a nuclear magnetic resonance imaging).

HT represents a therapeutic procedure used to destroy a tumoral tissue at temperatures over 43°C [38]. It has been observed that tumoral cells have an increased thermal sensitivity in comparison to healthy cells; this feature is the result of an increased metabolism [44, 45]. Apoptosis is the result of cytotoxic effects that depend on physiological cell parameters (hypoxia or acidity) at temperatures over 43°C. 43°C is the temperature limit over which the expression of HSPs is stimulated, which leads to antitumor immunity and apoptosis [46]. The antitumor immunity increases as a result of an enhanced presentation of tumoral antigenic peptide to a major histocompatibility complex (MHC). HSP70 expression reaches its maximum 24 h after heating. The increased MHC class I surface expression is slower, so it starts 24 h after applied hyperthermia and the peak is after 48 h [38]. Two mechanisms have been suggested.

One of the possible mechanisms is that the heat induces the enhancement of antigenic peptide presentation through MHC class I antigens of tumor cells. Another possible mechanism is the cross-presentation of antigenic peptides by dedicated antigen-presenting cells (APCs) [46].

The advantage of magnetic hyperthermia is that it restricts the heating to the tumoral area, which presents both grand opportunities and challenges for the non-invasive treatment of tumors. Therefore, by combining this characteristic of the tumoral tissue with the MNPs property, it is obvious that the administration of MNPs (with the purpose of delivering toxic amounts of thermal energy to the tumoral tissue) will produce a more effective destruction of the tumoral tissue.

For clinical practice, MNPs must meet several criteria: they must be small enough to remain in the circulation after injection and pass through the capillary; they must not be an embolic agent; they must be non-toxic and non-immunogenic; they must maintain the initial structure; and they must be biodegradable. Another important property of these particles is to be highly magnetized in order for their movement to be controlled with a magnetic field so that they can be immobilized near the targeted tumoral area [47]. The most important factors, which determine the biocompatibility and toxicity of these materials, are the nature of the magnetically responsive component, the final size of the particles, their core, and their coatings [39]. The most utilized MNPs are magnetite (Fe3O4) or its oxidized form, maghemite (γ-Fe2O3). Magnetite is easier to obtain than maghemite; therefore, most of the studies utilized magnetite [38]. In order to avoid the constitution of large aggregates, the modification from the original form and biodegradation, the MNPs are coated with a biocompatible polymer during or after the synthesis [39]. The particles' size influence the stability, tissular diffusion, effective surface areas (easier attachment of ligands), and the power of absorption at tolerable altering current magnetic fields. Therefore, only subdomain magnetic particles (nanometer-sized), especially particles smaller than 100 nm (so-called nanoparticles), can be utilized [48, 49]. Also, it is important to highlight that the heating potential is dependent on particle size and shape, and thus the use of uniform particles is essential for a rigorous control in temperature [39]. Therefore, the magnetic particles used may modify the energy, absorption rate, mode of energy deposition, application, and focusing. For this technique, the sizes of the particles are as follows: seeds (rods of several millimeter size), multidomain particles (1–300 mm), nanoparticles (1–100 nm), and subdomain particles (below 20 nm) [41].

Gilchrist was the first author that showed promising results obtained after selective heating that followed the direct injection of a suspension of magnetic particles into draining lymph nodes from colon cancer [50]. In 2001, Moroz showed that hepatic arterial infusion of lipiodol containing ferromagnetic particles could result in an excellent targeting of liver tumors with hyperthermia on the subsequent application of an external alternating magnetic field [51]. The following years, encouraged by the results of the use of MNPs in animal studies (on mouse mammary carcinoma, glioblastoma, and prostate cancer), some authors focused on the improvement of HT techniques for clinical applications [52–56]. For in vivo delivery, the authors used thermosensitive liposomes, direct injection into the tumor, or the intravenous route.

An important progress has been made in improving the quality of the MNPs; therefore, for construction, high temperature crystallization or different coatings were used, such as dextran, polyethylene glycol (PEG), dopamine, silanes and gold [43].

Several authors introduced MNPs either in the core or in between the lipid bilayer of thermosensitive liposomes and, on alternating magnetic field AMF heating, the encapsulated drugs were released [43]. Shinkai utilized liposomes where he introduced magnetite nanoparticles (with a diameter of 10 nm). After administration, these nanoparticles increased the temperature of the tissue [57]. In another study, Ito injected magnetite cationic liposomes (MCLs) into the tumor tissue. They heated the tissue above 43°C and obtained a complete regression of mammary carcinomas in all mice [58]. Also, Jimbow [52] developed a particle with N-propionylcysteaminylphenol (NPrCAP) conjugated onto the surface of magnetite nanoparticles (NPrCAP/M). The result was the inhibition of melanoma cells growth as a result of the production of cytotoxic free radicals. In another study, a thermosensitive polymer was layered onto MNPs covalently coupled to doxorubicin with an acid-labile hydrazine bond that showed release on heating with AMF and a pH of 5.3 (the pH of endosomes) [59]. The authors combined via emulsification MNPs with a polyvinyl alcohol polymer and encapsulated hydrophobic/ hydrophilic drugs. The drugs were released after the heating with an alternative magnetic field [60].

Direct intratumoral injection was used in the first MNP HT clinical trial treating a patient with a recurrent prostatic tumor [61]. Through the use of transrectal ultrasound and fluoroscopy guidance, the authors performed a transperineal injection of the MNPs into the prostate. After the administration of MNPs, the particles were selectively heated in an externally applied alternative magnetic field. The conclusions of these trials were encouraging. Due to the low clearance of MNPs from tumors, serial heat treatments were possible after a single magnetic fluid injection. Another positive aspect was the fact that a low magnetic field was used to produce the necessary temperatures. Furthermore, this treatment does not cause discomfort or serious side effects. In these studies, the CT exam had an accuracy rate of 85% in evaluating the treatment-related parameters. The same good results were obtained later in human glioma trials [62, 63].

In 2008, Takamatsu et al. combined the intra-arterial selective HT with the transcatheter arterial embolization technique in a rabbit model for renal carcinoma [64]. For injection, they utilized a mixture of commercially available nano-sized magnetic particles (Ferucarbotran) and lipiodol as embolic material. The mixture was injected into the renal artery under fluoroscopic guidance. The intratumoral temperatures of 45ºC were obtained after the area was exposed to an external alternating-current magnetic field. Even the result was not spectacular (the treated tumor was hypovascular) the authors speculated that this method can be used only in hypervascular tumors. In another study, Huang HS injected IV MNPs (1.9 mg Fe/g tumor) in a subcutaneous squamous cell carcinoma mouse model. After the injection, they applied a field of 38 kA/m at 980 kHz; therefore, the tumors could be heated to 60°C in 2 min. The results were encouraging, showing an ablating with millimeter (mm) precision and a surrounding tissue intact [43].

Intravenous administration has several advantages compared to sowing such as: it assures a more precise cover even for an irregular tumor and small tumors; it can be used for the treatment of metastasis (after one injection more than one tumor can be treated simultaneously); the distribution is more overall (rather than the dotted distribution from sowing); and it is minimally invasive [43, 48].

The evaluation of the iron concentrations can be mapped with high accuracy by MRI, computed tomography or magnetorelaxometry [43, 65, 66].

The science of MNPs is still in its early stages. The recent results of magnetic HT in cancer therapy are very encouraging; but it is necessary to traverse the experimental stages into clinical practice to see the real applicability of this new technique.

5. NP-based thermal therapy using radiofrequency

5.1. Standard RF-mediated nanoablation

Standard RFA is an invasive procedure that requires the insertion of electrodes within the tumor. Tumor destruction occurs as a result of vibrations of ions within tumor tissue induced by radio waves, which give rise to friction and lethal heat. Although it is possible to achieve local control in liver tumors < 2.5 cm, in larger lesions local tumor recurrence is common [67, 68].

Initially, in order to increase the efficacy of RFA, the ablation guidance methods were improved (contrast-enhanced ultrasound, fusion imaging, etc.), but this led only to a slight efficacy improvement. Because of the changes that occur after RFA (increased vascular and cellular membrane permeability), the periphery of the tumor becomes more susceptible to chemotherapy. Thus, the combination of thermal ablation and chemotherapy seemed to lead to promising results. The results of these methods did increase the efficacy of RFA, but it was not enough. Therefore, new treatments that will augment cytotoxicity at the margin of the ablation zone have been developed.

The efficiency of RFA can be significantly enhanced by administration of special thermal absorbing agents such as NPs, which are targeted into a tumor area (actively or passively) with the purpose to release locally the retained heat and thus enhance tumoral destruction.

The NPs in free form or those containing various anti-cancer agents may be administrated before, at the time, or after RFA [68, 69]. Administering CYT-6091, a TNF-labeled NP, 4 h prior to RFA yielded a significantly larger zone of central necrosis and a 23% increase in ablation volume in comparison to RFA alone [69]. Using this NP enhanced ablation, the partially ablated tissue at the periphery was replaced by completely ablated tissue [69].

The administration of NPs containing free doxorubicine at the time of RFA or after leads to an increased diameter of coagulated tumor tissue (and increased concentration of doxorubicine in the ablated tumor) [68]. The NPs accumulate in the region of ablation both in the treated tumor (as result of an increased leakage) and in the peripheral region with thermal induced inflammation. This is known as the enhanced permeability and retention (EPR) effect [70].

The liposomes were the first NPs that have been utilized in combination with RFA. The studies of Ahmed and Goldberg demonstrated that the use of lipid NPs as carriers of a drug combined with ARF was associated with an increased accumulation of doxorubicin in the tumor, while non-encapsulated free doxorubicin did not have increased tumor uptake following RFA [71]. Since then, an important number of investigators improved the lipid layer of liposomes that has contributed to enhanced tumor damage secondary to formation of lipid hydro-peroxide leading to enhanced oxidative stress. Also, the investigators demonstrated that NPs size could influence the intratumoral drug accumulation and tissue coagulation [68].

5.2. Non-invasive RF nanoablation

As a negative relationship between the frequency of the waves and the depth of penetration exists, radio waves may be used as an alternative to heat tumors that are deeply located. The heating rate of a certain tissue is described by the formula HR = SAR/69.77 CH where SAR is the specific absorption rate and CH the specific heat capacity of the tissue (kcal/kg °C). As SAR (W/kg) depends on the dielectric conductivity of the tissue, an enhanced conductivity provided by AuNPs or carbon nanotubes may increase the heat delivered to the tissue [72].

These low-frequency electromagnetic waves have the advantage to penetrate human tissues and pass through the entire body with minimal perturbations until the RF fields interact with metal. The metal particles absorb RF energy and release heat to the adjacent region. Several reports suggested that tumoral hyperthermia may be improved through the use of targeted nanomaterials, which produce an intracellular hyperthermia and act as RF-thermal transducers, leaving the surrounding healthy tissue intact [68].

The delivery of RF generated heat in deep structures may be achieved either by RF needle inserted into the tumor (standard RFA) or by an external device that generates an RF field [68, 72].

If standard RF ablation produces a hyperthermic region of 2–4 cm diameter around the probe's tip, the nanoparticle-mediated RF field induces a hyperthermic area of approximately 100 μm. The heating mechanism of NPs in an RF field is a complex phenomenon that is still under debate [73]. Most of the RF field devices produce shortwave RF fields (13.56 MHz), allowing them to be used in the medical field. Several reports have shown that Joule heating of the background ionic suspension where the NPs are suspended can be the main source of RF heat production [74]. A relative high variety of NPs as AuNPs, carbon nanotubes (SWNTs), quantum dots (cadmium-selenide and indium-gallium-phosphide), silicon nanoparticles (Si NPs), and La0.7Sr0.3MnO3 (Dex-LSMO) have been associated with RF field [74, 75]. The use of NPs seems to improve the standard RFA by increasing the specificity of tumor destructions and affording a relative target therapy. Between these NPs are several differences, such as the SWNTs are heated faster than AuNPs unlike quantum dots that are heated in a similar manner to AuNPs [73].

SWNTs showed that they can be activated from a distance by RF field to produce thermal cytotoxicity [75]. The SWNTs have been injected in Vx2 tumors and induced the necrosis of all tumors within 5 min of RF field exposure. Regions of necrosis were identified with 2–5 mm borders. It is important to highlight that SWNTs alone or RF field exposure alone did not induce any measurable tumor necrosis or liver injury. In another study, the authors demonstrated that SWNTs injected into malignant cells may allow noninvasive RF field treatments to produce lethal thermal injury to the malignant cells. In a similar study conducted by Raoof, Hep3B and HepG2 cells were injected to kentera modified SWNT and were exposed to an 800 W RF field. Significant thermal cytotoxicity was demonstrated with 2 min of RF exposure in a concentration-dependent manner [75]. Also the group conducted by Cardinal obtained similar results after they exposed a rat model (with HepG2 cells) into an RFA field following the administration of AuNPs [76]. In a study conducted by Glazer ES, AuNPs utilized cetuximab-conjugated AuNPs in nonionizing RF radiation to investigate human pancreatic xenograft destruction in a murine model [73]. The result showed an increased apoptosis with decreased viability of tumoral cells after treatment with cetuximab-conjugated AuNPs and RF field exposure. Another important observation was the lack of injury to other organs.

It becomes a reality the fact that nanotechnologies will play a major role in new antitumoral therapies. In the last years, the thermal approach using nanoparticles, nanoemulsion, pH responsive nanoparticles, nanoparticles combined with radiation, and nanovectors for drug delivery have been the most evaluated nanoparticle-based cancer treatment methods. The ability of SWNTs to convert NIR laser radiation into heat, due to the photon–phonon and electron interactions, provides the opportunity to create a new generation of immunoconjugates for cancer phototherapy. In 2011, Iancu et al. demonstrated that the HepG2 cells treated with multi-walled carbon nanotubes (HSA–MWCNTs) following laser irradiation had a higher necrotic rate compared with normal cells [77].

5.3. Thermosensitive liposomes currently in advanced clinical trials

Discovered in 1964 by Alec Bangham, liposomes are self-assembling, biocompatible, biodegradable, and nonimmunogenic nanovesicles consisting of a lipid bilayer enclosing an aqueous phase [78]. The features of liposomes allow for a wide range of drug delivery; consequently, hydrophilic drugs can be trapped in the liposome's aqueous compartments while the lipid bilayer can be utilized to incorporate hydrophobic drugs. Due to the discontinuous endothelial lining and the lack of efficient lymphatic drainage of the tumor, the extravasations of liposomes into the interstitial space is increased and the liposomes can accumulate in the tumoral tissue; therefore, they will function as a sustained drug-release formula [79]. Immordino mentioned for the first time this process and named it as EPR effect [80]. Moreover, the combination (liposome–chemotherapy) changes drug pharmacokinetic properties and minimizes its systemic toxicity. Furthermore, the drug prevents the entrapped drug from premature inactivation in the circulation. The main issue of liposomes is that they are rapidly phagocytized by the mononuclear phagocyte (MP) and removed from the blood circulation after intravenous injection. To avoid this inconvenience, the authors developed a grafting poly-(ethylene glycol) (PEG) or oligoglycerol-moieties on the surface of the liposomal carrier. By reducing MP system uptake [80], long-circulating PEGylated liposomes can passively accumulate into solid tumors undergoing angiogenesis. Another improvement was the incorporation of additional lipid compounds that further enhance membrane permeability at the phase transition temperature of the lipid membrane (lysolipid or oligoglycerol-polyglycol) [79, 81–84]. The result was a long blood circulation time *in vivo*. These types of low temperature thermosensitive liposomes (LTSLs)[79] are injected just prior to or during the HT treatment, with immediate release of their contents upon arrival in the heated tumor area.

The main limit of this type of therapy remains the intimate relation between the biodisponibility of liposomes and the vascular permeability. It is important to underline that vascular permeability between different tumor types and even within tumors can be highly variable, resulting in unpredictable liposome extravasation into the tumor tissue [85, 86]. Due to the combination of sub-optimal drug release kinetics and unpredictable vascular permeability, only modest results in the therapeutic index of chemotherapy have been obtained using liposomes for target drug delivery [87].

An important progress in the use of liposomes was the invention of small, 100 nm-long circulating liposomes that have a long blood-residence time as their main characteristic. These favorable circulation properties resulted in an enhanced accumulation of liposomal drugs in the tumor area.

To date, several liposomal products have been approved for clinical use: liposomes with doxorubicin (Doxil/Caelyx, Myocet, and Lipo-Dox) for treatment of Kaposi's sarcoma, ovarian cancer, breast cancer, and multiple myeloma; liposomes with daunorubicin (DaunoXome) for treatment of Kaposi's sarcoma; and liposomes encapsulating vincristine (Marqibo) for acute lymphoblastic leukemia [88].

Hyperthermia represents the heating of tumors to temperatures of up to 43°C. The main effect consists of an increased tissue perfusion, oxygenation and blood flow velocity, and microvessel permeability contributing to increased antibodies, drug, or nanoparticles levels in tumors at clinically tolerated temperatures [89–92]. Nowadays, hyperthermia for triggering TSLs is applied locally and in a noninvasive way from an external source to a targeted area using focused ultrasound technology (FUS) and high-intensity focused ultrasound (HIFU), or invasively using ARF or MWA [93, 94]. For superficial tumors, the authors used regional HT and external antennas or applicators that emit microwaves or radio waves. Localized HT is used to destroy deeply located tumors. The antennas (microwave antennas, radiofrequency electrodes) are inserted directly within the tumor. The major limit of this heating method is the tumor diameter (less than 5 cm). Focused ultrasound is used to heat small lesions (mm). In a recent study Dromi et al. combined LTSLs with hyperthermia from FUS [95]. They obtained an increased drug discharge at the tumoral area and the most important tumor had a delayed growth.

The newest heating method is magnetic resonance guided focused ultrasound technology (MRgFUS). These combinations allow simultaneous treatments, imaging to guide the treatment and MR thermometry to noninvasively monitor temperature changes and assure feedback in real-time [87]. In two recent studies, the authors used MRgFUS and drug-loaded liposome in rat [96] and rabbit [97] models. The results showed that the combination MRgFUS with drug loaded liposome assured the greatest uptake of the drug when compared to controls (liposome only and/or free drug). Several studies have analyzed the combination of RFA and the non-thermally sensitive liposomal doxorubicin, showing larger ablation zones compared with RFA alone, both at the preclinical and clinical levels. The suggested mechanisms for the synergistic effect of liposomal doxorubicine and RFA are as follows: increased markers of DNA breakage, oxidative stress and apoptosis, increased heat-shock protein 70 in the areas surrounding the ablation zone after combination treatment [98, 99]. In addition, Ahmed and colleagues observed that after combining RFA with Doxil, the intratumoral drug uptake increased, while the dose of doxorubicin necessary for tumor destruction decreased [100].

In order to optimize the effects of liposomes, the use of TSLs that trigger the release of the drug at the edge of the heated zone was suggested [101–103]. These TSLs contain thermosensitive lipids in their bilayer, undergoing a gel-to-liquid phase transition at the desired temperature (usually between 41°C and 43°C), after which the drug enters tumor cells in free form. This conversion is the consequence of a conformational change in the alkyl chains of the lipids, which leads to an increase in the volume occupied by the hydrocarbon chains in the membrane and thus an increase in the permeability of the lipid bilayer [79]. Common TSLs have been composed from 1, 2-dipalimitoyl-sn -glycero-3-phosphocholine (DPPC) as the primary lipid, because its phase transition temperature (Tm) occurs at 41.5°C.

In 2009, TSLs containing Dox known as ThermoDox®, became the first heat-triggered release formula of the anthracycline doxorubicin that reached pharmaceutical development (Celsion Corporation, Columbia, Maryland, USA) and clinical application [104–105]. Thermodox® is composed of DPPC:MSPC:DSPE-PEG2000 (86:10:4 molar ratio) and in combination with mild was used in the Phase III clinical trial to treat hepatocellular carcinoma and the Phase II trial in combination with local mild for patients with recurrent breast cancer of the chest wall and colorectal liver. After intravenous administration, Thermodox® concentrates in the liver where it rapidly permeates HCC lesions and their vasculature. Regarding safety and tolerability, in Phase I ThermoDox® was associated with low side effects and the maximum tolerated dose was established at 50 mg/m2. According to the Phase I trial, RFA and ThermoDox® may be used as a front-line therapy for HCC > 3 cm [106]. Unfortunately, in 2013 Celsion Corp. was unable to demonstrate the effectiveness of ThermoDox® in the improvement of free survival [79]. It seemed that the temperature of drug release is different between *in vivo* and *in vitro*. In a study conducted by Hossann, about 90–100% Dox release from LTSLs in plasma or serum at 39–40°C resulted in 2°C below the theoretical temperature [107]. Therefore, it might be that all drug content is released from the LTSLs below 41–42°C, which means that the drug is discharged in blood circulation before the accumulation of LTLS in the target heated tumoral area [79]. In a recent study, after the incorporation of lysophosphatidylcholines (lyso-PC, e.g. 1-stearoyl-2-hydroxy-sn-glycero-3-phosphocholine, MSPC) into the liposomal membrane, it was possible to further accelerate the encapsulated drug at Tm [108].

Fine tunings in drug release kinetics of LTSLs was demanded to assure an improved dug release [109]. In 2014, Chen J evaluated [79] high temperature triggered TSLs (HTSLs) composed of DPPC and hydrogenated soy phosphatidylcholine (HSPC). For these types of liposomes, the theoretical temperature of discharge of HTSLs was set at 44°C; thus, the body temperature had less influence on the drug release from the vesicles. The result of this study was encouraging. Compared to conventional LTSLs, the new formula of HTSLs was associated with higher stability and less content discharge to the heated tumor area.

Several authors recommended the attaching of targeting ligands to the nanoparticles to assure a more specific localization and retention of the liposomal drug in tumors. Another reason to utilize these ligands is the capacity of promoting active cellular uptake of the drug-containing nanoparticles through binding to targeted internalizing receptors [110-112].

The cationic TSLs, called CTSLs (cationic thermosensitive liposome) is a new class of LTSL that contains a cationic lipid in its membrane. The CTSLs are absorbed by vascular endothelium and tumor cells; afterwards, they release their contents upon applying a temperature trigger [113]. It seems that, once accumulated, rapid drug release by intracellular cationic liposomes may achieve high intracellular concentrations of drug, thereby maximizing damage to both the endothelial cell and tumor cell compartments [113]. To evaluate tumoral accumulation of liposomes, radionuclides and nuclear imaging may be used. Even if the authors have obtained good results, in the future these types of treatment will have to demonstrate their therapeutic potential in clinical practice.

6. Conclusions and future perspectives

As we have already seen, there are several types of thermal-based therapies that have shown modest efficacy in HCC treatment. Unfortunately, simple heating techniques have trouble discriminating between tumors and surrounding healthy tissues. Moreover, the use of thermal therapies in large HCC is of limited value. In order to overcome these limitations many groups have investigated the use of NPs to increase the tumor ablation zone.

There are many types of NPs, each type with its own major advantages and disadvantages. Based on currently available literature, we could not say which of the above-described NPs is better for the long-term management of HCC. Unfortunately, there are no studies comparing AuNPs with carbon nanoparticles or magnetic nanoparticle. The use of NPs such as AuNPs, carbon nanoparticles, and magnetic nanoparticles have shown great promise as light absorbers for cancer therapy, demonstrating an ability to destroy cancerous lesions both in vivo and in vitro [31].

We believe that an ideal NP should be a good light absorber in order to achieve complete ablation of the tumor tissues. To avoid systemic toxicity, the NPs should show selective accumulation in target tissue with minimal nonspecific distribution. Not at least, they should be rapidly cleared from the body after their mission to prevent redistribution into off-target sites [38].

Future research should focus on the development of multifunctional NP. For instance, theranostic agents could improve both the diagnostic accuracy and therapy of HCC. Small HCC means better outcomes. The majority of NPs are functionalized to target the tumor cells, leaving the tumor stroma unaffected. A pro-tumorigenic stroma or better said a pro-tumorigenic microenvironment could lead to tumor recurrence, therefore dual targeting of both tumor cells and tumor stroma could overcome these limitations.

Specific targeting in HCC is still a major problem. There are many molecular pathways involved in HCC development. Moreover, not all HCC express the same receptors on the cell surface. In order to specifically deliver NP in the tumor area, immunohistological staining must be performed. This is hard to perform, particularly in HCC, since liver biopsy is no longer recommended for HCC diagnosis. Maybe it is time to go back where we started and reconsider the role of liver biopsy in HCC management.

In the last 50 years, despite tremendous advances in our knowledge of the molecular mechanism of cancer, there has been no change in the age-adjusted mortality from cancer [39]. This data clearly suggests that what we are doing now is wrong and an individualized treatment could bring new hopes for HCC patients.

Acknowledgements

This material was financed by the partnership program in priority areas – PN II, implemented with support from the National Authority of Scientific Research (ANCS), CNDI – UEFISCDI, project nr. 2011-3.1-0252 (NANO- ABLATION).

Author details

Zeno Sparchez[1*], Tudor Mocan[2] and Pompilia Radu[2]

*Address all correspondence to: zsparchez@yahoo.co.uk

1 Iuliu Hatieganu University of Medicine and Pharmacy, Cluj Napoca, Romania

2 Institute for Gastroenterology and Hepatology, Cluj Napoca, Romania

References

[1] Kim YS, Lim HK, Rhim H, Lee MW. Ablation of hepatocellular carcinoma. Best Pract Res Clin Gastroenterol. 2014;28(5):897-908.

[2] Gillams AR. Liver ablation therapy. Br J Radiol. 2004;77(92):713-723.

[3] Shiina S, Tateisshi R, Imamura M, Teratani T, Koike Y, Sato S, et al. Percutaneous ethanol injection for hepatocellular carcinoma: 20-year outcome and prognostic factors. Liver Int. 2012;32(9):1434-1442.

[4] McWilliams JP, Yamamoto S, Raman SS, Loh CT, Lee EW, Liu DM, et al. Percutaneous ablation of hepatocellular carcinoma: current status. J Vasc Interv Radiol. 2010;21(8 Suppl):S204-213.

[5] Lin SM, Lin CJ, Lin CC, Hsu CW, Chen YC. Randomised controlled trial comparing percutaneous radiofrequency thermal ablation, percutaneous ethanol injection, and percutaneous acetic acid injection to treat hepatocellular carcinoma of 3 cm or less. Gut. 2005;54(8):1151-1156.

[6] Chen MS, Li JQ, Zheng Y, Guo RP, Liang HH, Zhang YQ, et al. A prospective randomized trial comparing percutaneous local ablative therapy and partial hepatectomy for small hepatocellular carcinoma. Ann Surg. 2006;243(3):321-328.

[7] Brunello F, Veltri A, Carucci P, Pagano E, Ciccone G, Moretto P, et al. Radiofrequency ablation versus ethanol injection for early hepatocellular carcinoma: aA randomized controlled trial. Scand J Gastroenterol. 2008;43(6):727-735.

[8] Seror O. Percutaneous hepatic ablation: what needs to be known in 2014. Diagn Interv Imaging. 2014;95(7-8):665-675.

[9] Skinner MG, Iizuka MN, Kolios MC, Sherar MD. A theoretical comparison of energy sources—microwave, ultrasound and laser—for interstitial thermal therapy. Phys Med Biol. 1998;43(12):3535-3547.

[10] Yu H, Burke CT. Comparison of percutaneous ablation technologies in the treatment of malignant liver tumors. Semin Intervent Radiol. 2014;31(2):129-137.

[11] Shibata T, Iimuro Y, Yamamoto Y, Maetani Y, Ametani F, Itoh K, et al. Small hepatocellular carcinoma: cComparison of radio-frequency ablation and percutaneous microwave coagulation therapy. Radiology. 2002;223(2):331-337.

[12] Zhang L, Wang N, Shen Q, Cheng W, Qian GJ. Therapeutic efficacy of percutaneous radiofrequency ablation versus microwave ablation for hepatocellular carcinoma. PLoS One. 2013;8(10):e76119.

[13] Christophi C, Muralidharan V. Treatment of hepatocellular carcinoma by percutaneous laser hyperthermia. 2001;16:548-552.

[14] Rapaccini GL. Percutaneous ablative treatments of hepatocellular carcinoma. Hepatology. 2014. doi: 10.1002/hep.27615.

[15] Ferrari FS, Megliola A, Scorzelli A, Stella A, Vigni F, Drudi FM, et al. Treatment of small HCC through radiofrequency ablation and laser ablation. Comparison of techniques and long-term results. Radiol Med. 2007;112(3):377-393.

[16] Di Costanzo GG, Tortora R, D'Adamo G, De Luca M, Lampasi F, Addario L, et al. Radiofrequency ablation versus laser ablation for the treatment of small hepatocellular carcinoma in cirrhosis: A randomized trial. J Gastroenterol Hepatol. 2015;30(3): 559-565.

[17] Maccini M, Sehrt D, Pompeo A, Chicoli FA, Molina WR, Kim FJ. Biophysiologic considerations in cryoablation: aA practical mechanistic molecular review. Int Braz J Urol. 2011;37(6):693-696.

[18] Wang C, Wang H, Yang W, Hu K, Xie H, Hu KQ, et al. A multicenter randomized controlled trial of percutaneous cryoablation versus radiofrequency ablation in hepatocellular carcinoma. Hepatology. 2014. doi: 10.1002/hep.27548.

[19] Lee EW, Thai S, Kee ST. Irreversible electroporation: A novel image-guided cancer therapy. Gut Liver. 2010;4(Suppl 1):S99-S104.

[20] Scheffer HJ, Nielsen K, de Jong MC, van Tilborg AA, Vieveen JM, Bouwman AR, et al. Irreversible electroporation for nonthermal tumor ablation in the clinical setting: aA systematic review of safety and efficacy. J Vasc Interv Radiol. 2014;25(7):997-1011.

[21] Bardhan R1, Lal S, Joshi A, Halas NJ. Theranostic nanoshells: fFrom probe design to imaging and treatment of cancer. Acc Chem Res. 2011;44(10):936-946.

[22] Hwang S, Nam J, Jung S, Song J, Doh H, Kim S. Gold nanoparticle-mediated photothermal therapy: Current status and future perspective. Nanomedicine (Lond). 2014;9(13):2003-2022.

[23] Kennedy LC, Bickford LR, Lewinski NA, Coughlin AJ, Hu Y, Day ES, et al. A new era for cancer treatment: gGold-nanoparticle-mediated thermal therapies. Small. 2011;7(2):169-183.

[24] Liu SY, Liang ZS, Gao F, Luo SF, Lu GQ. In vitro photothermal study of gold nanoshells functionalized with small targeting peptides to liver cancer cells. J Mater Sci Mater Med. 2010;21(2):665-74.

[25] You J, Zhang R, Xiong C, Zhong M, Melancon M, Gupta S, et al. Effective photothermal chemotherapy using doxorubicin-loaded gold nanospheres that target EphB4 receptors in tumors. Cancer Res. 2012;72(18):4777-4786.

[26] Gupta S, Stafford RJ, Javadi S, Ozkan E, Ensor JE, Wright KC, et al. Effects of near-infrared laser irradiation of biodegradable microspheres containing hollow gold nanospheres and paclitaxel administered intraarterially in a rabbit liver tumor model. J Vasc Interv Radiol. 2012;23(4):553-561.

[27] Zhenglin Li, Yongyi Zeng, Da Zhang, Ming Wu, Lingjie Wu, Aimin Huang, et al. Glypican-3 antibody functionalized Prussian blue nanoparticles for targeted MR imaging and photothermal therapy of hepatocellular carcinoma. J. Mater. Chem. B. 2014;2:3686-3696.

[28] Zhao J, Vykoukal J, Abdelsalam M, Recio-Boiles A, Huang Q, Qiao Y, et al. Stem cell-mediated delivery of SPIO-loaded gold nanoparticles for the theranosis of liver injury and hepatocellular carcinoma. Nanotechnology. 2014;25(40):405101. doi: 10.1088/0957-4484/25/40/405101.

[29] Singh R, Torti SV. Carbon nanotubes in hyperthermia therapy. Adv Drug Deliv Rev. 2013;65(15):2045-20460.

[30] Robinson JT, Welsher K, Tabakman SM, Sherlock SP, Wang H, Luong R, et al. High performance in vivo near-IR (>1 μm) imaging and photothermal cancer therapy with carbon nanotubes. Nano Res. 2010;3(11):779-793.

[31] Manthe RL, Foy SP, Krishnamurthy N, Sharma B, Labhasetwar V. Tumor ablation and nanotechnology. Mol Pharm. 2010;7(6):1880-1898.

[32] Asharani PV, Hande MP, Valiyaveettil S. Anti-proliferative activity of silver nanoparticles. BMC Cell Biol. 2009;10:65.

[33] Mironava T, Hadjiargyrou M, Simon M, Jurukovski V, Rafailovich MH. Gold nanoparticles cellular toxicity and recovery: eEffect of size, concentration and exposure time. Nanotoxicology. 2010;4(1):120-137.

[34] Kang B, Mackey MA, El-Sayed MA. Nuclear targeting of gold nanoparticles in cancer cells induces DNA damage, causing cytokinesis arrest and apoptosis. J Am Chem Soc. 2010;132(5):1517-1519.

[35] Ziyad S, Iruela-Arispe ML. Molecular mechanisms of tumor angiogenesis. Genes Cancer. 2011;2(12):1085-1096.

[36] Danhier F, Vroman B, Lecouturier N, Crokart N, Pourcelle V, Freichels H, et al. Targeting of tumor endothelium by RGD-grafted PLGA-nanoparticles loaded with paclitaxel. J Control Release. 2009;140(2):166-173.

[37] Lunov O, Syrovets T, Büchele B, Jiang X, Röcker C, Tron K, et al. The effect of carboxydextran-coated superparamagnetic iron oxide nanoparticles on c-Jun N-terminal kinase-mediated apoptosis in human macrophages. Biomaterials. 2010;31(19): 5063-50671.

[38] Kobayashi T. Biotechnol J. Cancer hyperthermia using magnetic nanoparticles. 2011;6(11):1342-1347.

[39] Tartaj P, Puerto Morales P, Veintemillas-Verdaguer S, Carre T, Carlos J Serna J. The preparation of magnetic nanoparticles for applications in biomedicine Phys. D: Appl. Phys. 2003;36:182-197

[40] Batlle X, Labarta A. Finite-size effects in fine particles: mMagnetic and transport properties J. Phys. D: Apply. Phys. 2002;35:R15.

[41] Johannsen M, Gneveckow U, Thiesen B, Taymoorian K, Cho CH, Waldöfner N, et al. Thermotherapy of prostate cancer using magnetic nanoparticles: fFeasibility, imaging, and three dimensional temperature distribution. Eur Urol 2007;52(6):1653-1661.

[42] Rosensweig RE. Heating magnetic fluid with alternating magnetic field. J Magn Magn Mater. 2002;252(1-3):370-374.

[43] Huang HS, Hainfeld JF. Intravenous magnetic nanoparticle cancer hyperthermia. Int J Nanomedicine. 2013;8:2521-253.

[44] Jordan A, Scholz R, Wust P, Schirra H, Thomas Schiestel, Schmidt H, Felix R. Endocytosis of dextran and silan-coated magnetite nanoparticles and the effect of intracellular hyperthermia on human mammary carcinoma cells in vitro. Journal of Magnetism and Magnetic Materials 1999;194:185-196.

[45] Moroz P, Jones SK, Gray BN. Magnetically mediated hyperthermia: Current status and future directions. Int J Hyperthermia. 2002;18(4):267-284.

[46] Srivastava PK1, Menoret A, Basu S, Binder RJ, McQuade KL. Heat shock proteins come of age: Primitive functions acquired new roles in an adaptive world. Immunity. 1998;8(6):657-665.

[47] Jordan A, Scholz R, Maier-Hauff K, Johannsen M, Wust P, Nadobny J, et al. J. Magn. Magn. Mater. 2001;225.

[48] Hilger I, Frühauf K, Andrä W, Hiergeist R, Hergt R, Kaiser WA. Heating potential of iron oxides for therapeutic purposes in interventional radiology. Acad Radiol. 2002;9(2):198-202.

[49] Hyeon T. Chemical synthesis of magnetic nanoparticles. Chem Commun. 2003;8:927-934.

[50] Gilchrist RK, Medal R, Shorey WD, Hanselman RC, Parrott JC, Taylor CB. Selective inductive heating of lymph nodes. Annals of surgery. 1957;146(4):596-606.

[51] Moroz P, Jones SK, Winter J, Gray BN. Targeting liver tumors with hyperthermia: fFerromagnetic embolization in a rabbit liver tumor model. J Surg Oncol 2001;78(1): 22-29.

[52] Jimbow K, Takada T, Sato M, Sato A, et al. Melanin biology and translational research strategy; melanogenesis and nanomedicine as the basis for melanoma-targeted DDS and chemothermoimmunotherapy. Pigm. Cell Melanoma Res. 2008:21:243-244.

[53] Jordan A, Scholz R, Maier-Hauff K, van Landeghem FK, Waldoefner N, Teichgraeber U, et al. The effect of thermotherapy using magnetic nanoparticles on rat malignant glioma. J Neurooncol. 2006;78(1):7-14

[54] Johannsen M, Jordan A, Scholz R, Koch M, Lein M, Deger S, et al. Evaluation of magnetic fluid hyperthermia in a standard rat model of prostate cancer. J Endourol. 2004;18 (5):495-500.

[55] Johannsen M, Thiesen B, Jordan A, Taymoorian K, Gneveckow U, Waldöfner N, et al. Magnetic fluid hyperthermia (MFH) reduces prostate cancer growth in the orthotopic Dunning R3327 rat model. Prostate. 2005;64:283-292.

[56] Johannsen M, Thiesen B, Gneveckow U, Taymoorian K, Waldöfner N, Scholz R, et al. Thermotherapy using magnetic nanoparticles combined with external radiation in an orthotopic rat model of prostate cancer. Prostate. 2006;66:97-104.

[57] Shinkai M, Yanase M, Honda H, Wakabayashi T, Yoshida J, Kobayashi T. Intracellular hyperthermia for cancer using magnetite cationic liposome–in vitro study. Jpn. J. Cancer Res. 1996:87;1179.-183.

[58] Ito A, Tanaka K, Honda H, Abe S et al., Complete regression of mouse mammary carcinoma with a size greater than 15 mm by frequent repeated hyperthermia using magnetite nanoparticles. J. Biosci. Bioeng. 2003;96:364-369.

[59] Zhang J, Misra RD. Magnetic drug-targeting carrier encapsulated with thermosensitive smart polymer: core-shell nanoparticle carrier and drug release response. Acta Biomater. 2007;3(6):838-850.

[60] Hu SH, Liao BJ, Chiang CS, Chen PJ, Chen IW, Chen SY. Core-shell nanocapsules stabilized by single-component polymer and nanoparticles for magneto-chemotherapy/hyperthermia with multiple drugs. Adv Mater. 2012;24(27):3627-3632.

[61] Johannsen M, Gneveckow U, Taymoorian K, Cho CH, Thiesen B, Scholz R, et al. Thermal therapy of prostate cancer using magnetic nanoparticles. Actas Urol Esp. 2007;31(6):660-667.

[62] Maier-Hauff K, Rothe R, Scholz R, Gneveckow U, Wust P, Thiesen B, et al. Intracranial thermotherapy using magnetic nanoparticles combined with external beam radiotherapy: rResults of a feasibility study on patients with glioblastoma multiforme. J Neurooncol. 2007;81(1):53-60.

[63] van Landeghem FK, Maier-Hauff K, Jordan A, Hoffmann KT, Gneveckow U, Scholz R, et al. Post-mortem studies in glioblastoma patients treated with thermotherapy using magnetic nanoparticles. Biomaterials. 2009;30(1):52-57.

[64] Takamatsu S, Matsui O, Gabata T, Kobayashi S, Okuda M, Ougi T, et al. Selective induction hyperthermia following transcatheter arterial embolization with a mixture of nano-sized magnetic particles (ferucarbotran) and embolic materials: Feasibility study in rabbits. Radiat Med. 2008;26:179-187.

[65] Yuan Y, Wyatt C, Maccarini P, et al. A heterogeneous human tissue mimicking phantom for RF heating and MRI thermal monitoring verification. Phys Med Biol. 2012;57(7):2021-2037.

[66] Wiekhorst F, Steinhoff U, Eberbeck D, Trahms L. Magnetorelaxometry assisting biomedical applications of magnetic nanoparticles. Pharm Res. 2012;29(5):1189-1202.

[67] Widmann G, Schullian P, Haidu M, Bale R. Stereotactic radiofrequency ablation (SRFA) of liver lesions: tTechnique effectiveness, safety, and interoperator performance. Cardiovasc Intervent Radiol. 2012;35(3):570-580.

[68] Phillips WT, Bao A, Brenner AJ, Goins BA. Image-guided interventional therapy for cancer with radiotherapeutic nanoparticles. Adv Drug Deliv Rev. 2014, 30;76: 39-59.

[69] Shenoi MM, Anderson J, Bischof JC. Nanoparticle enhanced thermal therapies. Conf Proc IEEE Eng Med Biol Soc. 2009;2009:1979-1982.

[70] Torchilin V. Tumor delivery of macromolecular drugs based on the EPR effect. Adv. Drug Deliv. Rev. 2011;63:131-135.

[71] Ahmed M, Goldberg SN. Combination radiofrequency thermal ablation and adjuvant IV liposomal doxorubicin increases tissue coagulation and intratumoural drug accumulation. Int J Hyperthermia. 2004;20(7):781-802.

[72] Day ES, Morton JG, West JL. Nanoparticles for thermal cancer therapy. J Biomech Eng. 2009;131(7):074001.

[73] Glazer ES, Curley SA. Non-invasive radiofrequency ablation of malignancies mediated by quantum dots, gold nanoparticles and carbon nanotubes. Ther Deliv. 2011;2:1325-1330.

[74] Corr SJ, Cisneros BT, Green L, Raoof M, Curley SA. Protocols for assessing radiofrequency interactions with gold nanoparticles and biological systems for non-invasive hyperthermia cancer therapy. J Vis Exp. 2013;28:(78).

[75] Raoof M, Curley SA. Non-invasive radiofrequency-induced targeted hyperthermia for the treatment of hepatocellular carcinoma. Int J Hepatol. 2011;676957. doi: 10.4061/2011/676957.

[76] Cardinal J, Klune JR, Chory E, Jeyabalan G, Kanzius JS, Nalesnik M, Geller DA. Non-invasive radiofrequency ablation of cancer targeted by gold nanoparticles. Surgery. 2008;144(2):125-132.

[77] Iancu C, Mocan L, Bele C, Orza AI, Tabaran FA, Catoi C, Stiufiuc R, Stir A, Matea C, Iancu D, Agoston-Coldea L, Zaharie F, Mocan T. Enhanced laser thermal ablation for the in vitro treatment of liver cancer by specific delivery of multiwalled carbon nanotubes functionalized with human serum albumin. Int J Nanomedicine. 2011;6:129-141.

[78] Bangham AD, Horne RW. Negative staining of phospholipids and their structural modification by surface-active agents as observed in the electron microscope. J. Mol. Biol. 1964;8:660-668.

[79] Chen J, He CQ, Lin AH, Gu W, Chen ZP, Li W, Cai BC. Thermosensitive liposomes with higher phase transition temperature for targeted drug delivery to tumor. Int J Pharm. 2014;475(1-2):408-415.

[80] Immordino ML, Dosico F, Cattel L. Stealth liposomes: review of the basic science, rationale, and clinical applications:, existing and potential. Int. J. Nanomed. 2006;1:297-315.

[81] Needham D, Anyarambhatla G, Kong G, Dewhirst MW. A new temperature sensitive liposome for use with mild hyperthermia: cCharacterization and testing in a human tumor xenograft model. Cancer Res. 2000;60(5):1197-1201.

[82] Unezaki S, Maruyama K, Takahashi N, Koyama M, Yuda T, Suginaka A, Iwatsuru M. Enhanced delivery and antitumor activity of doxorubicin using long-circulating thermosensitive liposomes containing amphipathic polyethylene glycol in combination with local hyperthermia. Pharm Res. 1994;11(8):1180-1185.

[83] Lindner LH, Eichhorn ME, Eibl H, Teichert N, Schmitt-Sody M, Issels RD, Dellian M. Novel temperature-sensitive liposomes with prolonged circulation time. Clin Cancer Res. 2004;10(6):2168-2178.

[84] Li T, Zhang M, Han Y, Zhang H, Xu L, Xiang Y. Targeting therapy of choroidal neovascularization by use of polypeptide- and PEDF-loaded immunoliposomes under ultrasound exposure. J Huazhong Univ Sci Technolog Med Sci. 2010;30(6):798-803.

[85] Seynhaeve AL, Hoving S, Schipper D, Vermeulen CE, de Wiel-AmbagtsheerGa, van Tiel ST, et al. Tumor necrosis factor alpha mediates homogeneous distribution of liposomes in murine melanoma that contributes to a better tumor response. Cancer Res. 2007;67(19):9455-9462.

[86] Harrington KJ, Mohammadtaghi S, Uster PS, Glass D, Peters AM, Vile RG, Stewart JS. Effective targeting of solid tumors in patients with locally advanced cancers by radiolabeled pegylated liposomes. Clin Cancer Res. 2001;7(2):243-254.

[87] Ta T, Porter TM. Thermosensitive liposomes for localized delivery and triggered release of chemotherapy. J ControlRelease. 2013;10 169(1-2):112-125.

[88] Allen TM, Cullis PR. Liposomal drug delivery systems: From concept to clinical applications. Adv Drug Deliv Rev. 2013;65:36-48.

[89] Horsman MR, Overgaard J. Can mild hyperthermia improve tumour oxygenation? Int J Hyperthermia. 1997;13(2):141-147.

[90] Karino T, Koga S, Maeta M. Experimental studies of the effects of local hyperthermia on blood flow, oxygen pressure and pH in tumors. Jpn J Surg. 1988;18(3):276-283.

[91] Fujiwara K, Watanabe T. Effects of hyperthermia, radiotherapy and thermoradiotherapy on tumor microvascular permeability. ActaPathol Jpn. 1990;40(2):79-84.

[92] Li L, ten Hagen TL, Bolkestein M, Gasselhuber A, Yatvin J, van Rhoon GC, Eggermont AM, Haemmerich D, Koning GA. Improved intratumoral nanoparticle extravasation and penetration by mild hyperthermia. J ControlRelease. 2013;28 167(2): 130-137.

[93] Kennedy JE. High-intensity focused ultrasound in the treatment of solid tumours. Nat Rev Cancer. 2005;5:321-392.

[94] Clement GT. Perspectives in clinical uses of high-intensity focused ultrasound. Ultrasonics. 2004;42:1087-1093.

[95] Dromi S, Frenkel V, Luk A, Traughber B, Angstadt M, Bur M, et al. Pulsed-high intensity focused ultrasound and low temperature-sensitive liposomes for enhanced targeted drug delivery and antitumor effect. Clin Cancer Res. 2007;13(9):2722-2727.

[96] de Smet M, Heijman E, Langereis S, Hijnen NM, Grüll H. Magnetic resonance imaging of high intensity focused ultrasound mediated drug delivery from temperature-sensitive liposomes: an in vivo proof-of-concept study. J. Control. Release 2011;150(1):102-110.

[97] Ranjan A, Jacobs GC, Woods DL, Negussie AH, Partanen A, Yarmolenko PS, et al. Image-guided drug delivery with magnetic resonance guided high intensity focused ultrasound and temperature sensitive liposomes in a rabbit Vx2 tumor model. J. Control. Release 2012;158:487-494.

[98] Ahmed M, Moussa M, Goldberg SN. Synergy in cancer treatment between liposomal chemotherapeutics and thermal ablation. Chem Phys Lipids. 2012;165(4):424-437.

[99] Solazzo SA, Ahmed M, Schor-Bardach R, Yang W, Girnun GD, Rahmanuddin S, Levchenko T, Signoretti S, Spitz DR, Torchilin V, Goldberg SN. Liposomal doxorubicin increases radiofrequency ablation-induced tumor destruction by increasing cellular oxidative and nitrative stress and accelerating apoptotic pathways. Radiology. 2010;255(1):62-67.

[100] Ahmed M, Monsky WE, Girnun G, Lukyanov A, D'Ippolito G, Kruskal JB, Stuart KE, Torchilin VP, Goldberg SN. Radiofrequency thermal ablation sharply increases intratumoral liposomal doxorubicin accumulation and tumor coagulation. Cancer Res. 2003;63(19):6327-6333.

[101] Yatvin MB, Weinstein JN, Dennis WH, Blumenthal R. Design of liposomes for enhanced local release of drug by hyperthermia. Science. 1998;202:1290-129.

[102] Mills JK, Needham D. The materials engineering of temperature-sensitive liposomes. Methods Enzymol. 2004;387:82-113.

[103] Needham D, Anyarambhatla G, Kong G, Dewhirst MW. A new temperature sensitive liposome for use with mild hyperthermia: cCharacterization and testing in a human tumor xenograft model. Cancer Res. 2000;60(5):1197-1201.

[104] Poon RTP, Borys N. Lyso-thermosensitive liposomal doxorubicin: aA novel approach to enhance efficacy of thermal ablation of liver cancer. Expert Opin Pharmacother. 2009:10;333-342.

[105] Landon CD, Park J, Needham D, Dewhirst MW. Nanoscale drug delivery and hyperthermia: tThe materials designand preclinical and clinical testing of low temperature-sensitive liposomes used in combination with mild hyperthermia in the treatment of local cancer. Open Nanomed J. 2011;3:38-64.

[106] Poon RT, Borys N. Lyso-thermosensitive liposomal doxorubicin: An adjuvant to increase the cure rate of radiofrequency ablation in liver cancer. Future Oncol. 2011;7(8):937-945.

[107] Hossann M, Syunyaeva Z, Schmidt R, Zengerle A, Eibl H, Issels RD, Linder, LH. Proteins and cholesterol lipid vesicles are mediators of drug release from thermosensitive liposomes. J Control. Release 2012:162;400-406.

[108] Mills J.K, Needham D. Lysolipid incorporation in dipalmitoylphosphati-dylcholine bilayer membranes enhances the ion permeability and drug release rates at the membrane phase transition. Biochim Biophys Acta. 2005:1716;77-96.

[109] Park K. Lessons learned from thermosensitive liposomes from improved chemotherapy. J Control.Release 2014;174:219.

[110] Park JW, Hong K, Carter P, Asgari H, Guo LY, Keller GA, Wirth C, Shalaby R, Kotts C, Wood WI, et al.. Development of anti-p185HER2 immunoliposomes for cancer therapy. Proc Natl Acad Sci USA. 1995;92(5):1327-1331.

[111] Kullberg M, Mann K, Owens JL. A two component drug delivery system using Her-2-targeting thermosensitive liposomes. J Drug Target. 2009;17(2):98-107.

[112]] Negussie AH, Miller JL, Reddy G, Drake SK, Wood BJ, Dreher MR. Synthesis and in vitro evaluation of cyclic NGR peptide targeted thermally sensitive liposome. J Control. Release 2010;143(2): 265-273.

[113] Dicheva BM, ten Hagen TL, Li L, Schipper D, Seynhaeve AL, van Rhoon GC, Eggermont AM, Lindner LH, Koning GA. Cationic thermosensitive liposomes: aA novel dual targeted heat-triggered drug delivery approach for endothelial and tumor Cells. Nano Lett. 2013;13(6):2324-2331.

Chapter 10

Diagnostic and Therapeutic Challenges in Nonparasitic Liver Cysts

Mirela Patricia Sîrbu Boeți, Mirela Boroș,
Vlad Herlea, Amalia Petrișor and Irinel Popescu

Additional information is available at the end of the chapter

http://dx.doi.org/10.5772/61057

Abstract

Nonparasitic hepatic cysts constitute a heterogeneous group of disorders. A proper diagnosis of hepatic cyst is necessary in order to adopt the best treatment. The term hepatic cyst usually refers to simple hepatic cysts. Nonparasitic hepatic cysts are also linked to genetic disorders such as polycystic liver disease (PLD) with/without autosomal dominant polycystic kidney disease (ADPKD) or Caroli disease. Generally, patients with nonparasitic hepatic cysts less than 3 cm are asymptomatic. These cysts become symptomatic when are large, multiple, or complicated. Percutaneous abdominal ultrasound is the best imaging modality to diagnose hepatic cysts but must be completed by other imaging and serological tests. It is important to differentiate simple hepatic cyst from hydatid cyst, cystadenoma, and cystadenocarcinoma before proceeding with the treatment. Sometimes the diagnosis is very challenging. Asymptomatic single liver cysts need only surveillance, but symptomatic and complicated ones require therapeutic intervention. Percutaneous aspiration of the cyst under ultrasound guidance is a mini-invasive procedure generally associated with sclerotherapy. The highest success rates were reported for laparoscopic or open cyst fenestration. Liver transplantation is indicated for patients with severe PLD.

Keywords: Simple hepatic cyst, serous hepatic cyst, nonparasitic hepatic cyst, polycystic liver disease

1. Introduction

Nonparasitic hepatic cysts encompass a heterogeneous group of disorders, which differ in etiology, prevalence, and manifestations. The term hepatic cyst usually refers to solitary nonparasitic cysts of the liver, also known as simple cysts. Generally, hepatic cysts are incidentally found during surgery and more frequently during imaging examinations for other reasons. Nowadays, due to the imaging procedures, prevalence of nonparasitic hepatic cysts is found increased up to 18% in adult population [1]. The incidence is higher in females older than 50 years.

2. Classification and etiology

2.1. Serous/simple hepatic cyst

Hepatic serous or simple cysts may be single or multiple and are considered to be congenital. They are derived from aberrant bile ducts that have apparently lost communication with the biliary tree and continue to secrete intramural fluid [2]. Microscopically, they are lined by a single layer of cuboid, columnar, flattened (Figure 1) or pseudostratified (Figure 2), or by stratified epithelial cells (Figure 3), resembling biliary epithelial cells.

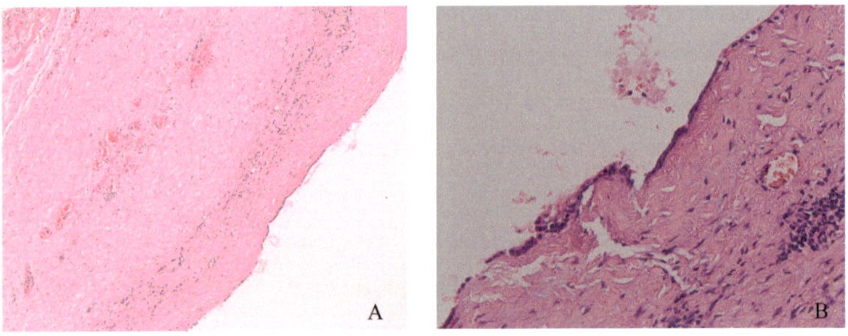

Figure 1. Serous cyst with flattened epithelium. (A) Hematoxylin and eosin staining ×100. (B) Hematoxylin and eosin staining ×400.

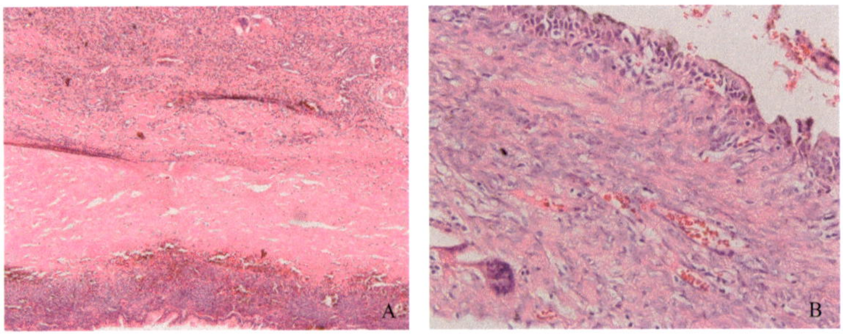

Figure 2. Serous cyst with pseudostratified epithelium. (A) Hematoxylin and eosin staining ×100. (B) Hematoxylin and eosin staining ×400.

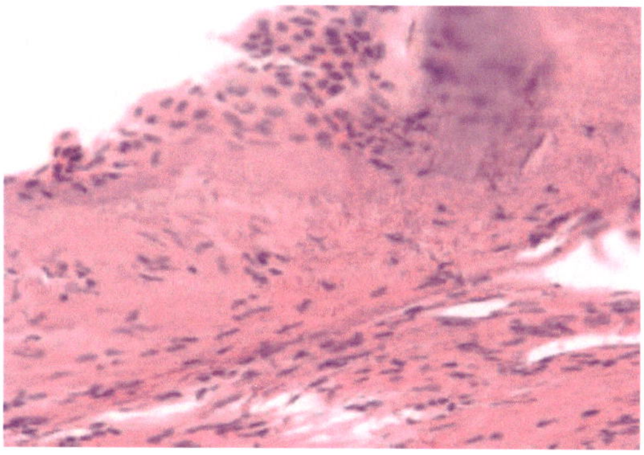

Figure 3. Serous simple cyst with stratified cuboidal epithelium. Hematoxylin and eosin staining ×200.

2.2. Polycystic liver disease

Serous hepatic cysts are also linked to genetic disorders such as polycystic liver disease (PLD) with/without autosomal dominant polycystic kidney disease (ADPKD) or Caroli disease. Isolated PLD is associated with heterozygous mutations in PRKCSH or SEC63 genes. PLD associated with ADPKD is linked with mutations in the PKD1 or PKD2 gene [3]. Overall prevalence is similar for both genders, but females develop a more severe liver disease. Pregnancy, multiparity, and use of steroids increase the risk for severe hepatic cystic disease.

Gigot and collaborators have described a classification for patients with polycystic liver disease based on the number and size of hepatic cysts and residual normal liver parenchyma between the cysts. This description is based on preoperative computed tomography (CT) [4]. Also, this classification can delineate the therapeutic strategy [5].

- Type I—less than 10 large cyst (7–10 cm) with large areas of noncystic parenchyma
- Type II—diffuse involvement of liver parenchyma by medium-sized cysts (5–7 cm) with remaining large areas of noncystic parenchyma
- Type III—massive, diffuse involvement of liver parenchyma by small- and medium-sized cysts (less than 5 cm) and only a few areas of normal liver parenchyma between cysts [2, 4, 5]

It is of exquisite importance to differentiate hepatic cyst from hydatid hepatic cyst, hepatic cystadenoma, and hepatic cystadenocarcinoma before proceeding with the treatment. In certain situations, it can be very challenging to properly diagnose a hepatic cystic mass [6, 7]. There are also rare hepatic cystic lesions that must be taken into consideration [8]. In pediatric population, the surgeon should be aware of the wide range of other types of liver cysts to ensure appropriate treatment [9].

2.3. Localized Caroli disease or solitary dilatation of intrahepatic biliary duct

Caroli disease is an autosomal recessive inheritance linked to mutation in PKHD1 gene. It is classified as type V choledochal cyst by the Todani classification [10]. The cystic lesions are depicted as irregular in shape, fusiform, or saccular (Figures 4A). On MRCP they are seen to communicate with biliary tree (Figure 4B). On gross examination of the operative specimen, the cystic cavity contains biliary sludge and even gallstones (Figure 5).

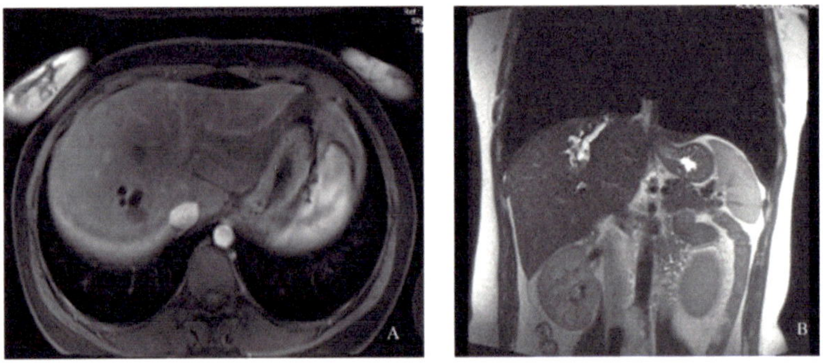

Figure 4. Localized Caroli disease. (A) MRI, axial section: group of cysts in hepatic segment VIII. (B) MRCP, coronal section: group of cysts that communicate with biliary tree.

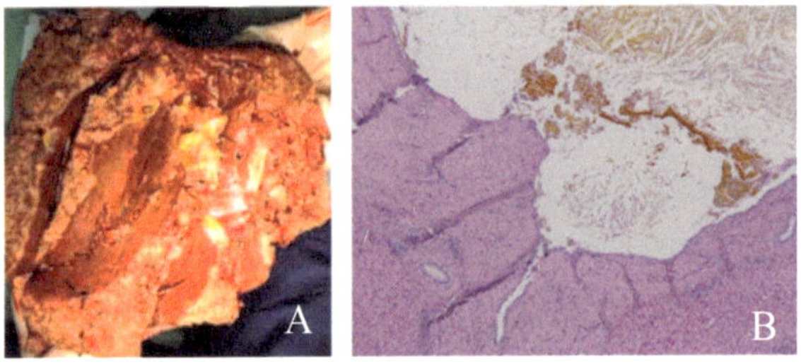

Figure 5. Localized Caroli disease. (A) Resected specimen with biliary cysts filled with bile sludge. (B) Histological examination with hematoxylin and eosin staining ×100.

2.4. Intrahepatic biliary papilloma

Biliary papilloma represents a tumorous growth of the bile duct epithelia in the bile duct lumen and can cause a localized dilatation of the intrahepatic bile duct. If native and contrast enhanced CT fail to observe the biliary papilloma, the bile duct dilatation may be confused with a hepatic serous cyst. ERCP can demonstrate the communication between the cystic lesion and the bile duct [11].

2.5. Biliary cystadenoma and cystadenocarcinoma

Biliary cystadenoma is a very rare cystic lesion of the liver that usually occurs in middle-aged woman. The exact etiology of this insidiously progressive tumor is unknown. This cyst may originate from a congenitally aberrant bile duct or directly from a primitive hepatobiliary stem cell.

http://dx.doi.org/10.5772/61057

Cystadenoma of the liver is characterized by multilocular cysts with internal septation and epithelial lining composed of columnar to cuboidal cells capable of mucin production. They usually contain clear mucinous fluid and rarely the fluid may be bilious, purulent, proteinaceous, or hemorrhagic. Bloody fluid often signifies a malignant component [12]. The septa may show calcifications.

Two subgroups are distinguished by presence or absence of mesenchymal (ovarian like) stroma between an inner epithelial lining and an outer layer of collagenized connective tissue (Figure 6).

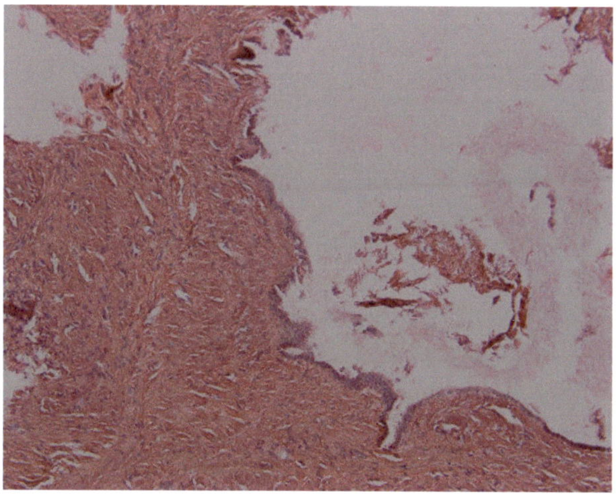

Figure 6. Cystadenoma without mesenchymal stroma. Hematoxylin and eosin staining ×200.

The mesenchymal stroma resembles primitive mesenchyme, and cell differentiation varies from smooth muscle or fibroblasts to adipocytes or capillaries. Cystadenoma with mesenchymal stroma occurs exclusively in women (Figure 7) possibly as a consequence of the female milieu influence, while cystadenoma without mesenchymal stroma predominates in men [13].

Mesenchymal stroma may give rise to both cystadenocarcinoma and sarcomas. Intrahepatic biliary cystadenoma cannot be clearly differentiated from cystadenocarcinoma before operation. Some authors consider the diagnostic value of the analysis of serum and aspirated cyst fluid for tumor markers. However, elevated carbohydrate antigen CA 19-9 and carcinoembryonic antigen CEA has been associated both with cystadenoma and cystadenocarcinoma [14]. Only histopathologic exam can certainly differentiate it from malignant degeneration. Being considered a premalignant lesion, surgical excision seems to be a wise decision in patients with intrahepatic biliary cystadenoma. If not completely resected, the recurrence in biliary cystadenoma is greater than 90% [12]. Moreover, if malignancy is not recognized, a simple fenestration may prove catastrophic to patient. Patients with cystadenocarcinoma with mesenchymal stroma have a good prognosis, whereas cystadenocarcinoma in men, which is not associated with mesenchymal stroma, has a worse prognosis, even after complete excision [15].

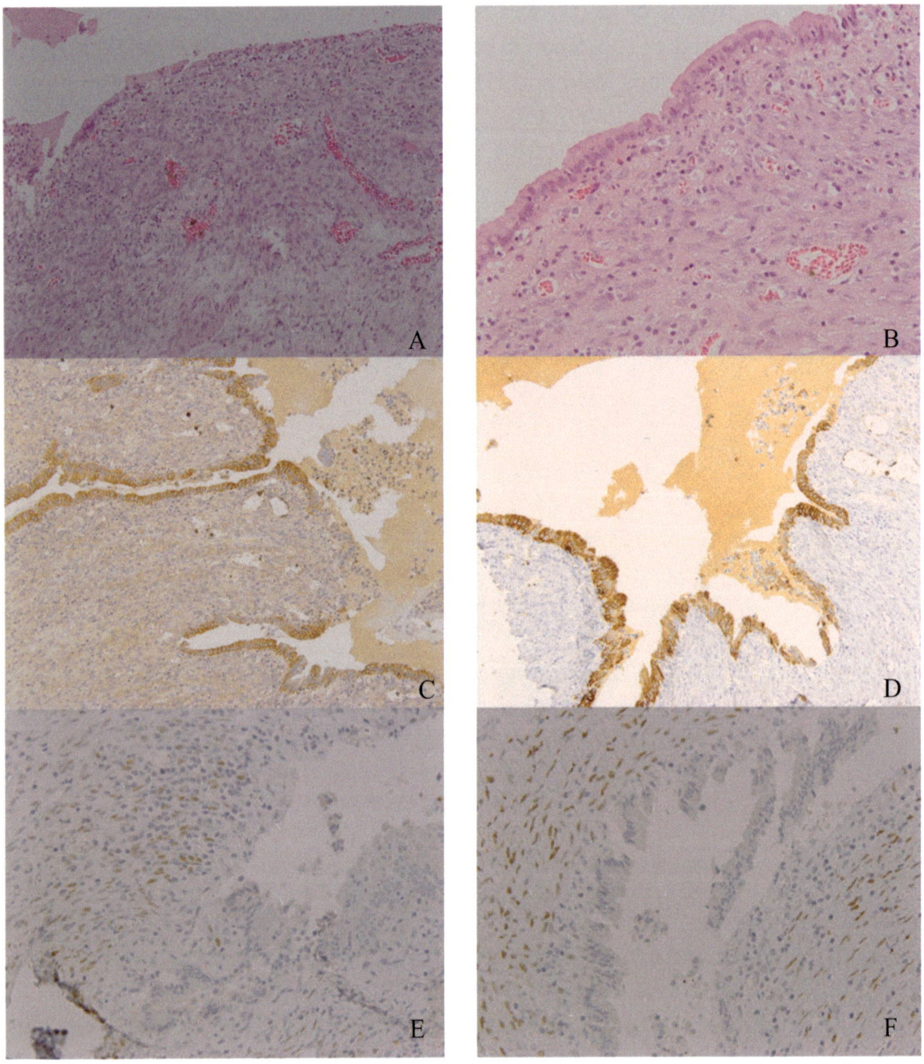

Figure 7. Cystadenoma with mesenchymal stroma. (A) Hematoxylin and eosin staining ×200. (B) Hematoxylin and eosin staining ×400. (C) Immunohistochemical staining CK7 ×200. Cyst epithelium is positive for CK7. (D) Immunohistochemical staining CK8-18 ×200. Cyst epithelium is positive for CK8-18. (E) Immunohistochemical staining ER ×400. Mesenchymal stroma contains cells (brown cells) that are positively stained for estrogen receptors. (F) Immunohistochemical staining PgR ×400. Mesenchymal stroma contains cells (brown cells) that are positively stained for progesterone receptors.

2.6. Bile duct hamartoma

Bile duct hamartomas, also called von Meyenburg complexes, originate from embryonic bile ducts that fail to involute. Generally, they are encountered as an incidental finding at imaging, laparotomy, or autopsy. Macroscopically, they are cyst-like, grayish-white nodular lesions of 0.1-1.5 cm diameter that do not communicate with the biliary tree. Sometimes they are associated with Caroli's disease, PLD and congenital fibrosis. In case of intraoperative discovery, they may be misdiagnosed as liver metastases.

2.7. Ciliated hepatic foregut cyst

Ciliated hepatic foregut cysts are rare foregut developmental malformation usually solitary and unilocular. Generally, these are situated in the central segments of the liver (Figure 8). These cysts are characterized by the typical microscopic finding of four layers (the inner ciliated, pseudostratified, columnar epithelium; subepithelial connective tissue; smooth muscle layer; and an outer fibrous layer at microscopic examination). Squamous metaplasia may be present with potential transformation into squamous cell carcinoma. Malignant transformation to squamous cell carcinoma with aggressive behavior has been reported in 3% of adult cases [4, 16].

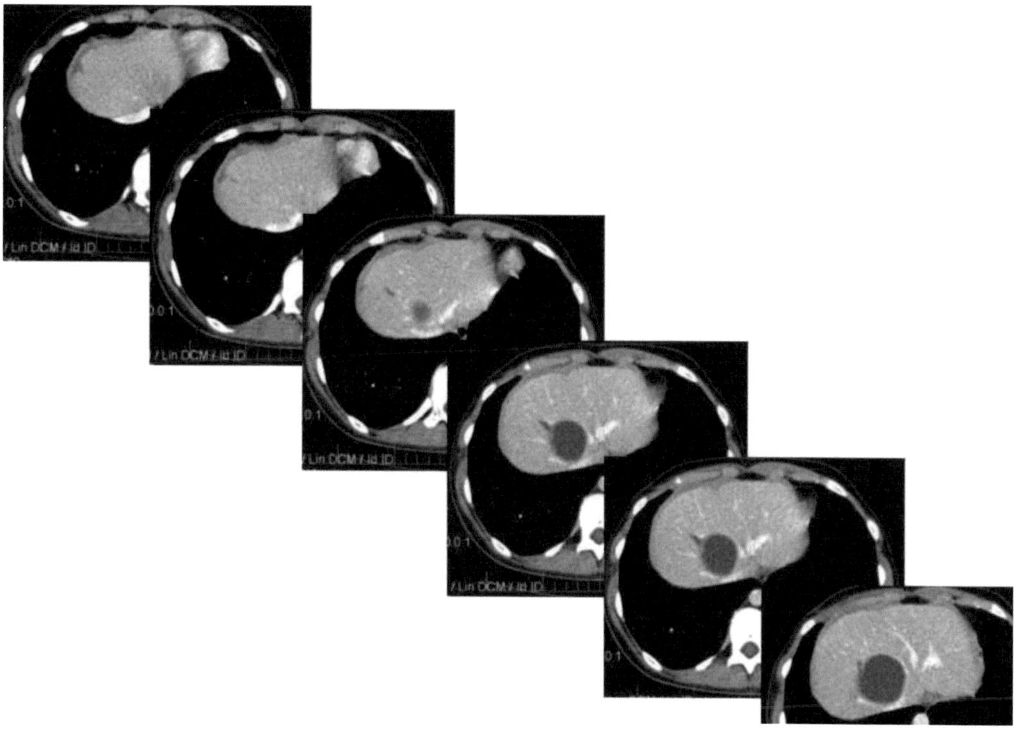

Figure 8. CT series showing a hepatic cyst situated in segment VIII, with an extension that is traced on the hepatic surface, raising the question of ciliated hepatic foregut cyst in a 14-year-old girl. The patient was submitted to open surgery due to the close proximity with the inferior vena cava and hepatic vein.

2.8. Intrahepatic pancreatic pseudocyst

Hepatic pseudocyst secondary to acute pancreatitis is extremely rare and is generally situated in the left lobe. A high level of amylase in the aspirated fluid confirms the diagnosis. Asymptomatic intrahepatic pseudocyst can be treated conservatively, and symptomatic intrahepatic pseudocyst can be managed either percutaneously or surgically [17].

2.9. Posttraumatic hepatic cyst

Only those symptomatic or of uncertain nature need treatment.

2.10. Biloma

Biloma appears as a cystic mass. It is caused by spontaneous, traumatic, or iatrogenic rupture of the biliary system.

2.11. Peribiliary cysts

Peribiliary cysts are mostly encountered in cirrhotic patients with portal hypertension or after liver transplantation. The cysts are located along the portal pedicles. Usually they are small and asymptomatic.

2.12. Liver hematoma

Liver hematomas are cystic lesions that develop after trauma, liver biopsy, or surgery.

2.13. Hepatic epidermoid cyst

Liver epidermoid cysts are extremely rare. These malformations have been diagnosed in pediatric patients, with the youngest one being 5 months years old. The importance of resection of such cystic lesions in pediatric population resides in the need of elimination of a lesion lined by squamous epithelium with possible squamous metaplasia that can potentially undergo malignant transformation, resulting in squamous cell carcinoma.

2.14. Postcholecystectomy hepatic cystic mass

The term of gossypiboma derived from the Latin term gossypium is used to define a forgotten surgical material in the body after surgery. Sometimes gossypiboma has a cyst-like appearance on imaging tests.

2.15. Hepatic endometriosis

So far only 22 cases of hepatic endometrioma have been reported in the literature [18]. Hepatic endometriosis should be considered in women of any age presenting with a hepatic cystic mass, with or without previous endometriosis history. Frozen sections of intraoperative transhepatic biopsy are necessary to avoid radical hepatectomy in order to decrease postoperative morbidity and mortality. However, the diagnosis is confirmed through histological immunostaining. Complete pericystectomy is necessary to avoid recurrence.

http://dx.doi.org/10.5772/61057

2.16. Hepatic vascular tumors

There are hepatic vascular tumors with predominantly solid appearance at gross examination but with cyst-like appearance on imaging examinations due to the high water content. Histopathological diagnosis must differentiate between lymphangioma, hemangioma, hemangiopericytoma, or undifferentiated embryonal sarcoma (Figure 9).

2.17. Liver metastases

Liver metastases from ovarian, pancreatic, colon, renal, or neuroendocrine cancer may have cyst-like appearance on imaging tests.

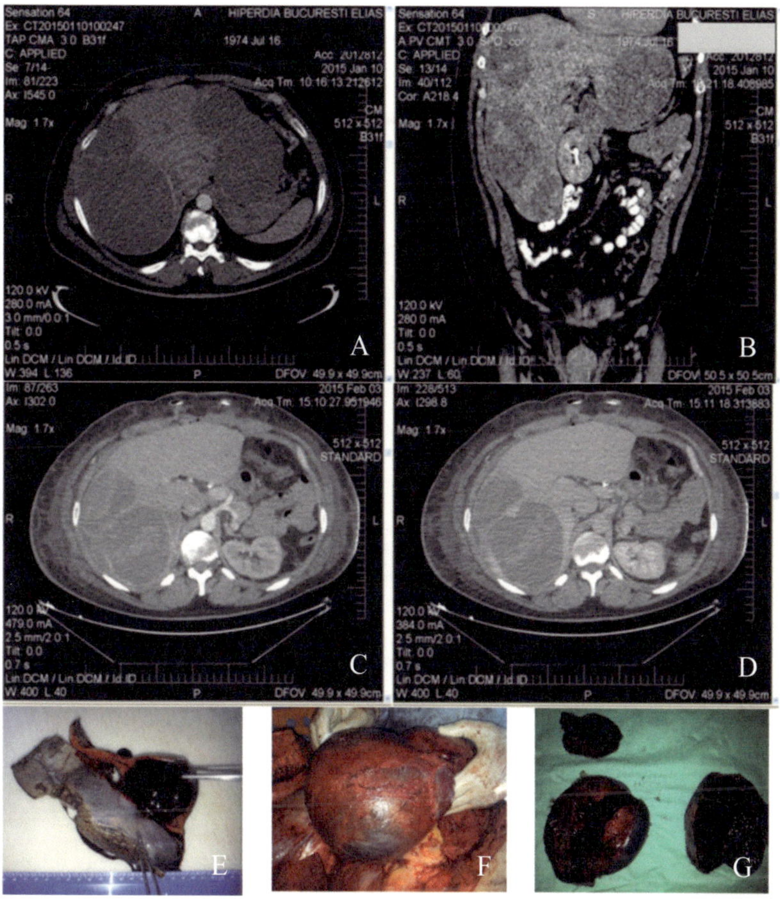

Figure 9. Hepatomegaly caused by multiple bilateral liver vascular tumors with cystic features on CT and operative specimen. (A) CT, axial view. (B) CT, coronal view. (C) CT with i.v. contrast, axial view, after left lateral sectionectomy. (D) CT without contrast, axial view after left lateral sectionectomy. (E) Resected specimen after left lateral sectionectomy with hemorrhagic cystic feature on section. (F) Intraoperative aspect of the hepatic vascular tumor. (G) Resected specimen after atypical hepatectomies for the tumors located in the right lobe, with hemorrhagic cystic feature on section.

3. Clinical manifestations

Generally, patients with nonparasitic hepatic cysts less than 3 cm are asymptomatic [2]. Cysts are classified as "large" when they are greater than 4 cm in the longest diameter. If the diagnosis of hepatic serous cyst is clear, there is no need of treatment, unless it becomes symptomatic, has a diameter more than 5 cm, or if the cyst grows rapidly within a short period of time [19].

Around 15% of patients with liver cysts develop symptoms at some stage in life. When the patients start complaining, the most common symptom is pain in the right upper quadrant. Other encountered symptoms are nausea, vomiting, abdominal meteorism, shoulder or lumbar pain, dyspnea, and/or postprandial fullness. Hepatic cysts become symptomatic when they are large, fast growing, multiple, or complicated.

3.1. Complications

Complications occur in approximately 10% of patients [20]. Obstructive jaundice, portal hypertension, intracystic hemorrhage, infection, intraperitoneal and/or intrahepatic rupture, torsion, and inflammation represent complications of nonparasitic hepatic cysts [21–24]. The compression exerted by a large hepatic cyst on the adjacent structures can manifest as cardiac arrhythmia or inferior vena cava thrombosis [25, 26]. The vicinity with the cholecyst can cause its functional disturbance with consecutive gallstones.

Hemorrhage into a simple liver cyst is rather uncommon but poses issues regarding differential diagnosis. The differential diagnosis between intracystic hemorrhage, cystadenoma, and cystadenocarcinoma is difficult with the imaging studies currently available. One consequence is to assume a simple cyst with intracystic hemorrhage as being neoplastic lesion and perform an unnecessary hepatectomy. The other consequence is to assume a neoplastic lesion as being benign and perform laparoscopic fenestration with subsequent peritoneal dissemination of malignant cells.

There are situations when an intracystic hemorrhage occurs unrecognized. Even if no acute symptoms supervene, the hemorrhage causes a rapid enlargement of the cyst, raising suspicion of malignant degeneration.

Infection of hepatic cyst can occur through common bile duct or blood stream. The most common encountered microorganisms are *Escherichia coli* and *Klebsiella pneumoniae. Proteus, Bacteroides*, and *Clostridium* are also incriminated in infection of hepatic cysts. The most likely source of infection for simple liver cysts is the gastrointestinal tract. Diverticulitis of the sigmoid colon and gut manipulation during abdominal operations have been found to be the cause of infectious complications of hepatic cysts [27]. The patients with diabetes mellitus, undergoing chronic hemodialysis or immunosuppressive therapy (e.g., after kidney transplant in patient with polycystic liver and kidney disease), are prone to develop such infections.

The patient with infected liver cyst presents with acute onset of right upper quadrant abdominal pain, diarrhea, and/or fever. There are situations when pain is absent, and the only symptoms are fever and malaise that render a complete workup to rule out other causes.

The rupture of serous hepatic cyst is a rare complication that needs emergency intervention. The cyst rupture is generally secondary to trauma, but a spontaneous one is also possible. The cyst fluid can enter the pleural or peritoneal cavity, causing pain in right upper quadrant or even diffuse abdominal pain due to peritoneal irritation.

Granuloma degeneration is a rare complication of the hepatic cysts (Figure 10). In severe form, it can resemble malignant invasion into surrounding tissues. The differential diagnosis is difficult to make even intraoperatively. Extensive excision of involved tissues is sometimes necessary [28]. Eventually histology delineates the diagnosis.

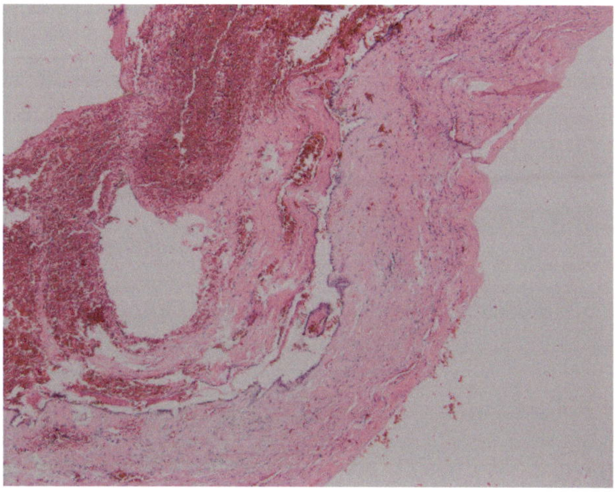

Figure 10. Serous cyst with granulomatous transformation, hyaline collagen fibrosis and focal, nonspecific chronic inflammation. Hematoxylin and eosin staining ×100.

4. Diagnosis

Percutaneous abdominal ultrasonography (US) is the best imaging modality for diagnosis of serous hepatic cysts. US is generally the first choice diagnostic procedure because it is sensitive, specific, noninvasive, and ready available. The typical appearance of simple cyst on US is as follows: round or oval anechoic mass, well circumscribed, with thin and smooth borders or indiscernible walls, strong posterior echo enhancement, without mural vegetations, calcifications, or septations (Table 1).

Although US can offer reliable data regarding relations of the hepatic cysts to the vascular and biliary tree, the standard diagnostic protocol in our clinic includes CT with i.v. contrast substance. MRI is also useful to establish a correct diagnosis (Algorithm 1) [29].

Intraoperative use of an ultrasound probe, where the abdominal wall thickness is not an issue, allows the placement of a higher MHz ultrasound transducer directly on the liver surface. Therefore, intraoperative ultrasound images are much sharper and well defined than those obtained through a transabdominal approach. Intraoperative US not only confirms the diagnosis but also adds important information to define the relation between the cysts and the surrounding structures (portal and hepatic veins, inferior vena cava, bile ducts), especially in deeply located cysts. Intraoperative US is also used to guide the surgeon for cyst approach in case no capsular expression is found. For laparoscopy, specially designed ultrasound probe and software are necessary.

	Simple cyst	**Cystic echinococcosis**	**Alveolar echinococcosis**	**Cystadenoma and cystadenocarcinoma**
Border	Sharp and smooth	Laminated, thick	Irregular	Irregular
Shape	Spherical or oval	Round or oval	Irregular	Round or oval
Echo pattern	Anechoic	Anechoic or atypical	Hyperechogenic outer ring and hypoechogenic centre	Hypoechogenic, with hyperechogenic floating material, fluid–fluid sedimentation
Appearance	No septa	Multiseptated	Multivesicular	Septations and/or papillary projections
Posterior acoustic feature	Relative accentuation of echoes	Dorsal shadowing (calcified areas)	Dorsal shadowing (calcified areas)	Dorsal shadowing (calcified areas)

Table 1. Ultrasonographic features for the diagnosis of monocystic diseases of the liver

CT and MRI can resolve the diagnosis of the doubtful cases and provide more information on the location of the cyst and relations with the great vessels and biliary tree. Thus, CT and/or MRI are mandatory for an appropriate treatment planning. US, CT, and MRI are complementary in evaluation of hepatic cysts. Based on imagistic examinations, parasitic cysts, neoplastic degeneration, and complications must be ruled out before pursuing any therapy decision.

On CT scan, simple hepatic cysts are well-defined, space occupying, round or oval-shaped, thin-walled, homogenous masses, with a density close to water (0–5 Hounsfield) and modest enhancement after contrast injection.

The presence of septa is not a common feature of the simple cyst, but multiple contiguous cysts can simulate it. For countries where hydatid disease is endemic, the differential diagnosis must include it because it is essential for therapeutic decision making.

The injection of intravenous contrast allows the manifestation of a possible communication between the cyst and the biliary tree on CT and MRI [29]. The communication of the hepatic cyst with the bile ducts can also be visualized using cystography, intraoperative cholangiography, and ERCP.

The mural calcifications are nonspecific but are usually present in echinococcal cysts and malignant lesions.

MRI provides valuable information concerning the nature of the cyst content and helps differentiating between blood and mucin [12]. MRI can identify a hypointense pseudocapsule characteristic of the echinococcal cyst. MRI, especially associated with MRCP, is helpful for the diagnosis of biliary cysts, localized Caroli disease (Figure 4), intrahepatic biliary cystadenoma, and cystadenocarcinoma.

A liver cyst with intracystic hemorrhage appears as a heterogeneous echogenic cyst on US. For improved US imaging, an ultrasound contrast substance (e.g., Levovist, Bayer Australia Limited; SonoVue, Bracco International B.V.) can be used. The procedure is known as contrast-enhanced ultrasound (CEUS) and uses a microbubble agent that produces multiple small (approximately 3 μm) stabilized air bubbles when suspended in water. After intravenous injection of Levovist, Doppler enhancement of the blood pool is observed for 2–5 min, followed by a late hepatosplenic phase that lasts for more than 30 min. If no enhancement of the intracystic structures but an enhanced smooth cyst wall is observed on Levovist US, then an intracystic clot is suspected. On plain CT, the hemorrhagic cyst appears heterogeneous low-density (Figure 11). On MRI, T1-weighted images reveal the clot as low intensity and the fluid as high intensity, whereas T2-weighted images show the clot as low intensity and the fluid as high intensity [30].

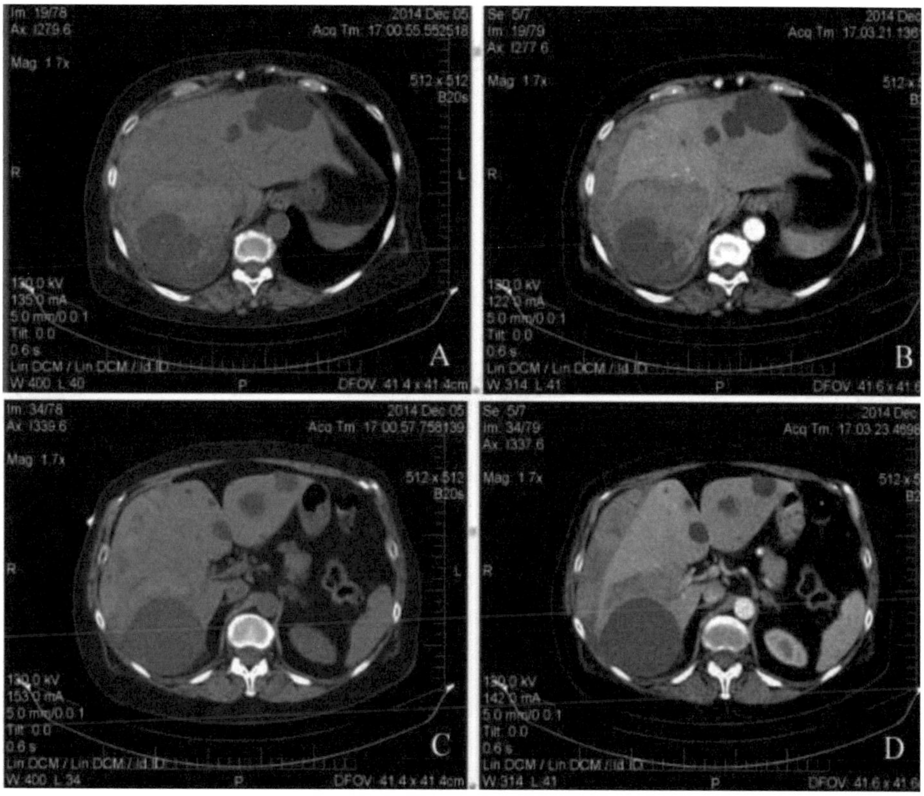

Figure 11. CT, axial view: multiple hepatic cysts, the largest cyst, located in segment VI–VII is ruptured in hepatic parenchyma; intracystic hematoma and extensive subcapsular hematoma are visible on the right hepatic lobe. (A, C) Native examination; (B,D) Examination with i.v. contrast administration.

On US, the differential diagnosis between intracystic hemorrhage and neoplastic degeneration may be challenging when intracystic parietal protrusions are identified (Figure 12). If no Doppler signal exists, these protrusions may be interpreted as sedimentations of hematin on the cyst wall. On macroscopic examination during operation, these protrusions have the equivalent of the blackish-brown deposits that stain the cyst wall. If Doppler signal is certified in the intracystic mural protrusions, then malignancy is highly considered.

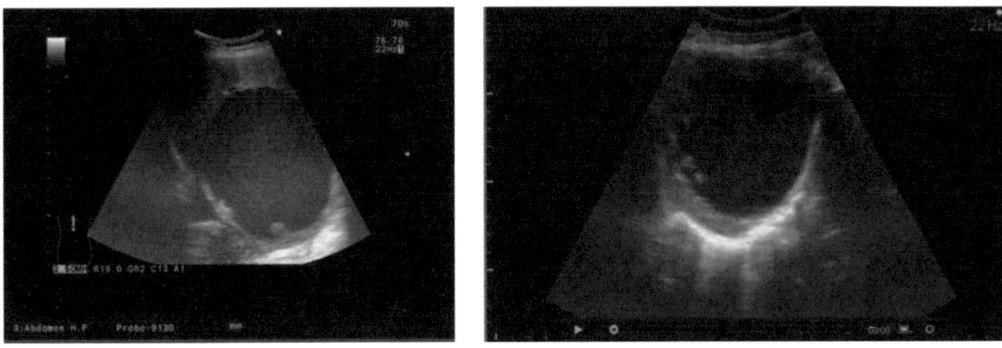

Figure 12. Transabdominal US for a cystic mass in the liver: the mass is anechoic, homogenous, with thin border, without calcifications, but with small hyperechoic parietal protrusions that do not change with patient's position. On Doppler examination, these protrusions are avascular and on CT are not visible. The intraoperative and histological diagnosis was serous hepatic cyst with hemorrhagic content. Cystadenocarcinoma had to be ruled out. Patient was submitted to open surgery.

Gallium scintigraphic study can be used to search for the site of infection in a patient with a previous diagnosis of simple hepatic cyst [27]. 18-F-fluorodeoxyglucose is helpful for the detection of cyst infection using positron emission tomography in patients with multiple liver and renal cysts [31]. In a patient diagnosed with hepatic cyst, any febrile status should raise the question of its possible infectious complication.

In case of cyst rupture, on imaging scans, irregularities of the partially evacuated cyst wall, heterogeneous content, fluid under the liver capsule, or free liquid in the peritoneal or pleural cavity are depicted.

Nonparasitic hepatic cysts may coexist with other hepatic lesions, bringing out the issue of correlation the lesion with the patient's symptoms and also of adopting the right management decision.

Nonparasitic cysts may coexist with parasitic ones (Figure 13). Even if the size of nonparasitic cyst does not justify its fenestration, it is recommended to solve both types of cysts in the same operation in order to avoid future misdiagnosis between the nonparasitic and parasitic cyst.

Nonparasitic hepatic cysts may coexist with other benign or malignant liver tumors. When a benign tumor lesion (e.g., hepatic hemangioma) is diagnosed besides hepatic cyst, there is an issue regarding which lesion should be treated to elevate the pain in the right upper quadrant (Figure 14).

http://dx.doi.org/10.5772/61057

Algorithm 1. Diagnostic decision

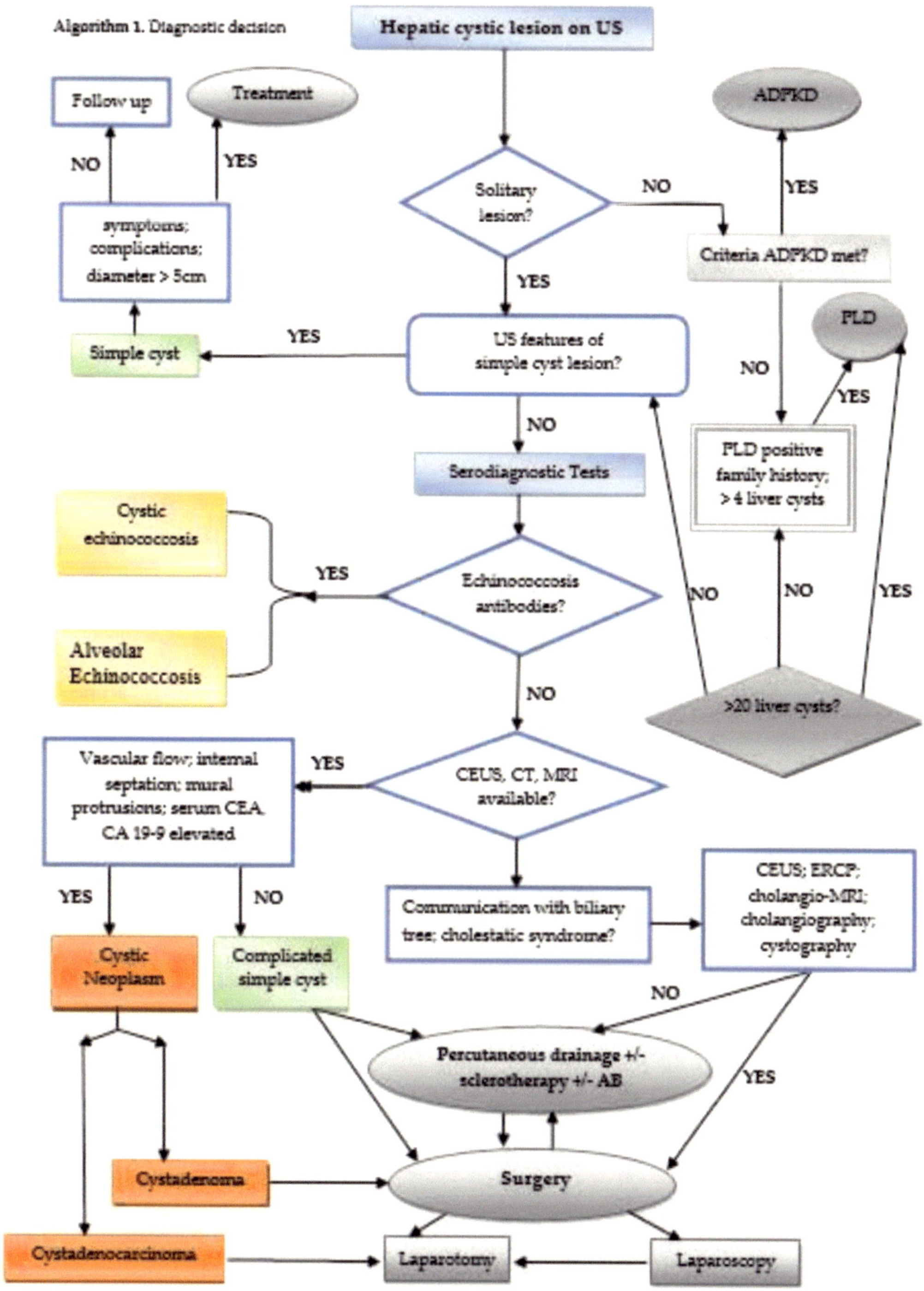

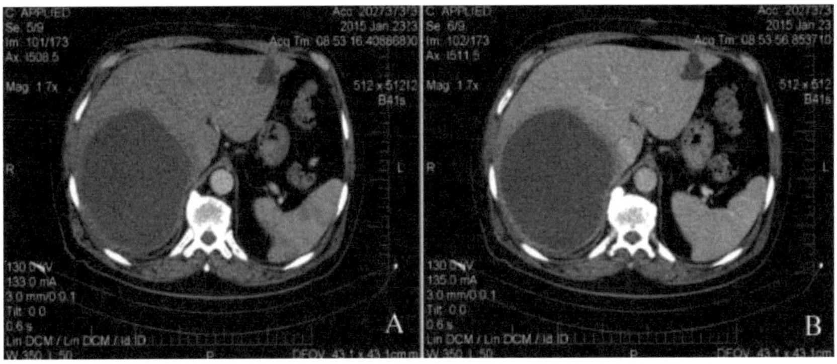

Figure 13. CT, axial view: voluminous hydatid cyst in the right hepatic lobe and small cyst mass in segment II-III. (A) Native; (B) after administration of i.v. contrast.

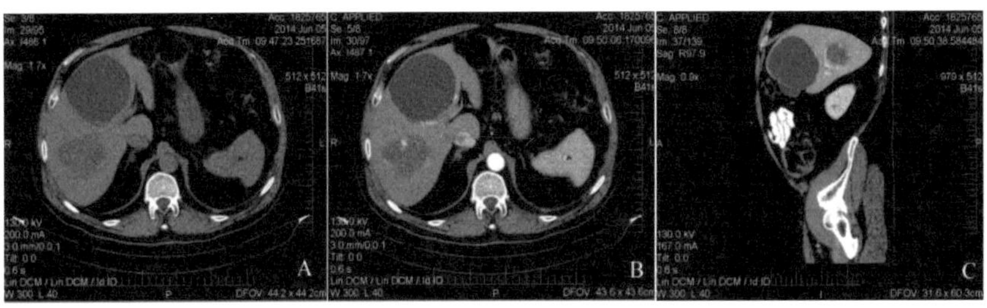

Figure 14. CT showing coexistence of two hepatic lesions: central simple hepatic cyst, in close proximity with gallbladder, and hepatic hemangioma in segment VI. (A) Axial view, native; (B) axial view, after i.v. contrast, arterial phase; (C) sagittal view, after i.v. contrast, arterial phase. Patient was submitted to laparoscopic fenestration of the hepatic cyst. The operation was successful in abolishing the right quadrant pain.

Nonparasitic cysts can also coexist with peripheral cholangiocarcinoma. The association was found in patients with PLD after kidney transplantation. The presence of liver metastasis from colorectal cancer was also found in patients with PLD (Figure 15).

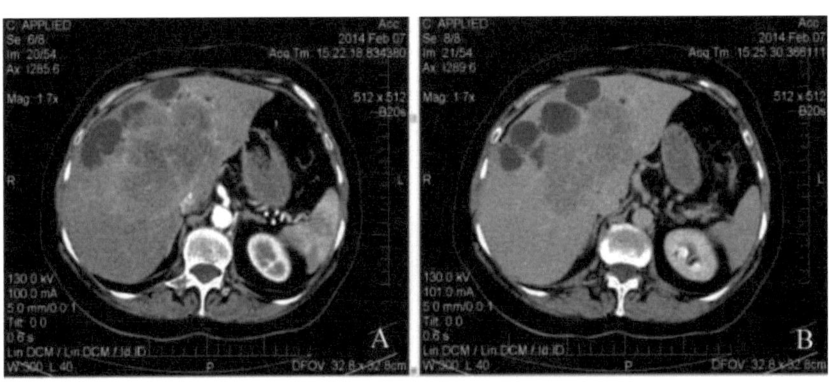

Figure 15. CT, axial view, with (A) and without (B) i.v. contrast showing coexistence of a bulk solid liver metastasis from colonic cancer in a patient with previously known PLD.

http://dx.doi.org/10.5772/61057

Serological tests for *Echinococcus* are electrosyneresis, hemagglutination, and ELISA (enzyme-linked immunosorbent assay) (the latter two being quantitative) [32]. The specific serology for *Echinococcus* has a sensitivity of 80% in the diagnostic process of parasitic cysts.

Serum tumor markers (e.g., CA 19-9 and CEA) must be checked to rule out neoplasia.

Right upper pain requires workup to exclude other associated pathology that may be the only or in addition responsible for causing the symptoms. Thus the surgeon should rule out cholelithiasis, gastroesophageal reflux disease, peptic ulcer disease, acute gastritis, or colorectal cancer. Upper and lower gastrointestinal endoscopy can reveal such pathologies and help avoiding misdiagnosis and mistreatment based solely on the pain supposedly caused by the hepatic cyst.

5. Treatment

Asymptomatic single liver cysts do not require treatment or surveillance. Symptomatic and complicated hepatic cysts require therapeutic intervention (Algorithm 2). It is considered that surgery is necessary for cyst of more than 5 cm in diameter. The primary indication for surgery is troublesome pain.

5.1. Percutaneous treatment

Percutaneous aspiration under ultrasound guidance of the cyst fluid is a mini-invasive procedure with a high recurrence rate if it is not associated with injection of a sclerosing agent in the remnant cavity.

Percutaneous treatment is performed on an inpatient basis under local anesthesia with lidocaine or sedation. For cyst puncture, an 18-gauge aspiration needle can be used. The puncture line must be chosen through normal hepatic parenchyma to avoid fluid leakage into peritoneal cavity. To prevent intracystic bleeding during evacuation caused by the sharp contact of the needle with the cyst wall, a 6- to 7-F catheter can be used instead. After complete evacuation of the cyst, the fluid is sent to cytological and bacteriological examination. Even in the absence of obvious signs of communication of the cyst with the biliary tree, this possibility must also be ruled out before injecting the sclerosant. Otherwise, an irreversible sclerosing cholangitis may supervene. There are available some imagistic methods to check the communication between liver cyst and biliary ducts. The most feasible and reliable method is the injection of a diluted US contrast agent (e.g., 2–4 drops of SonoVue, Bracco International B.V. in 40–200 ml 0.9% saline) in the evacuated cyst. The volume of contrast agent injected is the same or lower than the aspirated one [33]. Other alternative methods in ruling out cyst–biliary tree communication are cystography, ERCP, and bile duct scintigraphy [23].

Only after the absence of biliary communication is certified, the instillation of the sclerosant is allowed. One has to choose from a list of sclerosing agents that include ethanol [34–36], minocycline hydrochloride [37], tetracycline chloride [38], hypertonic saline solution [39], polidocanol [40], and ethanolamine oleate [41].

Ethanol has remained the most used sclerosing agent. It destroys the cell lining of the cystic cavity and discontinues the cystic fluid secretion. Different concentrations of ethanol (95–99%) and different volumes (10–50% of the cystic volume) have been reported. The exposure time varies from 10 min to 4 h. In order to minimize ethanol side effects, time exposure to ethanol should be less than 60 min. When using ethanol instillation, the cyst must be completely evacuated, a condition that is not necessary when using other sclerosing agents. After complete cyst evacuation, its walls collapse hampering the thorough distribution of sclerosant, with the risk of its subsequent lobulation. The other sclerosants are active in small concentration and do not need complete evacuation of the cystic fluid. When the cyst is only partially evacuated, the misplacement of needle tip is also avoided. The residual fluid is progressively resorbed through microscopic communication between the cyst and the surrounding liver parenchyma. Polidocanol needs only one application. Its application is painless and hence no intracystic anesthesia or sedation is required [33].

The percutaneous treatment can be repeated when necessary. Percutaneous drainage must be done under antibiotic prophylaxis. The recommended antimicrobial is ciprofloxacin because cephalosporins (e.g., cefazolin) were not found totally successful in preventing cyst infection after drainage [42]. Even if infection of the remnant cavity occurs, it can be remitted by oral Ciprofloxacin (500 mg twice daily) associated or not with clindamycin (300 mg three times daily) [42]. Oral ciprofloxacin is also indicated as the first line treatment in infected cysts [43].

5.2. Radiofrequency ablation

Radiofrequency ablation (RFA) for the treatment of hepatic cysts with the largest diameter up to 10 cm was reported to be efficient, safe, and free from complications [44].

5.3. Surgical treatment

High success rates in the treatment of hepatic cysts were reported being associated with laparoscopic or open deroofing [24].

5.3.1. Laparoscopic approach

Laparoscopic fenestration was first reported by Z'graggen in 1991 [45]. Being associated with low recurrence rate, reduced morbidity, and short hospital stay, laparoscopic fenestration tends to become the standard treatment for the simple hepatic cysts.

The indications for laparoscopic approach are determined not by the size but the location of the cysts, being limited to those located in the segments II, III, IV, V, and VI (Figure 16) [29]. However, some authors advocate that the use of a flexible laparoscope facilitates the laparoscopic approach of lesions located in the postero-superior segments of the liver (segments I, VII, and VIII) [46]. Hepatic cysts that cannot be entirely explored laparoscopy are not candidates for laparoscopic approach.

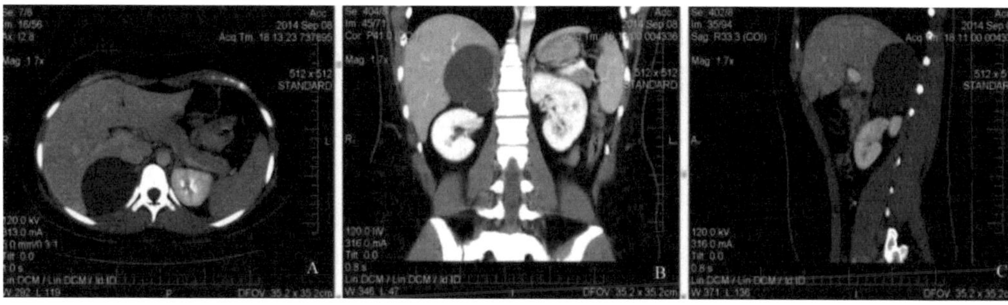

Figure 16. CT showing serous hepatic cyst in segment VI–VII. (A) Axial view, (B) coronal view, and (C) sagittal view. Laparoscopic approach is not indicated for such localization of the hepatic cyst.

Laparoscopy is not suitable for fenestration in case of close proximity of the cyst wall to the hepatic veins and inferior vena cava (Figure 17) [47].

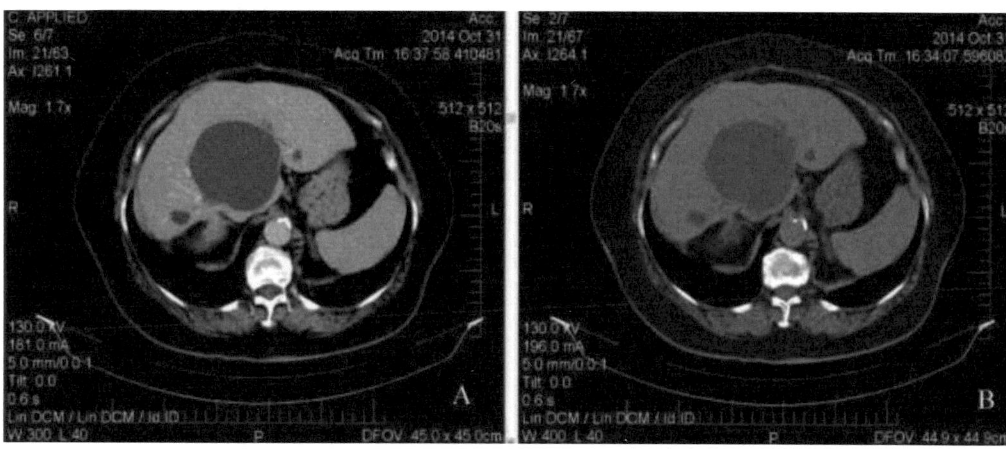

Figure 17. CT, axial view, with contrast (A) and without contrast (B): large simple hepatic cyst in contact with the inferior vena cava and hepatic veins and other two small cysts in proximity. Patient was submitted to open surgery.

Previous laparotomies or laparoscopies are not considered contraindications to the laparoscopic approach.

A 30° laparoscope is used. A medium CO_2 insufflation and an intra-abdominal pressure less than 12 mm Hg should be used to avoid gas embolism. Liver veins are little prone to collapse in the supine position. The effect of venous gas embolism depends on the rate of CO_2 infusion and its volume. For adults, the potentially lethal volume is estimated at 200–300 ml or 3–5 ml/kg [48]. Surgeons must routinely purge laparoscopic tubing systems with CO_2 gas. If the system is not adequately purged with CO_2 gas before, substantial amounts of air (containing 79% of the insoluble N_2) may be insufflated into the peritoneal cavity from the tubing and may cause air embolism [48].Generally, the patient lies in the supine position with/without abducted legs or lithotomy position on the operating table. A left side-lying position of the patient can help approaching liver cysts located in the segments V-VI.

The operative procedure in the standard operation of fenestration is performed using three or four ports. One 10-mm trocar is inserted into the abdominal cavity through the umbilicus as an observation port. The main operating hole is located under the xiphoid and is made to accommodate a 10- or 12-mm trocar. Another hole is placed in the right upper quadrant of the abdomen at the medioclavicular line for insertion of a 5-mm trocar. An additional port can be placed for exposure, depending on the cyst localization.

On video inspection, the liver mass appears exteriorized on the hepatic surface with a translucent wall. If the serous hepatic cyst has no complication, there are no tight adhesions to the surrounding tissues. Instead, if the cyst is complicated by inflammation, infection, or hemorrhage, the surface of the corticalized cyst may develop tight adhesions to the surrounding organs and the cyst wall appears thick and thus indistinguishable from other hepatic cysts (e.g., hydatid cyst, pyogenic abscess, and tuberculoma) (Figure 18).

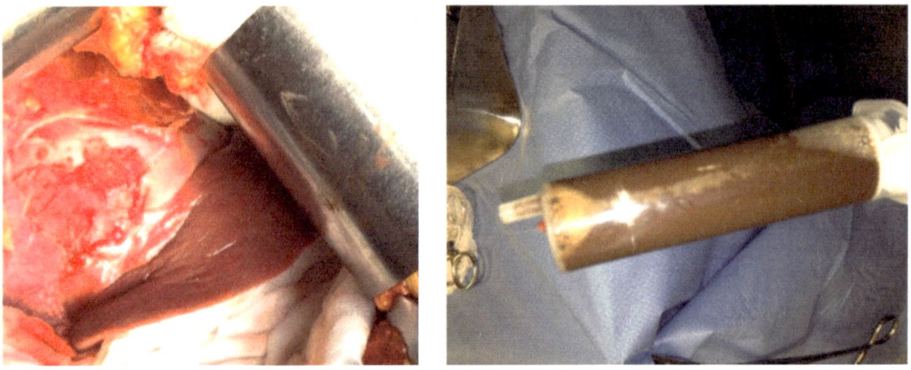

Figure 18. Serous cyst in the segments IV, V, and VIII. (A) Intraoperative aspect of the complicated hepatic cyst with adhesions to the diaphragm and with thick wall that make it undistinguishable from hydatid cyst. (B) Intraoperative aspect of the aspirated liquid. The brownish color is likely the result of an unrecognized intracystic hemorrhage.

After cyst evacuation, a large access to the cavity of the cyst should be obtained. The walls of the cyst are carefully inspected to identify possible indentation, vegetation, or thickness. Any suspicious lesion of the cyst wall must be biopsied and sent to frozen examination to rule out malignancy. If neoplastic changes are found, the laparoscopy is converted to open operation, and liver resection is performed. If mural nodules, intracystic septum, or honeycomb appearance are visualized, but there is no microscopic evidence of cystadenoma or cystadenocarcinoma on frozen sections, hepatectomy can be performed laparoscopically to clear all the affected segments.

Any suspected communication with the bile duct should be carefully investigated intraoperatively. Some authors consider the closure of the open bile duct under laparotomy to be a more rational choice [49]. Other authors advocate for laparoscopic closure of the communication with the bile duct [50].

Recurrence is low if wide cyst wall resection is accomplished. Fenestration can be carried out by electrocautery hook, bipolar scissors, high frequency bipolar electrocoagulation LigaSure™ (Valleylab, Tyco International Healthcare, Boulder, CO), Ethicon Ultracision Harmonic Scalpel LCS-5 (Ethicon, Cincinnati, Ohio), or cutting stapler. Argon beam coagulation may complete hemostasis. The cystic dome is resected up to 3–5 mm from the hepatic parenchyma to avoid hemorrhage and bile leakage from the cut edge of the liver parenchyma. The resected cyst is sent for frozen section and permanent histopathologic evaluation. If the cyst is not well corticalized on the liver capsule and the standard unroofing of the cyst is considered of inadequate size that can predispose to recurrence, then the cyst wall should be excised including a 3- to 4-mm rim of hepatic parenchyma. If the bile is spotted along the cystic edge, a hemostatic clip or a tie suture can be applied [46].

In case of aspiration of a straw-colored liquid and in the absence of bile staining of the cystic wall, intraoperative cholangiography is not indicated. However, in case of bile contamination of the cyst or compression of the biliary tree, intraoperative cholangiography is required to evaluate the biliary tree [51]. Intraoperatively missed biliary communication could lead to prolonged biliary fistula and even biliary peritonitis.

Sclerosant or alcohol application on the remnant wall of the cyst is recommended to prevent possible further fluid secretion by cyst epithelium and, hence, hepatic cyst recurrence. The great omentum should be packed into larger cavities to decrease dead space and prevent fluid collection. An omental flap transposition is recognized as an important aid in reducing the risk of cyst recurrence, but it is contraindicated in infected cysts.

The drainage of the remnant cavity must meet the declivity principle, especially for those cysts situated in the upper liver segments. The main reason for reconstitution of the cyst after operation is the coverage of the remnant cavity by the diaphragm. To establish a dry residual cavity after fenestration of liver cysts located in the segments VII and VIII, the vacuum effect of the respiratory movements of the diaphragm should be counteracted by an efficient external drainage. The drainage tube should be left in place until complete cessation of the secretion certified by ultrasound evaluation. The use of pigtail catheters for drainage is preferred to the usual drainage tubes for upper sited liver cysts. The realization of an efficient external drainage might be accomplished by transparenchymatous placement of the tube.

The atypical hepatic resections for large and/or multiple hepatic cysts that occupy more segments are laparoscopically feasible if performed by surgeons with advanced training in this technique. Most of these atypical hepatectomies involve the left lobe (Figure 19). Generally, the cut surface of the liver remains covered by the cyst wall.

5.3.2. Single-incision laparoscopy

Single-incision laparoscopic surgery can reach the effect of "no scar" and can be safely and effectively carried out in these patients. The operation is performed using a dedicated port such SILSTM Port (Covidien, MA, USA), GelPort® Laparoscopic System (Applied Medical, CA, USA), QuadPort+ (Olympus, PA, USA), or X-cone (Karl Storz, Germany). However, three trocars can also be used by their insertion into abdominal cavity through one 2.5-cm incision designed along the ventral midline on the upper edge of the umbilicus. The incision is sufficient to accommodate one 10-mm trocar and two 5-mm trocars [19]. The abdominal drainage tube can be appropriately placed through the same incision at the end of cyst fenestration. If the telescope cannot directly observe the liver cyst, the patient is not suited for single-incision laparoscopic surgery.

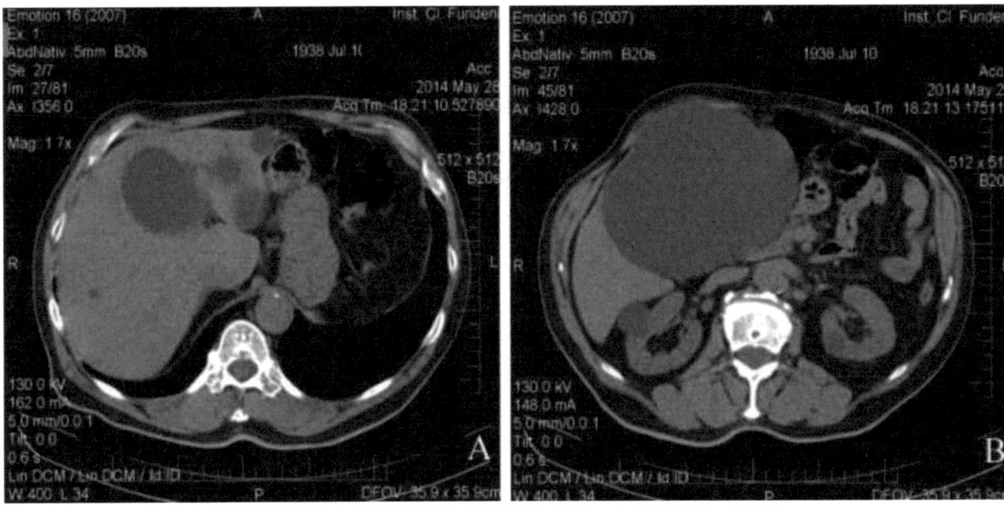

Figure 19. Patient with PLD and ADPKD operated by laparoscopic approach for hepatic cysts. CT in axial view shows small serous cysts grouped in segments II and III (A) and a large serous cyst in segment IV (B). Laparoscopic intervention was successfully performed.

Minilaparoscopic-assisted transvaginal approach is also mentioned [52].

5.3.3. Robotic approach

Robotic surgery is another possible approach, and it has been used in our clinic for nonparasitic hepatic cyst fenestration. The use of the Da Vinci robotic surgical system has certain technical advantages over the standard laparoscopic technique in case of the posterior location of the liver cysts [53]. However, conversion to laparoscopic or open surgery in case of difficulty is laborious and time consuming and could be life-threatening in a dire emergency.

5.3.4. Classic approach

The communication between cystic cavity and bile duct encountered during operation can be managed in different ways. The suture of the biliary communication is enough, but the means of doing that depend on different surgeons. Cystojejunostomy is mentioned by some authors [54], but it became history in our clinic. Biliary-enteric anastomosis is necessary if there is a concern of postoperative leak or intrahepatic biliary obstruction after suture control [55].

If cystadenoma is suspected, due to its malignant potential, the recommended therapy is laparoscopic or open cyst enucleation or liver resection. But if any suspicion of cystadenocarcinoma exists or especially if malignancy is proved by cytology of aspirated cyst fluid or frozen sections, the surgical decision should be open liver resection with tumor-free margins.

Enucleation is generally feasible due to the existence of a well-defined plane between the cyst wall and the normal liver parenchyma that is generally avascular (Figure 20). For cysts centrally situated, with an increased risk of intraoperative hemorrhage, Pringle maneuver

Algorithm 2. Therapeutic decision

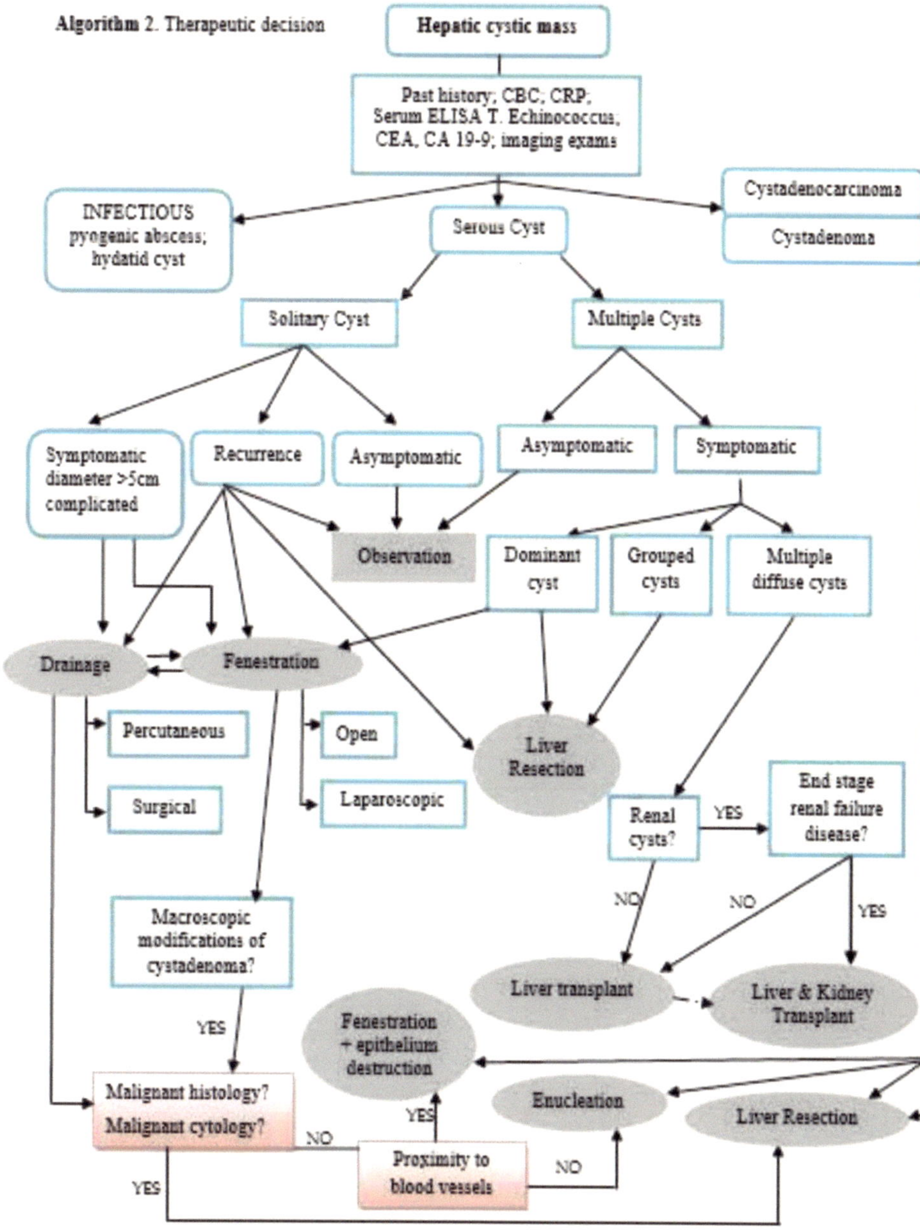

brings clear benefits. If there is a direct contact of the cyst wall with the portal pedicle, hepatic vein, or inferior vena cava, that portion of the wall can be abandoned if no malignancy is identified on frozen sections (Figure 21). However, there still remains the risk of abandoning malignant areas or malignant degeneration of the remnant cyst wall over time. For this reason, it is recommended to destroy the epithelium lining of the remnant cyst wall by electrofulguration or argon beam coagulation.

In case of malignant cytology and/or histopathology, the only potentially curative treatment is complete removal of the hepatic cyst, usually by a major liver resection with 1-cm free margin [15].

The elective treatment for the infected hepatic cysts is antibiotherapy combined with percutaneous drainage. It is thought that infection itself kills the inner epithelium, so the regular use of sclerosant injection into the cyst is not generally adopted by some authors. A shortening of time for sclerosant instillation is suggested by others [56]. In case of failure of the mentioned treatment, there is a need for surgery.

When intracystic or intraparenchymatous hemorrhage is certain, the active bleeding with negative hemodynamic impact imposes emergency operation. Otherwise, the percutaneous treatment can be the first option.

In dealing with cyst rupture, there is no standard therapy. In the presence of peritoneal irritation or internal hemorrhage signs, emergency operation is the rule. In the absence of such signs, the management may vary from conservatory treatment with close observation to surgical intervention [57].

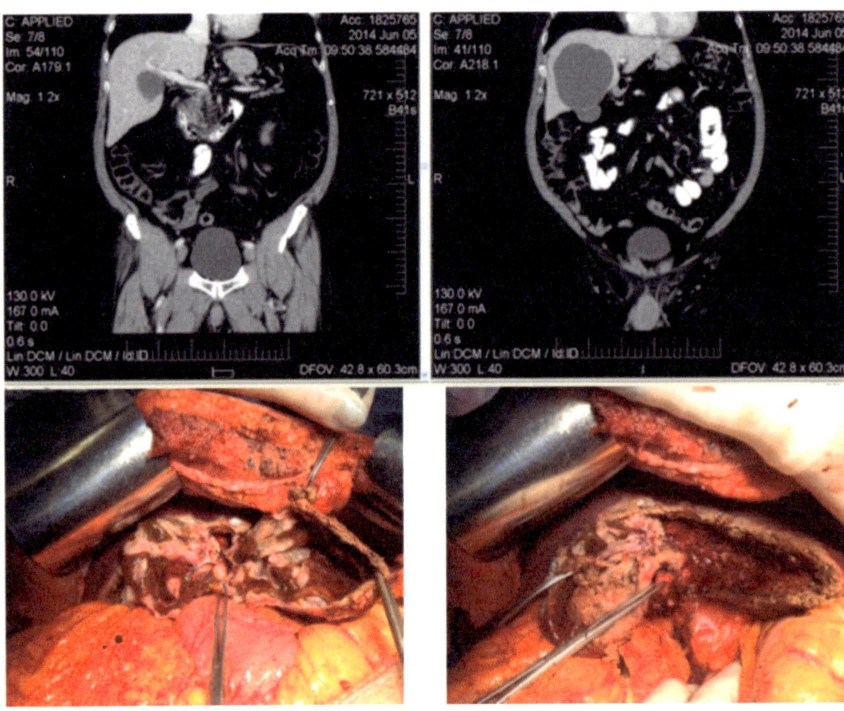

Figure 20. Recurrent cyst in segments IV–V with close proximity to the right portal pedicle (A) and gallbladder (B) on CT, coronal views. Intraoperative aspect of a thick cyst wall (C) and of hepatic parenchyma after cyst enucleation (D).

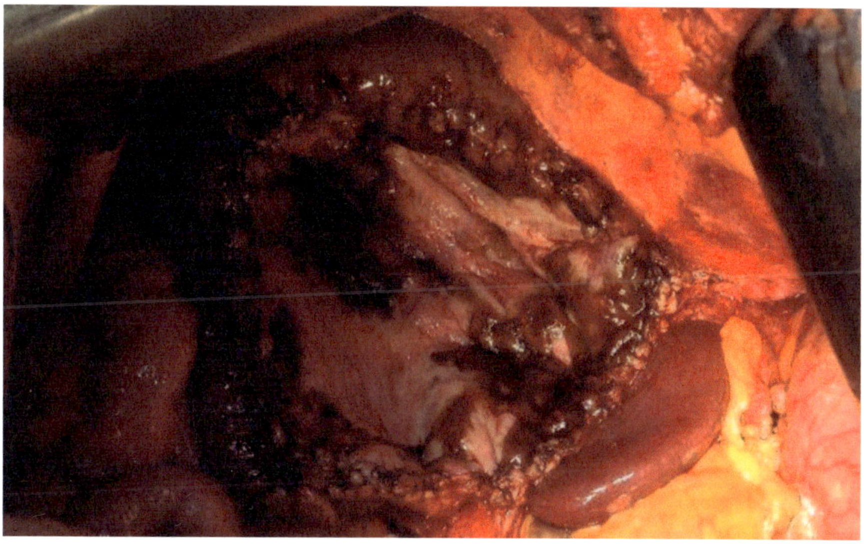

Figure 21. Intraoperative feature of the abandoned wall of a huge serous cyst that occupied segments IV and VIII and contained a chocolate-like fluid. The hemostasis on the hepatic rim was achieved by continuous suture.

5.3.5. Treatment of PLD

The appropriate treatment of PLD is based on Gigot's classification on CT findings. Most current therapies are invasive. However, the conservative management with lanreotide, a long-acting somatostatin analogue, is promising, being associated with a reduction of liver volume in PLD [58, 59]. Sclerotherapy is considered ineffective in the management of PLD. Laparoscopic fenestration is feasible only for PLD type I in Gigot's classification (Figure 22). For type II, open fenestration is indicated. For type III, only liver resection or liver transplantation is permitted in symptomatic patients. If liver transplantation is anticipated, fenestration or resection should be avoided to decrease postoperative morbidity and mortality.

5.3.6. Liver transplantation for PLD

Most of the patients with PLD have combined liver and kidney cystic disease. There are questions regarding whether kidney and liver transplantation must be performed and whether these transplants should be performed simultaneously or consecutively. The patients with advanced renal failure (dialysis or predialysis stage) need combined liver and kidney replacement. However, those patients who have normal renal function do not need a combined transplantation. It was reported that maximum 33% of the patients who first received a liver transplant alone needed a kidney transplant later [60]. In many patients, the renal function improves after orthotopic liver transplantation (OLT), possibly due to the release of compartment syndrome. Massive hepatomegaly causes an abdominal compartment syndrome that negatively affects renal function which can be reversed after OLT. Other authors argue that a combined liver and kidney transplantation should be performed even in patients with limited

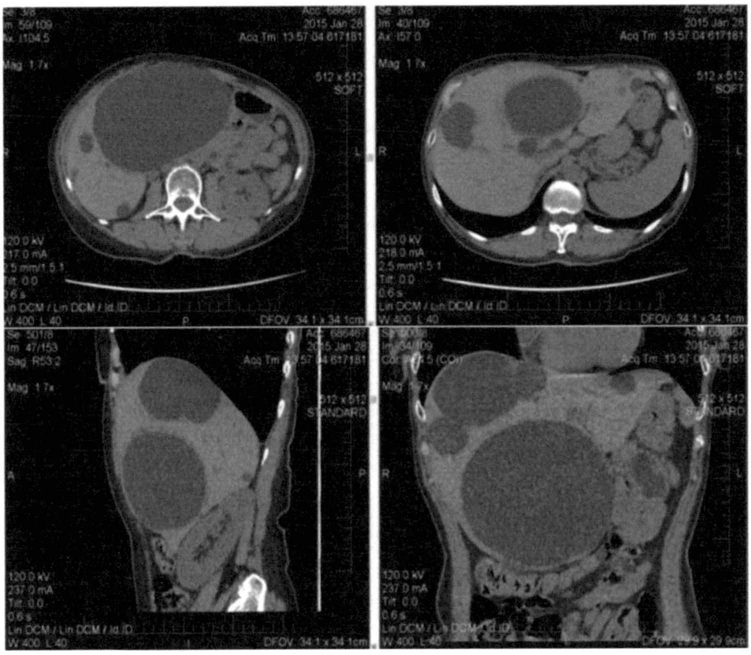

Figure 22. CT for a female patient with PLD submitted to laparoscopic fenestration of the largest cysts situated in the hepatic segments IV–V and VII–VIII. (A) Axial view of the upper liver. (B) Axial view of the lower liver. (C) Sagittal view of the liver. D. Coronal view of the liver.

renal dysfunction or even normal renal function. This strategy is justified by the progression of cystic renal disease after OLT and the immune advantage in transplanting both organs harvested from the same donor, rather than having to perform a third-party kidney transplantation later [61].

OLT is a rare procedure for PLD. It represents approximately 1% of all indications [62]. Total hepatectomy followed by OLT offers the chance of definitive treatment. The indication of OLT may be too drastic considering the absence of immediately life-threatening liver failure, the potential hazards associated with OLT procedure and postoperative immunosuppression, and the organ shortage. Indications for OLT in PLD are massive hepatomegaly, compartment syndrome, and clinically advanced malnutrition that produce severe physical and social handicap. Generally, these patients have preserved liver function and normal model for end stage liver disease (MELD) score if they do not have renal involvement [63].

Two drawbacks to OLT for patients with PLD are the susceptibility to infection caused by severe malnutrition and overimmunosuppression, and further degradation of renal function caused by immunosuppression. Therefore, the maintenance of immunosuppression in such patients must be lower than usual and the steroids should be discontinued after 3 months. It is also important not to delay OLT in these patients; otherwise, complications such portal vein thrombosis, portal hypertension, Budd–Chiari syndrome, peripheral cholangiocarcinoma, and liver failure may result in poorer tolerance of the patient to procedure, increased graft loss, and increased costs [62].

http://dx.doi.org/10.5772/61057

The first report of OLT for PLD was by Kwork and Lewin in 1988, but the patient died intraoperatively of intractable bleeding. In 1990, Starzl successfully performed OLT on 4 patients with PLD.

OLT in PLD is technically challenging because of the massive organomegaly (Figure 23). If OLT is anticipated on a patient with PLD, then any other surgical interventions should be withheld in order to avoid massive intraoperative bleeding and thus transfusion requirements.

The anatomic position of the vessels is not respected in patients with PLD. In total hepatectomy, dissection starts in the liver hilum because it is the only structure that lies at a near-normal anatomic position. Hepatic artery, portal vein, and principal biliary duct are identified. No attempt is made to control the suprahepatic vena cava at the beginning of dissection. Early attempts at controlling it may result in its laceration, fatal bleeding, and pulmonary air embolism. Patients with PLD have little portal hypertension and spontaneous portocaval shunts and thus poor tolerance of portal clamping [62]. The surgeons must be prepared for portal bypass if hypotension develops when portal vein is clamped. Other surgeons systematically use portal bypass. By dissecting portal vein for cannulation, a broad exposure of the intrahepatic vena cava is obtained. The decision of inferior vena cava resection is made based on the intraoperative conditions determined during the dissection phase [64]. Some surgeons choose to continue the dissection of the liver en bloc with the native vena cava and eventually safely control the suprahepatic vena cava. The en bloc resection of the liver with the native vena cava is justified by the fact that usually the cava vein is embedded within an extremely voluminous caudate lobe [62]. There are other surgeons who performed dissection of liver parenchyma from IVC. Cysts were aspirated to facilitate final access to the suprahepatic inferior vena cava. However, one should be prepared for vein control through transdiaphragmatic or transsternal approach.

Transcatheter embolization has been proposed to decrease arterial supply of the cysts and thus reduce the liver size and may be beneficial prior to liver transplantation [65].

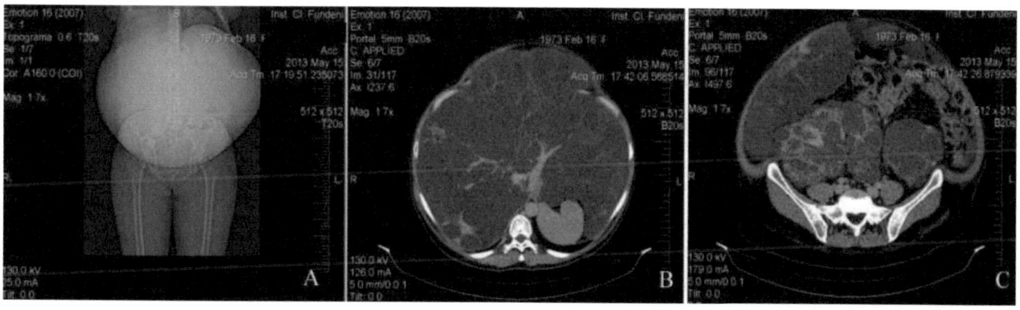

Figure 23. Female patient with PLD and ADPKD with indication for liver transplantation. (A) Body topography with huge abdomen volume. (B) CT, axial view: extensive hepatomegaly with multiple diffuse hepatic cysts entirely occupying the liver parenchyma. (C) CT, axial view: extensive hepatomegaly with the inferior border of the liver reaching the pelvis; multiple bilateral kidney cysts with both kidney displaced in the pelvis.

6. Outcomes

The most frequent complications encountered in the treatment of the simple hepatic cysts are hemorrhage and infection of the residual cavity. Recurrence of the hepatic cystic mass in the same location must be differentially interpreted based on the previous treatment, elapsed time from the treatment, histological type and size of the cyst, and existing symptoms.

In case of early recurrence of the hepatic cystic mass after percutaneous treatment, absence of malignancy criteria and symptoms, the treatment may vary from simple observation by US scan to surgical treatment, based on the patient's consent.

In case of early recurrence of hepatic cystic mass of similar size after percutaneous sclerotherapy or laparoscopic fenestration and malignancy criteria absence, the treatment may vary from percutaneous treatment to open surgery. An intracystic hematoma should be suspected as a cause of hepatic mass persistence especially when it is associated with inflammatory and/or internal hemorrhage symptoms. Percutaneous drainage is the first choice in the treatment of hematoma. In case of active bleeding and/or hemodynamic instability, emergency surgical intervention is indicated.

If the patient develops symptoms of infection associated with the persistence of hepatic cystic mass, hepatic abscess should be suspected as a complication and antibiotic treatment should be initiated empirically followed by further adjustments depending on bacterial cultures. If the symptoms persist and localization of the abscess permits, the percutaneous drainage is advisable. If the symptoms do not remit under antibiotics or the percutaneous drainage is not feasible, the patient must be referred to surgery.

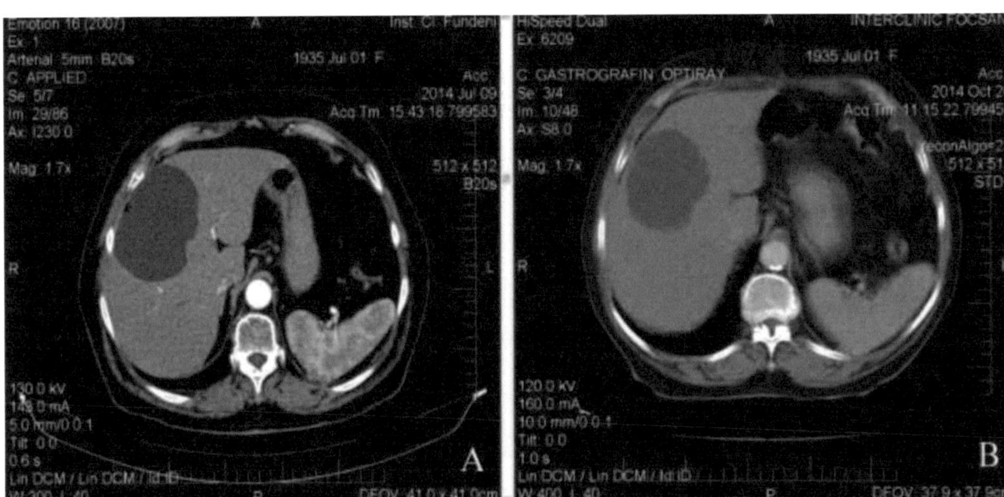

Figure 24. CT for central hepatic serous cyst (segments IV, V VII) (A) with recurrence after 3 months (B), having similar size and causing the same symptoms to the patient

In case of late recurrence after laparoscopic or classic fenestration for hepatic cyst, with documented US follow-up that initially attests the cyst remission, it should be reasonable to highly consider complete surgical removal of the recurrent cyst even if there are no serologic, imagistic, or histological criteria of malignancy (Figure 24).

The rate of symptomatic recurrence after percutaneous sclerotherapy is around 20%.

Laparoscopic unroofing or marsupialization can completely relieve symptoms from either simple lesions or PLD, with the procedure's morbidity, mortality, and recurrence rates being, respectively, 2%, 0%, and 2% for patients with simple cysts, and 25%, 0%, and 5% for patients with PLD. For infected cysts, the procedure of choice is percutaneous drainage, with morbidity, mortality, and recurrence rates for simple cysts being 0%, 0%, and 75%, respectively, and for PLD, 0%, 0%, and 20%, respectively [54]. The conversion rate from laparoscopy to laparotomy is less than 10% [66]. Postoperative morbidity in open deroofing of the hepatic cysts has been reported to be significantly higher than in laparoscopic procedure (33% versus 13%) but the difference may reflect the selection of more difficult cases for open surgery [66]. No mortality is acceptable for surgical therapy of hepatic cysts, unless liver transplantation is considered. Survival rate after OLT for PLD has been reported as high as 90% [67].

Abbreviations

AB—antibiotherapy

ADPKD—autosomal dominant polycystic kidney disease (ADPKD)

CA 19-9—carcinoma antigen 19-9

CBC—cell blood count

CEA—carcinoembryonic antigen

CEUS—contrast enhanced ultrasonography

CRP—C reactive protein

CT—computer tomography

ERCP—endoscopic retrograde cholangiopancreatography

MRCP—magnetic resonance cholangiopancreatography

MRI—magnetic resonance imaging

OLT—orthotopic liver transplantation

PLD—polycystic liver disease

US—ultrasonography

Acknowledgements

This study was supported by the Health, EEA-JRP-RO-NO-2013-1-0363 programme, through the project No. 4 SEE/30.06.2014, with the title "Hepatocellular carcinoma stratification based on noninvasive markers" and acronym HEPMARK.

Author details

Mirela Patricia Sîrbu Boeţi[1,2*], Mirela Boroş[3], Vlad Herlea[4,5], Amalia Petrişor[2] and Irinel Popescu[1,2]

*Address all correspondence to: paboet@yahoo.com

1 Department of Liver Transplantation and General Surgery, Fundeni Clinical Institute, Bucharest, Romania

2 Carol Davila University of Medicine and Pharmacy, Bucharest, Romania

3 Department of Radiology, Medical Imaging and Interventional Radiology, Fundeni Clinical Institute, Bucharest, Romania

4 Department of Pathology, Fundeni Clinical Institute, Bucharest, Romania

5 Titu Maiorescu University, Faculty of Medicine, Bucharest, Romania

References

[1] Carrim ZI, Murchison JT. The prevalence of simple renal and hepatic cysts detected by spiral computed tomography. *Clin Radiol.* 2003; 58: 626–9.

[2] Macedo FI. Current management of noninfectious hepatic cystic lesions: a review of the literature. *World J Hepatol.* 2013; 5: 462–9.

[3] Cnossen WR, Drenth JP. Polycystic liver disease: an overview of pathogenesis, clinical manifestations and management. *Orphanet J Rare Dis.* 2014; 1: 69.

[4] Russel RT, Pinson CW. Surgical management of polycystic liver disease. *World J Gastroenterol.* 2007; 13: 5052–9.

[5] Ramia JM, de La PR, Figueras J, Garcia-Parreno J. [Benign non-parasitic hepatic cystic tumours]. *Cir Esp.* 2011; 89: 565–73.

[6] Zhang YL, Yuan L, Shen F, Wang Y. Hemorrhagic hepatic cysts mimicking biliary cystadenoma. *World J Gastroenterol.* 2009; 15: 4601–3.

[7] Bakoyiannis A, Delis S, Triantopoulou C, Dervenis C. Rare cystic liver lesions: a diagnostic and managing challenge. *World J Gastroenterol.* 2013; 19: 7603–19.

[8] Miller JH. The ultrasonographic appearance of cystic hepatoblastoma. *Radiology.* 1981; 138: 141–3.

[9] Rogers TN, Woodley H, Ramsden W, Wyatt JI, Stringer MD. Solitary liver cysts in children: not always so simple. *J Pediatr Surg.* 2007; 42: 333–9.

[10] Ohmoto K, Shimizu M, Iguchi Y, Yamamoto S, Murakami M, Tsunoda T. Solitary cystic dilatation of the intrahepatic bile duct. *J Clin Pathol.* 1997; 50: 617–8.

[11] Aoki S, Okayama Y, Kitajima Y, *et al.* Intrahepatic biliary papilloma morphologically similar to biliary cystadenoma. *J Gastroenterol Hepatol.* 2005; 20: 321–4.

[12] Tsepelaki A, Kirkilesis I, Katsiva V, Triantafillidis JK, Vagianos C. Biliary cystadenoma of the liver: case report and systematic review of the literature. *Ann Gastroenterol.* 2009; 22: 278–83.

[13] Dixon E, Sutherland FR, Burak K, McKinnon G, May G. Cystadenoma of the liver without mesenchymal stroma in a female following hormonal therapy for acne. *HPB (Oxford)* 2001; 3: 183–6.

[14] Dixon E, Sutherland FR, Mitchell P, McKinnon G, Nayak V. Cystadenomas of the liver: a spectrum of disease. *Can J Surg.* 2001; 44: 371–6.

[15] Vogt DP, Henderson JM, Chmielewski E. Cystadenoma and cystadenocarcinoma of the liver: a single center experience. *J Am Coll Surg.* 2005; 200: 727–33.

[16] Khoddami M, Kazemi AM, Alvandimanesh A. Ciliated hepatic foregut cyst: two case reports in children and review of the literature. *Case Rep Med.* 2013; 2013: 372017.

[17] Balzan S, Kianmanesh R, Farges O, *et al.* Right intrahepatic pseudocyst following acute pancreatitis: an unusual location after acute pancreatitis. *J Hepatobiliary Pancreat Surg.* 2005; 12: 135–7.

[18] Hansman MF, Ryan JA, Jr., Holmes JH, *et al.* Management and long-term follow-up of hepatic cysts. *Am J Surg.* 2001; 181: 404–10.

[19] Wu S, Li Y, Tian Y, Li M. Single-incision laparoscopic surgery versus standard laparoscopic surgery for unroofing of hepatic cysts. *JSLS.* 2014; 18: 246–51.

[20] Murphy BJ, Casillas J, Ros PR, Morillo G, Albores-Saavedra J, Rolfes DB. The CT appearance of cystic masses of the liver. *Radiographics.* 1989; 9: 307–22.

[21] Poggi G, Gatti C, Delmonte A, Teragni C, Bernardo G. Spontaneous rupture of nonparasitic hepatic cyst. *Int J Clin Pract.* 2006; 60: 99–103.

[22] Takahashi G, Yoshida H, Mamada Y, Taniai N, Bando K, Tajiri T. Intracystic hemorrhage of a large simple hepatic cyst. *J Nippon Med Sch*. 2008; 75: 302–5.

[23] Terada N, Shimizu T, Imai Y, *et al.* Benign, non-parasitic hepatic cyst causing obstructive jaundice. *Intern Med.* 1993; 32: 857–60.

[24] Bistritz L, Tamboli C, Bigam D, Bain VG. Polycystic liver disease: experience at a teaching hospital. *Am J Gastroenterol.* 2005; 100: 2212–7.

[25] Ker J. The liver and right atrium-hepatic cyst as a cause of arrhythmia. *Clin Med Insights Cardiol.* 2010; 4: 63–7.

[26] Musielak MC, Singh R, Hartman E, Bernstein J. Simple hepatic cyst causing inferior vena cava thrombus. *Int J Surg Case Rep.* 2014; 5: 339–41.

[27] Mori E, Akai Y, Matsumoto T, *et al.* Hepatic cyst infection in a healthy older male. *BMJ Case Rep.* 2012; 2012.

[28] Kawashita Y, Kamohara Y, Furui J, *et al.* Destructive granuloma derived from a liver cyst: a case report. *World J Gastroenterol.* 2006; 12: 1798–801.

[29] Cappellani A, Zanghi A, Di VM, Menzo EL, Conti P. Nonparasitic cysts of the liver: laparoscopic treatment and long-term results. *Ann Ital Chir*. 2002; 73: 85–8.

[30] Akiyama T, Inamori M, Saito S, *et al.* Levovist ultrasonography imaging in intracystic hemorrhage of simple liver cyst. *World J Gastroenterol.* 2008; 14: 805–7.

[31] Bleeker-Rovers CP, de Sevaux RG, van Hamersvelt HW, Corstens FH, Oyen WJ. Diagnosis of renal and hepatic cyst infections by 18-F-fluorodeoxyglucose positron emission tomography in autosomal dominant polycystic kidney disease. *Am J Kidney Dis.* 2003; 41: E18–21.

[32] Beyrouti MI, Beyrouti R, Bouassida M, *et al.* [Hydatid cysts of the spigelian lobe (segment I) of the liver: clinical and therapeutic particularities]. *Presse Med.* 2007; 36: 1732–7.

[33] Sparchez Z, Radu P, Zaharie F, Al HN, Sparchez M. Percutaneous treatment of symptomatic non-parasitic hepatic cysts. Initial experience with single-session sclerotherapy with polidocanol. *Med Ultrason.* 2014; 16: 222–8.

[34] Moorthy K, Mihssin N, Houghton PW. The management of simple hepatic cysts: sclerotherapy or laparoscopic fenestration. *Ann R Coll Surg Engl.* 2001; 83: 409–14.

[35] Benzimra J, Ronot M, Fuks D, *et al.* Hepatic cysts treated with percutaneous ethanol sclerotherapy: time to extend the indications to haemorrhagic cysts and polycystic liver disease. *Eur Radiol.* 2014; 24: 1030–8.

[36] Blonski WC, Campbell MS, Faust T, Metz DC. Successful aspiration and ethanol sclerosis of a large, symptomatic, simple liver cyst: case presentation and review of the literature. *World J Gastroenterol.* 2006; 12: 2949–54.

[37] Ohhira M, Yamada M, Murazumi Y, *et al.* [Intracystic infusion therapy of minocycline hydrochloride for benign hepatic cysts]. *Nihon Ronen Igakkai Zasshi.* 1995; 32: 33–8.

[38] Lopes HM, Portela FA, Silva Pontes JM, Leitao MJ, Ribeiro JC, Freitas DS. Treatment of benign hepatic cysts by instillation of tetracycline hydrochloride. *Hepatogastroenterology.* 1998; 45: 496–9.

[39] Jusufovic R, Zerem E. Percutaneous treatment of symptomatic non-parasitic benign liver cysts with 20% NaCl solution. *Med Arh.* 2011; 65: 35–7.

[40] Spârchez Z, Radu P, Zaharie F, Al Hajjar N, Spârchez M. Percutaneous treatment of symptomatic non-parasitic hepatic cysts. Initial experience with single-sesion sclerotherapy with polidocanol. *Med Ultrason.* 2014; 16: 222–8.

[41] Yamamoto K, Sakaguchi H, Anai H, *et al.* Sclerotherapy for simple cysts with use of ethanolamine oleate: preliminary experience. *Cardiovasc Intervent Radiol.* 2005; 28: 751–5.

[42] Wijnands TF, Lantinga MA, Drenth JP. Hepatic cyst infection following aspiration sclerotherapy: a case series. *J Gastrointestin Liver Dis.* 2014; 23: 441–4.

[43] Lantinga MA, Geudens A, Gevers TJ, Drenth JP. Systematic review: the management of hepatic cyst infection. *Aliment Pharmacol Ther.* 2014.

[44] Du XL, Ma QJ, Wu T, Lu JG, Bao GQ, Chu YK. Treatment of hepatic cysts by B-ultrasound-guided radiofrequency ablation. *Hepatobiliary Pancreat Dis Int.* 2007; 6: 330–2.

[45] Z'graggen K, Metzger A, Klaiber C. Symptomatic simple cysts of the liver: treatment by laparoscopic surgery. *Surg Endosc.* 1991; 5: 224–5.

[46] Lee DH, Cho JY, Han HS, *et al.* Laparoscopic treatment of hepatic cysts located in the posterosuperior segments of the liver. *Ann Surg Treat Res.* 2014; 86: 232–6.

[47] Amendolara M, Bucca D, Barbarino C, *et al.* Surgical management of symptomatic simple hepatic cysts. *G Chir.* 2012; 33: 17–20.

[48] Kjeld T, Hansen EG, Holler NG, Rottensten H, Hyldegaard O, Jansen EC. Resuscitation by hyperbaric exposure from a venous gas emboli following laparoscopic surgery. *Scand J Trauma Resusc Emerg Med.* 2012; 20: 51.

[49] Cui W, Zhou HY, Zhang YH, Zhang T, Li Q. Surgical management of non-parasitic hepatic cyst with biliary communication: a case report. *Cancer Biol Med.* 2013; 10: 110–3.

[50] Masatsugu T, Shimizu S, Noshiro H, *et al.* Liver cyst with biliary communication successfully treated with laparoscopic deroofing: a case report. *JSLS.* 2003; 7: 249–52.

[51] Kaneya Y, Yoshida H, Matsutani T, *et al.* Biliary obstruction due to a huge simple hepatic cyst treated with laparoscopic resection. *J Nippon Med Sch.* 2011; 78: 105–9.

[52] Castro-Perez R, Dopico-Reyes E, Acosta-Gonzalez LR. Minilaparoscopic-assisted transvaginal approach in benign liver lesions. *Rev Esp Enferm Dig*. 2010; 102: 357–64.

[53] Berelavichus SV, Kriger AG, Starkov I, Shishin KV, Gorin DS, Poliakov IS. [Robotic-assisted and laparoscopic hepatic resections for nonparasitic cysts of posterior liver segments]. *Khirurgiia (Mosk)* 2013; 14–9.

[54] Mazza OM, Fernandez DL, Pekolj J, *et al*. Management of nonparasitic hepatic cysts. *J Am Coll Surg*. 2009; 209: 733–9.

[55] Koffron A, Rao S, Ferrario M, Abecassis M. Intrahepatic biliary cystadenoma: role of cyst fluid analysis and surgical management in the laparoscopic era. *Surgery*. 2004; 136: 926–36.

[56] Ishii K, Yoshida H, Taniai N, Moneta S, Kawano Y, Tajiri T. Infected hepatic cyst treated with percutaneous transhepatic drainage. *J Nippon Med Sch*. 2009; 76: 160–4.

[57] Ueda J, Yoshida H, Taniai N, Mineta S, Kawano Y, Uchida E. A case of spontaneous rupture of a simple hepatic cyst. *J Nippon Med Sch*. 2010; 77: 181–5.

[58] Gevers TJ, Chrispijn M, Wetzels JF, Drenth JP. Rationale and design of the RESOLVE trial: lanreotide as a volume reducing treatment for polycystic livers in patients with autosomal dominant polycystic kidney disease. *BMC Nephrol*. 2012; 13: 17.

[59] Temmerman F, Gevers T, Ho TA, *et al*. Safety and efficacy of different lanreotide doses in the treatment of polycystic liver disease: pooled analysis of individual patient data. *Aliment Pharmacol Ther*. 2013; 38: 397–406.

[60] Jeyarajah DR, Gonwa TA, Testa G, *et al*. Liver and kidney transplantation for polycystic disease. *Transplantation*. 1998; 66: 529–32.

[61] Benedetti E, Pirenne J, Troppmann C, *et al*. Combined liver and kidney transplantation. *Transpl Int*. 1996; 9: 486–91.

[62] Pirenne J, Aerts R, Yoong K, *et al*. Liver transplantation for polycystic liver disease. *Liver Transpl*. 2001; 7: 238–45.

[63] Smira G, Matei E, Gheorghe L, Popescu I. The MELD score exception for polycystic liver disease. *Chirurgia (Bucur.)* 2013; 108: 418–21.

[64] Kornasiewicz O, Dudek K, Bugajski M, Najnigier B, Krawczyk M. Choice of transplantation techniques and indications for liver transplantation in polycystic liver disease in patients with no signs of end-stage liver disease. *Transplant Proc*. 2008; 40: 1536–8.

[65] Takei R, Ubara Y, Hoshino J, *et al*. Intravascular embolization therapy in patients with enlarged polycystic liver. *Am J Kidney Dis*. 2014; 63: 937–44.

[66] 66. Scheuerlein H, Rauchfuss F, Franke J, *et al*. Clinical symptoms and sonographic follow-up after surgical treatment of nonparasitic liver cysts. BMC Surgery. 2013; 13:42-49

[67] Swenson K, Seu P, Kinkhabwala M, et al. Liver transplantation for adult polycystic liver disease. Hepatology. 1998; 28: 412–5.

Chapter 11

Experiences of 30 Years in Right Trisectionectomy for Huge Liver Tumor

Jing An Rui

Additional information is available at the end of the chapter

http://dx.doi.org/10.5772/61175

Abstract

Hepatocellular carcinoma (HCC) is the fifth most common cancer in the world and the third leading cause of cancer-related deaths. Up to now, surgery remains to be the main curative strategy for hepatocellular carcinoma. In this article the author summarizes his experiences of 30 years in right trisectionectomy for huge liver tumor. A total of 459 primary liver cancer patients were hepatomized in author's group. Among them, 33 cases of right trisectionectomies were performed under continuous single interruption of the porta hepatis. The 1-, 3-, and 5-year survival rates were 71.9%, 40.6%, and 34.4%, respectively. The longest cancer-free survival of right trisectionectomy in our group is 26 years. In the author's another cohort, 51 patients underwent hepatectomy without allogeneic blood transfusion. Compared with the control group containing 60 patients who underwent hepatectomy with allogeneic blood transfusion, the morbidity and recurrence rates in the group without allogeneic blood transfusion were significantly decreased ($P < 0.05$). Surgical anatomy study of the hepatic veins and case reports are also included in this article. Taken together, it is obvious that right trisectionectomy under continuous single interruption of the porta hepatis without allogeneic blood transfusion would benefit the patient with resectable huge HCC.

Keywords: primary liver cancer, right trisectionectomy, continuous single interruption of the porta hepatis, surgical anatomy of hepatic veins, major hepatectomy without allogeneic blood transfusion

1. Introduction

Hepatocellular carcinoma (HCC) is the fifth most common cancer in the world and the third leading cause of cancer-related deaths. More than 80% of HCC cases are from the Asian and African continents, and more than 50% of cases are from mainland China. It is estimated that more than 50% of liver cancers worldwide are attributable to HBV, and up to 89% of HBV-related HCC cases are from developing countries [1]. Recently, increasing trends in HCC incidence have been reported from several western countries, including France, Australia, and the United States, mainly because of the rising incidence of HCV [2]. At least one million new cases of HCC occur annually, and mortality from this disease remains high despite treatment. It was reported that 10–20% of newly diagnosed HCCs are >10 cm in diameter, which is commonly defined as huge HCC. Patients with huge HCC who survive more than 5 years were rarely reported in the literature. Recently, it is reported that a 5-year survival rate is less than 3–5% if without treatment. The mean overall survival rates via treatments at 1 year, 3 years, and 5 years are 66.1%, 39.7%, and 32.5%, respectively, 93.5%, 70.1%, and 59.1% for early-stage patients [1, 3–5]. Several novel strategies have been developed for the therapy of HCC in recent years, and the outcomes have taken marked progress. However, recurrence and metastasis rates remain high. Up to now, surgery, including hepatectomy and liver transplantation, remains to be the main curative strategy for hepatocellular carcinoma.

The developing history of hepatic surgery is strongly involved in the history of bleeding control during hepatic resections. In the early 1900s, a small but significant step forward was made in liver surgery by J. Hogarth Pringle [6], who in 1908 described a method for digital compression of the hilar vessels to control hepatic bleeding from traumatic injuries. Since the middle of the last century, right trisectionectomy (previous trisegmentectomy) has been used for huge hepatic neoplasms covering right and left medial section (Figure 1). In 1975, Starzl [7] described and clearly defined in detail a safe technique of right trisectionectomy (Figure 2). Then he reported his experience on 30 cases of the operation in 1980, including malignant and benign hepatic lesion [8]. Rui [9] reported his experience of 33 cases of primary liver cancer patients undergoing right trisectionectomy.

2. Selection of patients for right trisectionectomy of huge liver tumor

Up to now, the treatment of huge liver cancers is still very difficult due to poor outcomes and higher mortality and morbidity [9–11]. A number of reports have indicated that right trisectionectomy is effective for extensive hepatic malignancy, based on patients who have had long-term survival after this operation [9,12,13].

The situations of tumor were detected mainly by image examinations, including B-type ultrasonography, computed tomography (CT), magnetic resonance imaging (MRI), and angiography. To assess liver function of the patients before operation, we adopted the classic Child–Pugh classification, the ICGR test, and some concrete parameters, as described in standards [9].

The feasibility of right trisectionectomy for a given patient must be carefully evaluated according to the following criteria [9]: (1) tumor(s), including less than 2 satellite nodules, must be limited to the right lobe and left medial portion of the liver (there is no evidence of cancer invasion in left lateral segment); (2) tumor mass with clear borders or a pseudocapsule, and there is no tumor thrombus in the trunk of the portal vein and hepatic vein; (3) there is no evidence of distant metastasis; (4) compensatory enlargement of the left lateral section should

http://dx.doi.org/10.5772/61175

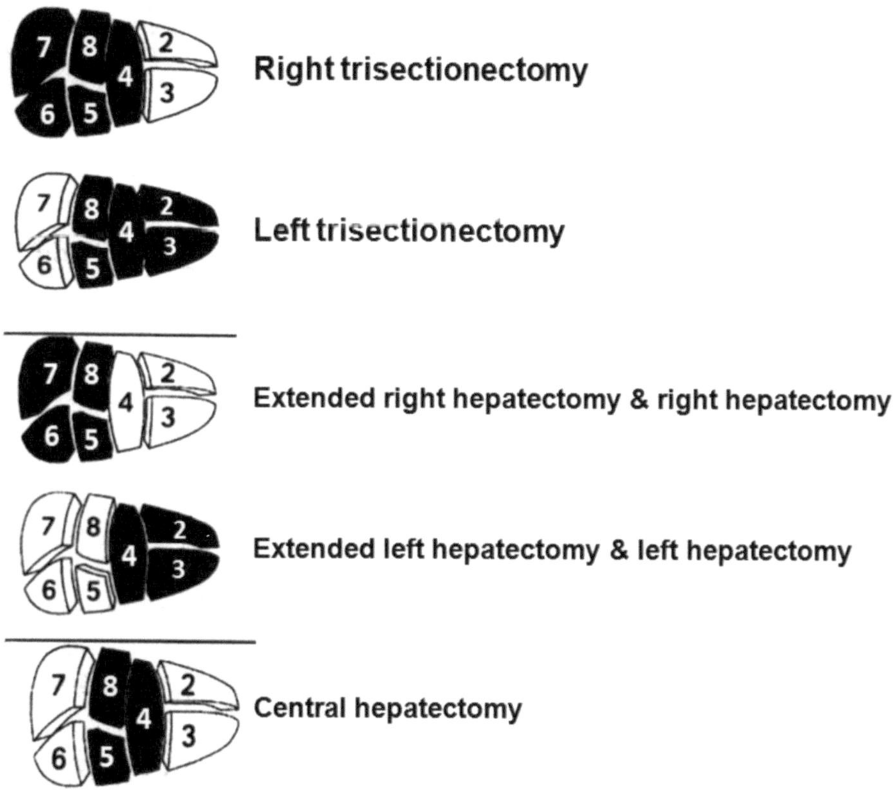

Figure 1. Photograph shows major hepatectomy. The regions in black color present the resected parts of the liver in various major hepatectomy.

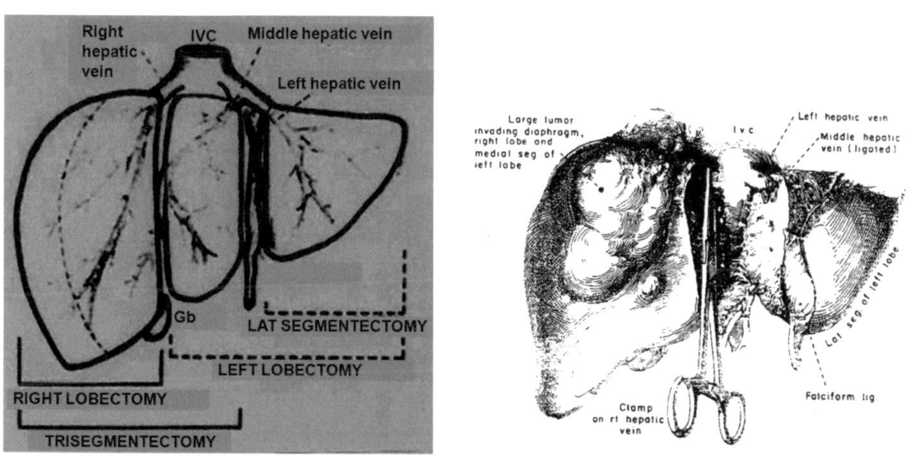

Figure 2. Photograph from Prof. TE Starzl shows right trisectionectomy.

be obvious; (5) the Child–Pugh classification of liver function must be grade "A" and the indocyanine green retention rate at 15 min (ICGR 15) should be lower than 15% before surgery; and (6) serum bilirubin is less than 34 mmol/L, serum albumin higher than 30 g/L, and serum prothrombin time larger than 60% before surgery.

A total of 459 primary liver cancer patients were hepatomized in our group. Among them, 33 cases of right trisectionectomies were performed. The patients included 24 males (72.7%) and 9 females (27.3%) with ages ranging from 15 to 69 years. Of the 33 cases, 28 (84.8%) were hepatitis B surface antigen (HBsAg) positive and 5 (15.2%) were negative. There were 8/33 cases (24.2%) with slight cirrhosis and 25/33 cases (75.8%) without cirrhosis; 22/33 cases (66.7%) were grade A in Child–Pugh classification, and 11/33 cases (33.3%) were grade B when the patients were hospitalized, but became grade A before surgical procedures through positive hepatic protective therapy; 27/33 cases (81.8%) with elevated serum α-fetoprotein (the highest value of AFP was 20,000 ng/ml) and 6/33 cases (18.2%) with normal α-fetoprotein. Sizes of tumor ranged from 8 to 20 cm. The stage of tumors was all IVa (T4N0M0). Pathological examination showed that 27 cases (81.8%) were hepatocellular carcinoma, 2 cases (6.1%) were cholangiocarcinoma, and 4 cases (12.1%) were mixed hepatocellular cholangiocarcinoma. Tumor thrombi were found in 17 cases (51.5%) in the right branch of the portal vein. Macroscopic satellite nodules were found in 15 cases (45.5%) and did not presented in left lateral section of the liver. All right trisectionectomies were performed under continuous single interruption of porta hepatis. The 1-, 3-, and 5-year survival rates after right trisectionectomy were 71.9%, 40.6%, and 34.4%, respectively [9]. The longest cancer-free survival of right trisectionectomy in our group is 26 years. This patient is still alive in Beijing. Recently, it is reported from The National Health and Family Planning Commission of The People's Republic of China that a mean of 5-year survival rate for HCC is 10.1% in China. It is obvious that right trisectionectomy would benefit the patients with resectable huge HCC.

3. Surgical procedures characterized by continuous single interruption of the porta hepatis for right trisectionectomy

Foster said (1989), "Surgical technique is an art form. It can be very personal, based mostly on experience, or it can take a cookbook approach. For many standard operations, we follow in the ruts created by our teachers, perhaps adding a nuance or two called forth by an unusual situation or by a creative mind. Unfortunately, many years ago when I needed help, there was no available to teach me to operate on the liver" [14].

Multiple intermittent hepatic inflow occlusion for hepatic resection had been proposed. The significance of intermittent hepatic inflow occlusion for hepatectomy had been generally accepted [15]. Belghiti et al. [16] demonstrated that the intermittent interruption of flow through the porta hepatis with periods of 15 min of clamping and 5 min of unclamping led to better parenchymal tolerance than continuous flow interruption, especially in patients with abnormal liver parenchyma. The total ischemic time under intermittent interruption of flow through the porta hepatis for hepatectomy was approximately 30–90 min (2–6 times of

http://dx.doi.org/10.5772/61175

clamping for 15 min each time). Nevertheless, in 1988, Rui reported his work on hepatectomy for primary liver cancer in Queen Mary Hospital (Hong Kong) titled *100 Cases of Hepatectomy under Normothermic Continuously Single Interruption of Porta Hepatis without Mortality*. We performed successfully major hepatectomy (Figure 1) for totally about 600 patients with HCC combined mostly with cirrhosis under normothermic continuous single interruption of porta hepatis. These studies were summarized in 20 cases of hemihepatectomy [17]; 4 cases of right trisectionectomy [18];179 cases of major hepatectomy, including 54 patients in elderly group and 125 in the nonelderly group [19]; and 33 cases of right trisectionectomy [9]. In the179 cases of major hepatectomy, the surgical procedures were shown in Tables 1 and 2. The postoperative complication rate was 10.6% (19/179), and the operative mortality was 1.1% (2/179). We noted that elderly HCC patients tend to presentations of significantly lower HBsAg positivity, smaller tumor sizes, less portal vein tumor thrombi (PVTT) and satellite nodule formation, earlier TNM staging, better differentiated tumors, less progressive, less aggressive, and less intrahepatically recurrence than that in the nonelderly. We found that Child–Pugh grading, PVTT, and Edmondson–Steiner grading independently predict postsurgical prognosis of elderly patients with HCC. In 2015, Uwatoko et al. [20] reported two cases of patients over 90 years old who underwent major hepatectomy for HCC, representing the oldest patients in the world to have done so. Generally, hepatectomy can be well tolerated for the elderly HCC patients, and a beneficial outcome similar to that of the nonelderly individuals can be expected, despite they had poorer liver function.

Surgical type	Elderly group (≥65 years) (n = 54)	Nonelderly group (≤65 years) (*n*= 125)
Right trisectionectomy	2	23
Left trisectionectomy	1	1
Extended right hepatectomy	2	11
Extended left hepatectomy		3
Right hepatectomy	9	20
Left hepatectomy	2	11
Central hepatectomy		4
Combined segmentectomy	20	34
Segmentectomy	8	6
Left lateral segmentectomy	5	7
Nonanatomical resection	5	5

Table 1. Summary of surgical type in 179 major hepatectomy under normothermic continuous single interruption of porta hepatis

In all of the major hepatectomy performed in our cohorts, the ischemic time under continuous single interruption of porta hepatis lasts generally 15 to 20 min, occasionally 40 min. The mean

Year	Overall survival rate	Cancer-free survival rate
1	82.0%	73.1%
2	56.7%	53.2%
3	51.1%	46.0%
4	46.2%	44.5%
5	40.2%	38.1%

Table 2. Survival rate of 179 cases of major hepatectomy for HCC under single time interruption of the porta hepatis

ischemic time in our cohorts is 20.6 min, which is much less than that of multiple intermittent hepatic inflow occlusion of the porta hepatic for major hepatectomy. The mean bleeding amount is 400 ml (400–2000 ml). The mortality and morbidity rates were 1.2% and 24.7%, respectively, indicating that the procedure can be carried out safely. In the process of hepatic resection under normothermic continuous single interruption of porta hepatis, the operative blood losing is much less, and the operating time is much shorter than that under multiple intermittent hepatic inflow occlusion. Capussotti et al. [21] reported their results of a prospective, randomized clinical trial from Italy that is similar to our experience. It is obvious that major hepatectomy under normothermic continuous single interruption of porta hepatis can be well performed if the surgeon has meticulous skill in liver surgery. Therefore, the intermittent interruption of the porta hepatis may not be generally necessary. It is now commonly agreed that compared with intermittent multiple hepatic inflow occlusions, continuous single interruption of porta hepatis can simplify procedures, shorten operating time, and reduce blood losing, especially during transaction of liver parenchyma. In addition, it is well known that reperfusion injury following ischemia is a clinically important process that contributes significantly to tissue damage [22,23]. Continuous single interruption of the porta hepatis during liver resection not only diminishes blood losing but also may attenuate reperfusion injury following ischemia as compared with multiple intermittent interruption of the porta hepatis.

Moreover, we have demonstrated via animal experiment on rats that intermittent or continuous clamping leads to similar extent of postischemic liver injury after a total 40 min clamping of porta hepatis [24]. The total 40 min interruption of porta hepatis, either intermittently or continuously, may cause reversible liver injury shown mainly by ALT and AST, and slightly by MDA and SOD in rats (Figure 3). Structural alteration was seen in liver tissue and hepatocytes but could recover gradually after blood perfusion was restored. Notably, no significant difference is seen in biochemical and structural injury between multiple intermittent and continuous single interruption, i.e., continuous single interruption of porta hepatis within 40 min would not significantly enhance the reversible injury of either liver structure detected by light and electron microscopy or liver functions detected by ALT and AST compared with the injury resulted from multiple intermittent interruption. Moreover, the levels of MDA, which is a marker for injury of peroxidation, resulted from ischemia/reperfusion, and SOD, which represents the scavenging potential for oxygen free radical, have no significant difference between continuous single interruption and intermittent interruption of porta hepatis for the total 40 min ischemia($p>0.05$). In addition, this experiment showed that GSH might be a protectant from liver injury that resulted from ischemia/reperfusion($p<0.05$) [22].

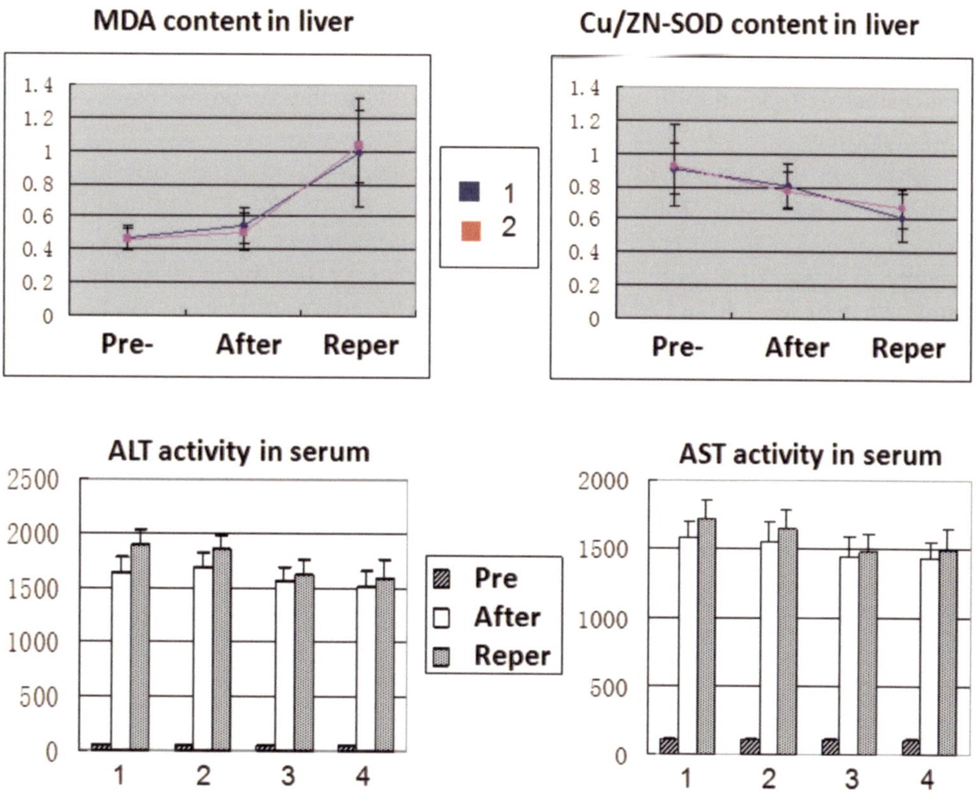

Figure 3. Comparison of liver injury induced by continuous single interruption and intermittent interruption of the porta hepatis via experiment on rats. Rats were divided into four groups ($n = 8$): (1) treated by intermittent interruption twice for 20 min each time with an interval of 5 min, (2) treated by continuous single interruption for 40 min, (3) treated by intermittent in administration of GSH (reduced glutathione), and (4) treated by continuous single interruption for 40 min in administration of GSH through portal vein. Malondialdehyde (MDA) and Cu/Zn superoxide dismutase (SOD) are used for the detection of injury induced by oxygen free radical in ischemia/reperfusion and protection level, respectively. Blue color curve: intermittent interruption; red color curve: continuous single interruption. Pre: preinterruption of porta hepatis; After: postinterruption of porta hepatis; Reper: reperfusion after interruption. 1 vs 2 & 3 vs 4 :$p>0.05$; 1 vs 3 &2 vs 4 : $p<0.05$.

4. Surgical anatomy study of the hepatic veins

Major hepatectomy under single interruption of porta hepatis requires fast operation in resection of liver lesion. It is most important for the liver surgeon to proficiently know the liver surgical anatomy. Hepatic vein is importantly related to the liver surgery. If hepatic vein is not treated perfectly in liver surgery, air embolization and bleeding may easily occur. Dai and Rui et al. [25] studied the anatomy of hepatic vein by perfusing ABS acetone solutions with various colors and then etching the liver parenchyma with HCl to show the draining variations of hepatic veins (Figure 4). We found that in 106 cases of livers from human fresh corpse, the draining variations of hepatic veins were rather popular. The variations appear mostly at Sg III, VI, and VII, least at Sg I, II, and VIII (Table 3). We also found that 80% (85/106) of middle vein and left vein join together into IVC (Figures 5 and 6), and 54.7% (58/106) middle vein is draining areas of VI, V, and VIII segments [25]. This work provides anatomic basis, especially when nonregular resection is performing and also warns to the liver surgeons to pay attention to the variations of hepatic veins. For example, during the execution of right trisectionectomy, the surgeons must carefully differentiate the middle hepatic vein (MHV) and the left hepatic vein (LHV) as well as their branch. In this case, the veins being taped must be MHV, as shown in Figure 6 (3,4), and RHV, as shown in Figure 6 (5,6), but not the HLV in Figure 6 (1,2) in the variants. As branches 1, 3, and 5 are rather thin, if any branch (such as 3 and 5 in Figure 6) of MHV and RHV is neglected and not taped, removing the liver being resected not only is impossible but also would subsequently lead to bleeding. Meanwhile, if the LHV or its branch (1,2) is taped, necrosis of the remnant liver parenchyma would happen. Any mistake would result in severe outcome.

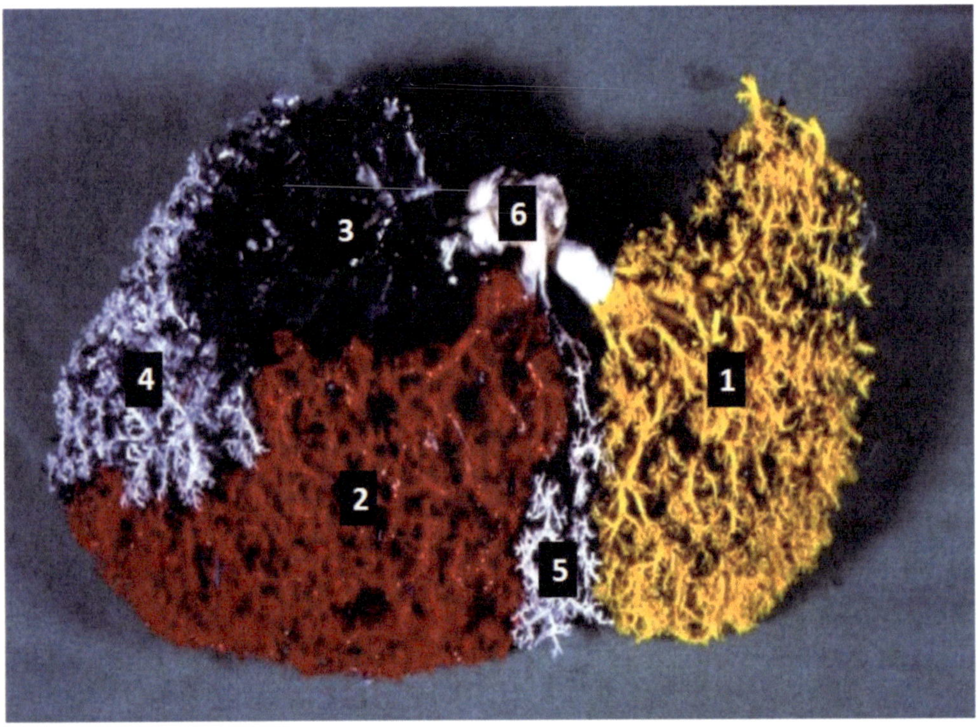

Figure 4. Surgical anatomy study of hepatic veins. (1) Left hepatic vein (LHV); (2) middle hepatic vein (MHV); (3) right hepatic vein (RHV); (4) right posterior and inferior vein; (5) left intersectional plane vein; (6) IVC.

http://dx.doi.org/10.5772/61175

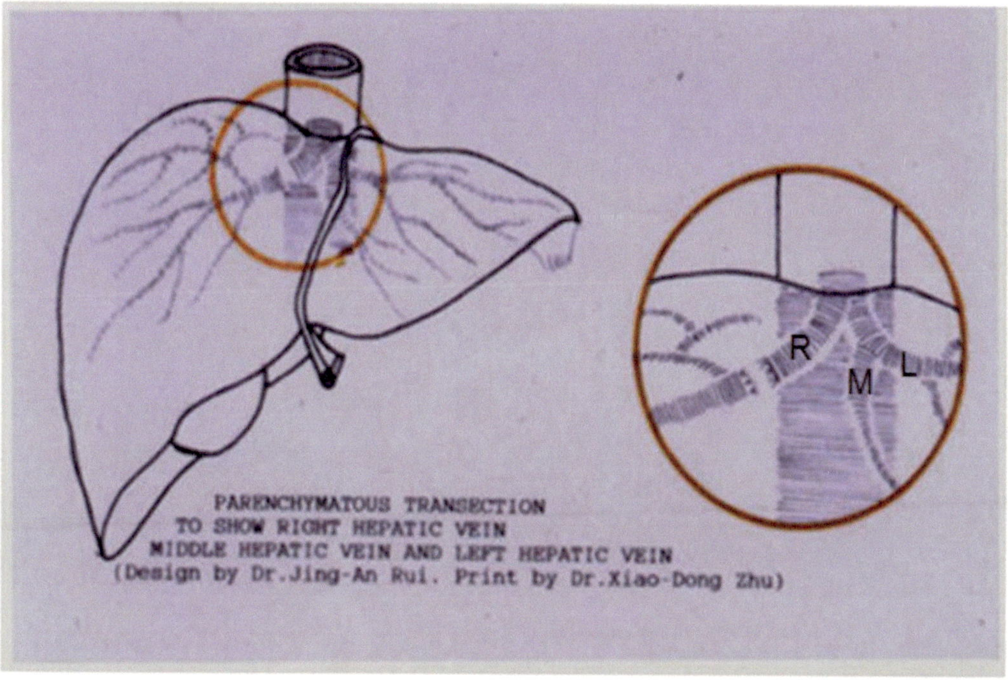

Figure 5. Photograph shows right hepatic vein (R), left hepatic vein (L), and Middle vein (M).

These veins run in the midplane of the liver (middle hepatic vein), the right intersectional plane (right hepatic vein), and the left intersectional plane (left hepatic vein). UV is the umbilical vein, which normally drains part of Sg 4 into the left hepatic vein.

Right hepatic vein (R)	Main type	49.0% (52/106)
	Disperse type	21.7% (23/106)
	Mix type	29.3% (31/106)
Middle hepatic vein (M)	Typical type	54.7% (58/106)
	Expand toward right type	19.8% (21/106)
	Expand toward left type	10.4% (11/106)
	Expand toward right and left type	8.5% (9/106)
	Contract type	6.6% (7/106)
Left hepatic vein (L)	Main type	69.8% (74/106)
	Disperse type	20.8% (22/106)
	Expand toward right type	9.4% (10/106)

Table 3. Variant rate of hepatic vein draining in 106 cases livers

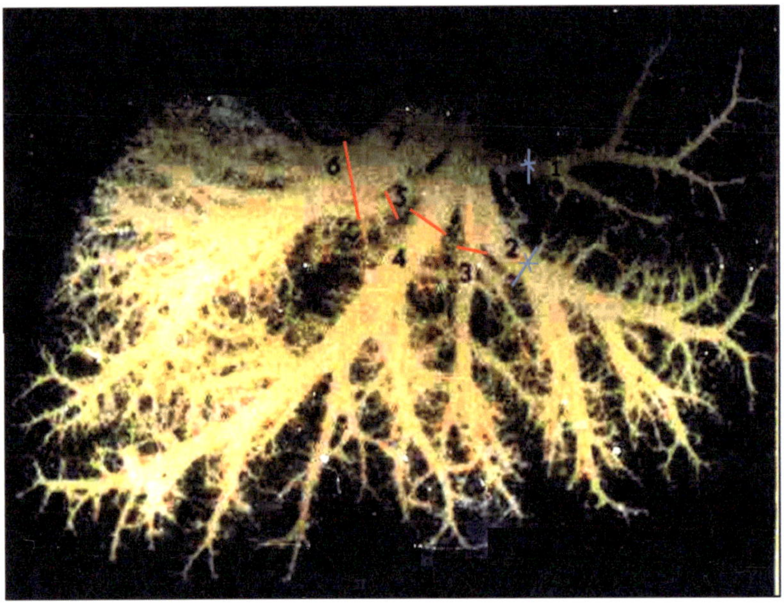

Figure 6. The taping veins for right trisectionectomy in one type of variant. This figure shows one type of variant, i.e., middle vein and left vein joined together into IVC, in which 1 and 2 are of LHV and 3 and 4 are of MHC. During the execution of right trisectionectomy on this variant, the taped veins must be RHV (5,6) and MHV (3,4), but not LHV (1,2).

5. Surgical arts of right trisectionectomy

The aim of liver resection in hepatocellular carcinoma is to remove the cancer with minimal operative risk. The major causes of hospital mortality associated with hepatectomy are postoperative hepatic failure, bleeding, and postoperative septic complications. It is obvious that surgical arts (skills) are extremely important for an ideal outcome of hepatectomy. The surgical arts of right trisectionectomy applied in my group are as follows:

1. Continuous single interruption of porta hepatis has been conventionally applied to attenuate bleeding. Based on the majority of HCCs company cirrhoses, the cirrhotic liver cannot tolerate liver ischemia as well as the normal liver. Compared with multiple intermittent hepatic inflow occlusion, continuous single interruption of porta hepatis significantly attenuates bleeding during hepatic resection. The author summarized a cohort of 459 cases hepatectomy for primary liver cancer patients. Among them, 33 cases of right trisectionectomies were performed. Continuous single interruption of porta hepatis has been applied for all of hepatectomy. The interruption of porta hepatis lasted 15 to 40 min. The operative mortality was 3.0% (1/33). These data suggested that continuous single interruption of the porta hepatis can be regarded as an effective and safe method to limit bleeding even if in right trisectionectomies [9].

http://dx.doi.org/10.5772/61175

2. Ultrasonic dissector (CUSA system 200) for dissecting hepatic parenchyma is applied, instead of previous finger fracture technique, introduced by Lin et al. [26]: The use of ultrasonic dissector makes the operative fields more clear.

3. Major hepatectomy without allogeneic blood transfusion has been advocated. Blood loss during liver resection is one of the most important factors affecting the perioperative outcomes of patients undergone hepatectomy. It has been accepted that infiltrative tumor type, surgical margin <10 mm and intraoperative blood transfusion are independent prognostic factors for overall survival [27,28]. Given that, cancer recurrence is the key factor related to overall survival. Besides the tiny tumor that was not able to be found and remains of cancer during surgical resection, the tumor recurrence after a curative hepatectomy generally resulted from the initiation and development of new lesion in the remnant liver, where apoptosis and proliferation of hepatocytes are both very active based on chronic hepatitis and cirrhoses. In other words, hepatocarcinogenesis in the remnant liver may occur *de novo*. It is well known that oncogenesis and development are tightly linked with immunosuppression. Perioperative transfusion of allogeneic blood would result in clinically significant effects on the recipient's immune system, including immunosuppression, and thus is associated with an increased rate of cancer recurrence, which has been confirmed in colorectal cancer, but is less known with other cancers [29,30]. We have demonstrated that major hepatectomy without allogeneic blood transfusion can reduce postoperative morbidity and recurrence rate of patients with hepatocellular carcinoma [25]. In this study, 51 patients were in the test group without allogeneic blood transfusion, and 60 patients were in the control group with allogeneic blood transfusion. In the text group the operative mortality and morbidity of major hepatectomy were 0% and 9.8%; the 1-, 2-, and 3-year recurrence rates were 24.1%, 27.6%, and 31.0%, respectively, as compared with the control group they were 3.3% and 28.3%; 43.5%, 54.3% and 58.7%, respectively. Statistically significant differences were seen in the morbidity and recurrence rates of patients with liver cancer between these two groups ($P < 0.05$). In the test group, 62.7% of patients underwent autotransfusion in hepatectomy for hepatocellular carcinoma. One potential risk of autotransfusion is considered to be linked with circulating tumor cells planting back to the remnant liver and leading to HCC recurrence. Hirano et al. [31] further demonstrated the safety and effective of autotransfusion: the cumulative 10-year survival rate in autotransfusion group and allotransfusion group were 20% versus 8%. Therefore, the bleeding control is most important in hepatectomy for avoiding perioperative transfusion of allogeneic blood. The mechanism of harmful effects resulted from allotransfusion on morbidity and recurrence of patients undergone hepatectomy have been discussed in another article from Rui et al. [27].

6. Adjuvant therapy and therapy after recurrence

Surgical therapy is best combined with appropriate adjuvant therapies based on individual situations of the patient. In case of tumor recurrence, the first choice is resection of the resectable tumor. Nevertheless, either surgical therapy or nonsurgical therapy, transcatheter arterial chemoembolization (TACE), radiofrequency ablation (RFA), percutaneous ethanol injection (PEI), cryotherapy coagulation therapy, ultrasound (US)-guided percutaneous microwave, high intensive focused ultrasound (HIFU), iodine^{125} brachytherapy, immunotherapy, cytotherapy, etc., can be considered according to individual situations of the patient to perform personalized therapy.

7. Case report

7.1. Case 1

The largest cancer-free survival time in our patients with huge HCC undergone right trisectionectomy has been more than 26 years. This patient is still alive in Beijing. The patient was a 57-year-old woman and diagnosed with hepatocellular carcinoma, and a right trisectionectomy was performed under continuous single interruption of the porta hepatic in 1988. The resected tumor weighted 2200 g (Figure 7, the left photograph).

7.2. Case 2

A 24-year-old man was diagnosed with hepatocellular carcinoma. A right trisectionectomy was performed under continuous single interruption of the porta hepatic. The intraoperation bleeding was 1500 ml. The patient accepted autologous blood transfusion (600 ml), and no allogeneic blood transfusion was administered. The resected tumor weighted 2500 g (Figure 7, the right photograph). The patient was discharged from hospital after recovery at 32 days after operation.

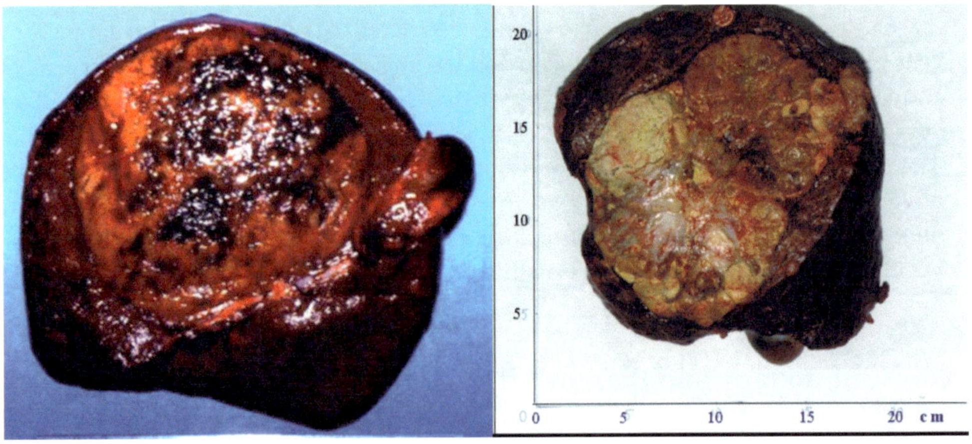

Figure 7. Tumors removed by right trisectionectomy.

7.3. Case 3

A 40-year-old male patient was suffering from hepatocellular carcinoma. The tumor diameter over 20 cm. One day, the tumor ruptured and the patient went into shock. Then the patient was urgently operated for right trisectionectomy. By follow-ups, the CT examination showed that no recurrence existed within 4 years after operation.

8. Conclusion

Right trisectionectomy is an effective and safe therapeutic strategy for huge HCC. Continuous single interruption of porta hepatis is an effective procedure in the attenuation of bleeding and shortening operation time based on skilled surgical manipulation and anatomical knowledge even in the treatment of huge tumor of primary liver cancers. Because of increasing morbidity and recurrence it is suggested to avoid allogeneic blood transfusion for patients undergone major hepatectomy. However, if necessary, autogeneic blood transfusion can be applied.

Author details

Jing An Rui

Address all correspondence to: drrlzhou@163.com

Department of Surgery, Peking Union Medical College Hospital, Chinese Academy of Medical Sciences, China

References

[1] Simonnetti, RG, Camma C, Fiorello, F, et al. Hepatocellular carcinoma. A worldwide problem and the major risk factors. Dig Dis Sci. 1991;36:962–972.

[2] McClune AC, Tong MJ. Chronic hepatitis B and hepatocellular carcinoma. Clin Liver Dis. 2010;14(3):461–476.

[3] Llovert JM, Burroughs A, Bruix J. Hepatocellular carcinoma. Lancet. 2003;362:1907–1917

[4] Munoz N, Bosch X. Epidemiology of hepatocellular carcinoma. In: Okuda K, Ishak KG, eds. Neoplasms of the liver 1988. Springer-Verlag, Berlin, Germany, pp. 3–19.

[5] Rustgi VK. Epidemiology of hepatocellular carcinoma. Gastroenterol Clin North Am. 1987;16:545–551.

[6] Pringle JH. Notes on arrest of hepatic hemorrhage due to trauma. Ann Surg. 1908;48:541–549.

[7] Starzl, TE, Bell RH, Beart RW. Hepatic trisegmentectomy and other liver resection. Surg Gynecol Obstet. 1975;141:429–437.

[8] Starzl TE, Koep LJ, Weil R 3rd, Lilly JR, Putnam CW, Aldrete JA. Right trisementectomy for hepatic neoplasms. Surg Gynecol Obstet. 1980;150:208–214

[9] Rui JA, Wang SB, Chen SG, Zhou L. Right trisectionectomy for primary liver cancer. World J Gastroenterol. 2003;9(4):706–709.

[10] Hanazaki K, Kajikawas S, Shimozawa N. Hepatic resection for large hepatocellular carcinoma. Am J Surg. 2001;181:347–353.

[11] Regimbeau JM, Farges O, Shen BY. Is surgery for large hepatocellular carcinoma justified? J Hepatol. 1999;31:1062–1068.

[12] Sugiura Y, Nakamura S, Lida S. Extensive resection of the bile ducts combined with liver resection for cancer of the main hepatic duct junction: a cooperative study of the keio Bile Duct Cancer Study Group. Surgery. 1994;155:445–451.

[13] Yamamoto M, Miura K, Yoshioka M. Disease-free survival for 9 years after liver resection for stage IV gallbladder cancer: report of a case. Surg Today. 1995;25:750–753.

[14] Foster JH. Liver resection techniques. Surg Clin North Am. 1989;69(2):235–249.

[15] Man K, Lo CM, Liu CL, et al. Effects of the intermittent Pringle manoeuvre on hepatic gene expression and ultrastructure in a randomized clinical study. Br J Surg. 2003;90:183–198.

[16] Belghiti J, Noun R, Malafosser R, et al. Continuous versus intermittent portal triad clamping for liver resection: a controlled study. Ann Surg. 1999;229:369–375.

[17] Rui JA, Wang K, Su Y, Li ZW, Wang CF, Wu JX, Zhao P. Right trisegmentectomy for primary liver cancer—a report of 4 cases with review of literature. Zhonghua Zhong Liu Za Zhi. 1991;13:37–39. Zhou Li, Rui JA, Wang SB. Outcomes and prognostic factors of cirrhotic patients with hepatocellular carcinoma after radical major hepatectomy. World J Surg. 2007;31:1782–1787.

[18] Rui JA, Qu JY, Su Y, Li ZW, Wang K, Zhu GJ, Wu JX, Chen GJ, Wang CF, Mao XW. Hemihepatectomy under hepato-portal interruption at normal temperature for liver malignancies: a report of 20 patients. Zhonghua Zhong Liu Za Zhi. 1987;9:221–223.

[19] Zhou L, Rui JA, Wang SB, et al. Clinicopathological features, post-surgical survival and prognostic indicators of elderly patients with hepatocellular carcinoma. EJSO. 2006;32:767–772.

[20] Uwatoko S, Yamamoto K, Sasaki T, Fukumori D, Igimi H, Yamamoto M, Yamamoto F, Yamashita Y. Age is no longer a limit: two cases of hepatectomy in patients over 90 years old. Case Rep Gastroenterol. 2015;9(1):49–55.

[21] Capussotti L, Nuzzo G, Polastri R, et al. Continuous versus intermittent portal triad clamping during hepatectomy in clinical trial. Hepatogastroenterology. 2003;50:1073–1077.

[22] Mitchell RN and Cotran RS. Cell Injury, Adaptation and Death. In: Basic pathology (7th ed.). Singapore: Elsevier; 2003. p. 9

[23] Lannan KL, Sahler J, Spinelli SL, Phipps RP, Blumberg N.Transfusion immunomodulation—the case for leukoreduced and (perhaps) washed transfusions. Blood Cells Mol Dis. 2013;50(1):61–8.

[24] Zhou Li, Rui JA, Zhou RL, Peng XM, Wang SB, Chen SG, Qu Q, Zhao YP. Liver injury after intermittent or continuous hepatic pedicle clamping and its protection by reduced glutathione. Hepatobiliary Pancreat Dis Int. 2004;3:209–213.

[25] Dai YH, Ji QY, Liu JH and Rui JA. Applied anatomy study on drainage of human segmental hepatic veins. Zhonghua Zhong Liu Za Zhi. 1988;26:568–571.

[26] Lin TY, Lee CS, Chen KM, Chen CC. Role of surgery in the treatment of primary carcinoma of the liver: a 31-year experience. Br J Surg. 1987;74:839–842.

[27] Rui JA, Zhou L, Chu QF, Wang SB, Chen SG, Qu Q, Wei X, Han K, Zhang N, Zhao HT. Major hepatectomy without blood transfusion: report of 51 cases. Chin Med J. 2004;117(5):673–676.

[28] Rui JA. Major hepatectomy without blood transfusion for hepatocellular carcinoma. In: Lau JWY. Hepatocellular Carcinoma-Clinical Research. Rijeka: InTech; 2011. pp. 197–208

[29] Refaai MA, Blumberg N. Transfusion immunomodulation from a clinical perspective: an update. Expert Rev Hematol. 2013;6(6):653–63.

[30] Cata JP, Wang H, Gottumukkala V, Reuben J, Sessler DI. Inflammatory response, immunosuppression, and cancer recurrence after perioperative blood transfusions. Br J Anaesth. 2013;110(5):690–701.

[31] Hirano T, Yamanaka J, Iimuro Y, Fujimoto J. Long-term safety of autotransfusion during hepatectomy for hepatocellular carcinoma. Surg Today. 2005;35(12):1042–1046.

Chapter 12

Liver Trauma

Hanan Alghamdi

Additional information is available at the end of the chapter

http://dx.doi.org/10.5772/61333

Abstract

The liver is the most frequently injured abdominal organ. Abdominal injuries occur in 31% of patients of polytrauma with 13 and 16% spleen and liver injuries respectively, and pelvic injuries in 28% of cases, making differential diagnosis between pelvic or intractable abdominal injury difficult.[1] Liver trauma is the most common cause of death after abdominal injury. The most common cause of liver injury is blunt abdominal trauma. Identification of serious intra-abdominal trauma is often challenging; many injuries may not manifest during the initial assessment and treatment period. Liver frequently injured following abdominal trauma and associated injuries contribute significantly to mortality and morbidity, and may mask the liver injury and causes delay in diagnosis. Management of hepatic injuries has evolved over the past 30 years. Prior to that time, a diagnostic peritoneal lavage (DPL) positive for blood, was an indication for exploratory celiotomy because of concern about ongoing hemorrhage and/or missed intra-abdominal injuries needing repair. The recognition that between 50 and 80 per cent of liver injuries stop bleeding spontaneously, coupled with better imaging of the injured liver by computed tomography (CT) and efficient ICU management, has led progressively to the acceptance of nonoperative management (NOM) with a resultant decrease in mortality rates.

Keywords: Blunt liver trauma, penetrating liver trauma, liver trauma grade, liver laceration, subcapsular hematoma, bile leak, hemobilia, biloma, parenchymal destruction, FAST, DPL, stab wound, hepatic artery embolization, nonoperative management

1. Introduction

Abdominal trauma is an emergency condition and, if not treated properly, is associated with significant morbidity and mortality. Today despite advancement in recognition, diagnosis, and management, the mortality remains high. Trauma is the second largest cause of hospital admission with 16% of global burden of all health cost. As per the estimate of the World Health Organization, by 2020, trauma will be the first or second leading cause of *years of productive life lost* for the entire world population [1].

The liver remains the most frequently and seriously injured abdominal organ due to trauma. About 31% patients of polytrauma have abdominal injuries. Almost 13% and 16% of cases have spleen and liver injuries, respectively, and pelvic injuries are seen in about 28% of cases. In close location of many organs, it is difficult to make differential diagnosis between pelvic or intractable abdominal injuries [2, 3].

In abdominal injuries, liver trauma is the leading cause of death. The most common way liver gets injured is in blunt abdominal trauma. By trauma, the identification of serious intra-abdominal injuries is a challenging task; many injuries may not be apparent during the initial assessment and treatment period. Since the liver gets frequently injured with other abdominal organs following abdominal trauma, associated injuries contribute significantly to mortality and morbidity and may cause the liver injury to be masked and diagnosis delayed. The management of hepatic injuries has evolved over the past 30 years. Previously, a diagnostic peritoneal lavage (DPL) was done to find out active bleeding and to diagnose missed intra-abdominal injuries needing surgical intervention. If DPL is positive for blood, it was an indication for exploratory celiotomy. Nowadays, it is recognized that between 50% and 80% of liver injuries stop bleeding spontaneously. In addition, there is better imaging of the injured liver by computed tomography (CT). Both these factors have led progressively to the acceptance of nonoperative management (NOM) and a resultant decrease in mortality rates [4, 5].

2. Mechanism of injury

Injury to liver ranges from major and serious to minor non serious injuries. It can extend from minor subcapsular hematomas and small capsular lacerations to major deep parenchymal lacerations, major crush injury, and vascular avulsion. Many factors contribute to the vulnerability of liver to injury in trauma. The liver is the biggest solid abdominal organ. It is surrounded by many organs and have attachments with peritoneal ligaments, giving it a relatively fixed position. Liver is anterior in the abdominal cavity in right upper quadrant. It is highly vascular in nature and has fragile parenchyma. The support of Glisson's capsule is easily disrupted making this organ vulnerable to injury. Motor vehicle accident is the most common cause of blunt liver injury.

Not surprisingly, even in the penetrating abdominal trauma, the liver is the second most commonly injured organ [6]. Most common cause of penetrating liver injury are due to knife assaults and gunshot wound. The severity of penetrating injury depends upon the trajectory of the missile or implements. The injuries can range from simple parenchymal injuries or serious and major vascular laceration [7].

During respiration, the liver margin, which can usually be palpated 2 to 3 cm below the right rib margin, rises and falls with the diaphragm. With expiration the dome of the liver rises as high as the level of nipple which is T4. This association with chest wall also makes liver vulnerable during injuries to chest. Furthermore, the penetrating injuries in the lower abdomen can cause serious trauma to liver as the inferior margin of the liver descends to as low as T12 with deep inspiration. [8].

http://dx.doi.org/10.5772/61333

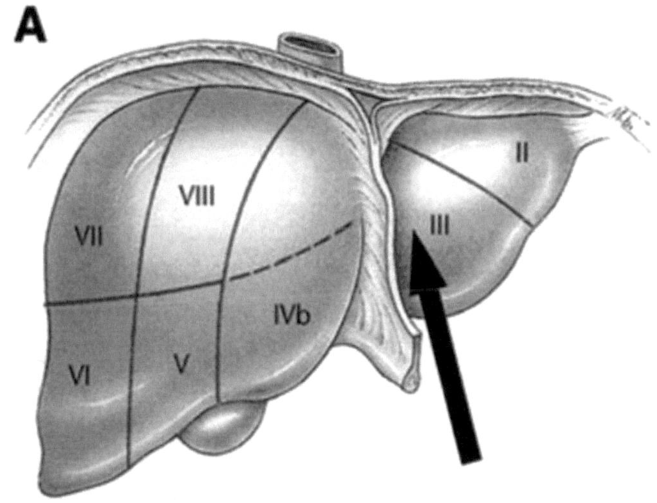

Type A injury: Patients suffer from rupture of the left liver lobe mostly along the falciform ligament, including segment II, III, or IV of the liver. This injury pattern is observed when the trauma has a direct frontal impact of the trauma energy.

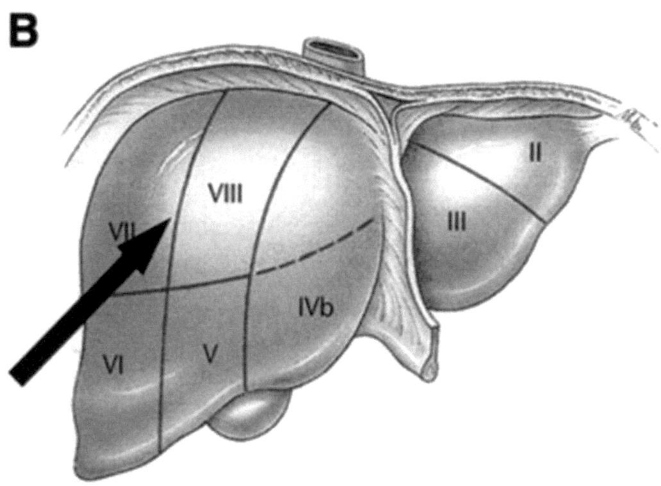

Type B injury: These injuries represent mechanisms of trauma with a more complex pattern of energy, with impacts coming from several directions, affecting segments V–VIII of the liver.

Figure 1. Mechanism of blunt liver trauma and the type of liver injury

The right liver lobe is more often involved, owing to its larger size and proximity to the ribs. Compression against the fixed ribs, spine or posterior abdominal wall generally result in predominant damage to posterior segments (segments 6, 7, and 8) of the liver (>85%). Inversely, a blow to the right hemithorax may propagate through the diaphragm producing contusion of dome of right lobe of liver. Liver's ligamentous attachments to diaphragm and posterior abdominal wall act as sites of shearing forces during deceleration injury. Liver injury can also occur as a result of transmission of excessively high venous pressure to remote body sites at the time of impact. Weaker connective tissue framework, relatively large size, and incomplete maturation and more flexible ribs account for higher chance of liver injury in children compared to adults. Deceleration injuries producing shearing forces may tear hepatic lobes and often involve the inferior vena cava and hepatic veins. While a steering column injury can damage an entire lobe. In general, liver trauma may result in subcapsular/intrahepatic hematomas, lacerations, contusions, hepatic vascular injury, and bile duct injury [9, 10].

Based on the mechanism and site of blunt liver trauma, the liver injury could be classified into two types, type A and B as described in (Figure 1) [11].

3. Assessment of liver trauma

The initial resuscitation and evaluation of the patient with blunt or penetrating abdominal or thoracic trauma is similar. Most commonly, the initial resuscitation, diagnostic evaluation, and management of the trauma patient with blunt or penetrating trauma are based upon protocols from the Advanced Trauma Life Support (ATLS) guidelines, established by the American College of Surgeons Committee on Trauma (Table 1) [12].

Primary examination	
	Airway
	Breathing
	Tension pneumothorax
	Open pneumothorax
	Flail chest
	Massive hemothorax
	Circulation
	Massive hemothorax
	Cardiac tamponade
Secondary examination (thoracic injury that endanger life)	
	Simple pneumothorax
	Pulmonary contusion
	Tracheobronchial lesions
	Closed cardiac injuries
	Traumatic aortic rupture
	Traumatic diaphragm injury
	Lesions crossing the mediastinum

Table 1. Systematic survey in ATLS

Accordingly, hemodynamically unstable trauma patients need to be transferred immediately to the operating room for emergency explore laparotomy for better life-saving evaluation and management. If the clinical setting allows, a Focused Assessment with Sonography for Trauma (FAST) exam, DPL, or CT may be performed [13].

Plain films obtained during the trauma evaluation are generally nonspecific but may demonstrate right-sided rib fractures, which increase the suspicion for liver injury [14].

3.1. History and physical examination

Trauma generally causes irritation of diaphragm and patient complaints of pain in the right upper abdomen, right chest wall, or right shoulder. The suspicion for liver injury increases if patient gives history of trauma to the right upper quadrant, right rib cage, or right flank. Clinically, most apparent findings like abdominal pain, tenderness, and distention are seen in cases of severe abdominal hemorrhage, including hemorrhagic shock.

Even though the most common findings indicative of intra-abdominal injury are abdominal tenderness and other peritoneal signs, these findings are not sensitive or specific for liver injury. Commonly seen physical findings due to liver injury include generalized abdominal tenderness or localized tenderness on right upper quadrant or lower chest wall, presence of abdominal wall contusion or hematoma (e.g., seat belt sign), or chest wall instability due to rib fractures. Sometimes significant liver damage can occur without a wound in close proximity to site of injury. Any penetrating injury to right chest, abdomen, flank, or back increases the seriousness of injury. A negative history and normal physical examination does not reliably exclude liver injury.

Many times, physical examination findings can be unreliable due to many reasons. Such mechanisms of injury often result in other associated injuries and that can divert the physician's attention from serious life-threatening intra-abdominal pathology. The injury can be underestimated due to nonspecific signs and symptoms, an altered mental state, drug and alcohol intoxication, and interpatient variability in reactions to intra-abdominal injury [1].

In about 80% of patients, other concurrent injuries can be present with blunt liver injury, which can include lower rib fractures, pelvic fracture, spinal cord injury, or combination of injuries. Such concurrent injuries can lead to rupture of vena cava, colon, diaphragm, right lung, duodenum, kidney, and extrahepatic portal structures [15].

4. Diagnosis

The physical stress of trauma is common in patients of liver injury, and this can cause disturbed biochemical blood test. Initial rise in white blood cell count and low red blood cell count is a nonspecific finding. The degree of anemia correlated to the volume of blood loss. Such loss can be from liver or other than the liver. Other causes include amount of crystalloids or colloids used during initial resuscitation. In posttraumatic hemorrhage, the duration and course of developing anemia is variable and as already explained related to the frequency, amount, and

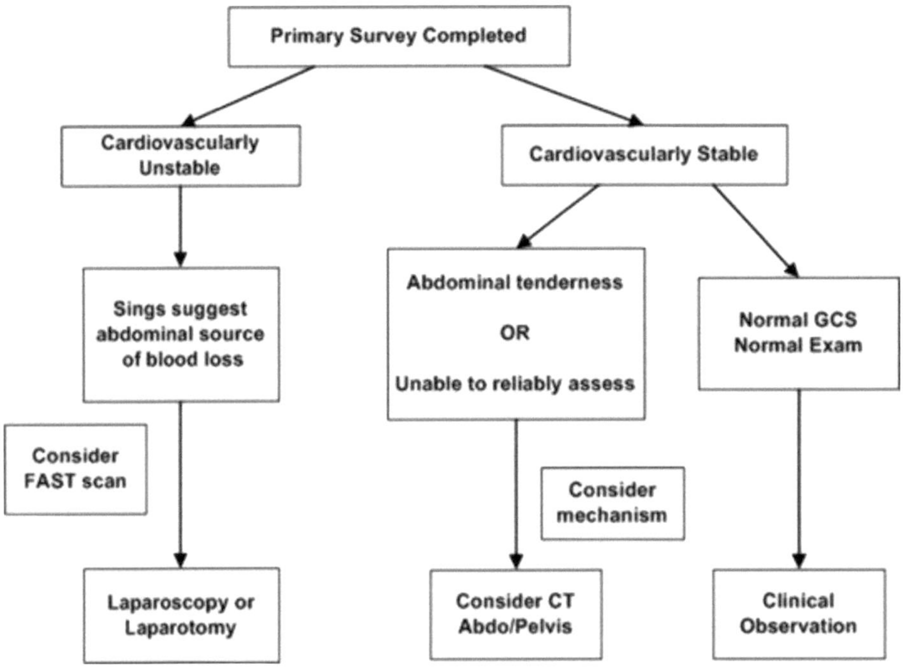

Figure 2. Assessment of trauma patient

rapidity of exogenous fluid administration and endogenous fluid shifts. Therefore, it is important to anticipate that significant liver trauma-related bleeding can happen irrespective of the presence or absence of anemia at the time of initial patient presentation.

In the hemodynamically stable patient, diagnosis of liver injury may be suspected based upon history of mechanism of injury, findings on physical examination, or laboratory findings of blood or other body fluids [16].

Imaging, especially using computed tomography (CT) with intravenous contrast of the abdomen, confirms the injury and also helps in defining the grade of injury. The characteristic pattern of pooling of intravenous contrast in or around the liver suggests ongoing bleeding and thus warrants the need for intervention. The imaging with the help of CT scan is also useful in identifying concurrent intra-abdominal and chest injuries [2, 17, 18].

The role of FAST examination comes when patient is hemodynamically unstable. However, in cases of intraparenchymal injuries, a negative FAST examination is not sufficient to exclude liver injury. Signs of liver injury on FAST examination include the presence of a hypoechoic (black) rim of subcapsular fluid, fluid in Morrison's pouch (hepatorenal space), or intraperitoneal fluid around the liver. The main objective of this investigation is quick bedside assessment for hemoperitoneum and hemopericardium. The primary utility of this investigation is identifying the presence of blood and bleeding and not the identification of or defining the degree of organ injuries [19, 20] (Table 2).

· It detects free fluid in the abdomen or pericardium
· It will not reliably detect less than 100 mL of free blood
· It does not identify injury to hollow viscus
· It cannot reliably exclude injury in penetrating trauma
· It may need repeating or supplementing with other investigations

Table 2. Value of The Focused Assessment with Sonography in Trauma (FAST)

Even if diagnostic peritoneal aspiration or lavage (DPL) has largely been replaced by the FAST examination, it may still be useful in selected patients, if the FAST is equivocal. In addition, the ATLS still includes DPL modality, and it remains one of the skills that physicians need to learn for ATLS certification. However, a recent Cochrane review has put a question mark on the reliability of ultrasonography for early diagnostic investigations in patients with suspected blunt abdominal trauma [21].

Detailed systematic abdominal ultrasound examination in the radiology suit and/or magnetic resonance imaging (MRI) is time consuming and not feasible in the setting of hemodynamic instability of trauma in the initial diagnosis of liver injury. Furthermore, it puts the patient in a location remote from trauma management area. However, MRI may be useful in a subset of hemodynamically stable patients who cannot undergo CT scan (e.g., IV contrast allergy), and patients with suspected bile ductal injury. Arteriography is generally reserved for patients who have indications for hepatic embolization to manage intrahepatic arterial hemorrhage [22, 23].

Recently, studies have tried to find out other markers that will help in grading the severity and deciding the conservative management of blunt hepatic injury. Koca et al. [24] found that liver transaminases can predict the hepatic injury with higher accuracy as the grade rises, and it can be superior to FAST in terms of determining the need for laparotomy.

Out of multiple modalities available for evaluating stable patients, CT scan along with hemodynamic stability are best in evaluating which patient requires surgery or in deciding which patient can be safely discharged from emergency. The main drawbacks of CT scan are its cost, low sensitivity in detecting bowel injuries, and hemodynamically unstable patients [1]. In

Table 3 some important summary points regarding investigation of blunt abdominal trauma [25].

· The diagnosis of abdominal injury by clinical examination alone is unreliable
· FAST is the investigation of choice in hemodynamically unstable trauma victim
· CT scan with IV contrast is the investigation of choice in hemodynamically stable trauma victim
· Solid organ injury in hemodynamically stable patients with no associated injuries (requiring urgent surgery) can often be managed without surgery

Table 3. Investigation of blunt abdominal trauma: key points

5. Hepatic injury grading

One of the most widely accepted injury grading scale to grade hepatic injuries is the American Association for the Surgery of Trauma (AAST) classification system. A study done using the National Trauma Data Bank (NTDB) in 2008 about the solid organ injuries showed that about 67% of hepatic injuries are Grade I, II, or III [26].

The nonoperative management (NOM) can give rise to higher successful outcome for low-grade injuries (Grades I, II, and III) and less success in cases of high-grade injuries (Grades IV and V). The major benefit of AAST grading system is for predicting the likelihood of success with NOM (see Figure 3).

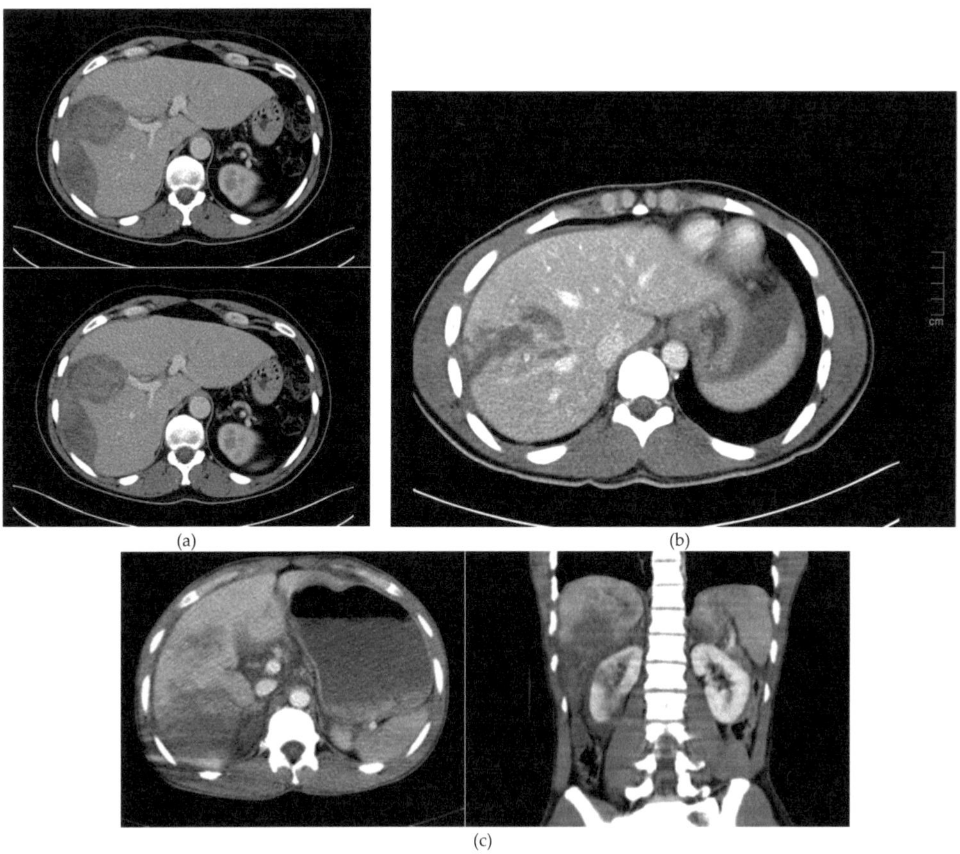

Figure 3. CT scan images show (A) Grad II Subcapsular, nonexpanding, 10-50% surface area; intraparenchymal nonexpanding <10 cm diameter; (B) Grad III liver injury with >3 cm laceration in the left lobe; (C) CT showing Grade IV liver injury with parenchymal disruption involving more than 25% of the liver.

Patients with Grade VI injuries are universally hemodynamically unstable and surgical intervention is required. The grades of hepatic injury are described in Table 4 [27-29].

Grade	Type	Injury Description
I	Hematoma	Subcapsular, nonexpanding, <10 cm surface area
	Laceration	Capsular tear, nonbleeding, <1 cm parenchymal depth
II	Hematoma	Subcapsular, nonexpanding, 10-50% surface area; intraparenchymal nonexpanding <10 cm diameter
	Laceration	Capsular tear, active bleeding, 1-3 cm parenchymal depth <10 cm in length
III	Hematoma	Subcapsular, >50% surface area or expanding; ruptured subcapsular hematoma with active bleeding; intraparenchymal hematoma >10 cm or expanding
	Laceration	>3 cm parenchymal depth
IV	Hematoma	Ruptured intraparenchymal hematoma with active bleeding
	Laceration	Parenchymal disruption involving 25-75% of hepatic lobe or one to three Couinaud's segments within a single lobe
V	Hematoma	Parenchymal disruption involving >75% of hepatic lobe or >3 Couinaud's segments within a single lobe
	Laceration	Juxtahepatic venous injuries (i.e., retrohepatic vena cava/central major hepatic veins)
VI	Hematoma	Hepatic avulsion

Table 4. Grading of liver injury based on the American Association of Surgery for trauma (AAST; 1994 revision) (data adopted from Moore EE, Cogbill TH, Gregory JJ, Shackford SR, Malangoni MA, Howard CR. Organ injury scaling: spleen and liver. J Trauma 1995;38:323-4)

In high-grade liver injury patients, liver-related complication rates are 11-13%. These can be predicted by the volume of packed red blood cells transfused at 24 hours post-injury and the grade of liver injury [30, 31].

6. Management

In the last 30 years, the management of liver injury has evolved significantly. The advancement of imaging studies has played an important role in the conservative approach for management. A shift from operative to nonoperative management for most hemodynamically stable patients with hepatic injury has been prompted by the speed and sensitivity of diagnostic imaging, particularly due to CT scanning and by advances in critical care monitoring [32, 33].

The operative versus NOM strategy depends upon presence of other injuries and medical comorbidities, hemodynamic status of the patient, and grade of liver injury (Table 5).

A positive FAST scan and DPL in hemodynamically unstable liver trauma patient promotes emergency abdominal exploration to establish the source of intraperitoneal hemorrhage. If the source is liver itself, an exploratory laparotomy is performed. The bleeding is control may be achieved through a damage-control approach or by using specific techniques for liver hemostasis. The approach depends upon the extent of the liver injury and presence and extent of associated injuries.

Hemodynamically "normal"	Investigation can be completed before treatment is planned.
Hemodynamically "stable"	Investigation is more limited. It is aimed at establishing whether the patient can be managed nonoperatively, whether angioembolization can be used or whether surgery is required.
Hemodynamically "unstable"	Investigations need to be suspended as immediate surgical correction of the bleeding is required.

Table 5. Classification of patients as per their physiological conditions after abdominal trauma

Hemodynamically stable patients with blunt liver injury who do not have other indications for abdominal exploration can be kept under observation. Patients with right-sided penetrating thoracoabdominal injuries, which can lacerate the liver, can remain hemodynamically stable. Such patients can also be kept under observation provided there are no associated intra-abdominal injuries. Nonoperative management generally fails in patients with higher-grade injuries than those with lower-grade injuries. Still such patients should be treated with NOM as long as they are hemodynamically stable. Other patients who suffer extra-abdominal injuries but requiring intervention can also be kept under observation. Nonoperatively managed patients who continue to bleed, and even with ongoing blood transfusion have hemodynamic instability need surgical exploration. It is also indicated in those patients who manifest a persistent systemic inflammatory response syndrome (SIRS), like presence of ileus, fever, tachycardia, and oliguria. Grade III and higher injuries often requires a combined angiographic and surgical management [34].

6.1. Nonoperative management

Nonoperative management (NOM) is widely accepted as the treatment of choice for hemodynamically stable patients with hepatic injury and with no other associated injuries indicating urgent intervention. Nonoperative management (NOM) consists of repeated assessment, close monitoring, and supportive intensive

2e care management with utilization of indicated arteriography and hepatic embolization. Furthermore, NOM is now recommended for penetrating injury (stab wound) as well as low-velocity gunshot wound to right upper quadrant in stable patients after exclusion of other injuries requiring urgent laparotomy. Most of the injuries that fall in this category are Grade I and II liver injuries [35].

In the positive response of trauma victim to initial fluid resuscitation with stable hemodynamic status, allows for further better imaging by CT scan of abdomen and pelvis. Angiogram and angioembolization are part of the management of all NOM algorithms if contrast extravasation is demonstrated to improve the success rate of NOM. Operative intervention is currently reserved to hemodynamically unstable patients, associated injuries requiring laparotomy, and failure of NOM [36].

The grade of liver injur4y alone and the volume of hemoperitoneum are not considered definitive criteria for selecting operative versus NOM [37].

Large retrospective reviews reported that more than 80% of patients with blunt hepatic injury could be treated by NOM with success rates more than 90% [38-40].

A recent Cochrane review also supported nonoperative management by concluding that currently there is no evidence to support the use of surgery over NOM for patients with abdominal trauma [41].

Some of the contraindications to nonoperative management of liver injury are listed in Table 6.

· Hemodynamic instability after initial resuscitation
· Other indication for abdominal surgery (e.g., peritonitis)
· Gunshot injury (relative contraindication)

Table 6. Contraindications to nonoperative management

Patients with isolated penetrating hepatic injuries due to abdominal stab wounds has been managed using nonoperative approach but management of patients with gunshot wounds remains controversial. Up to one third of patients of gunshot wound, who are treated using NOM approach, showed failure due to continuous bleeding and development of abdominal compartment syndrome. One of the most important concerns is missed injuries to the gastro-intestinal tract [42].

Patients that are managed by NOM needs to be admitted in hospital, placed on bed rest, and monitored continuously. If patients have a normal abdominal examination and stable hemoglobin for at least 24 hours, they can be discharged from hospitals. Large observational studies support this practice of discharging patients with liver injury regardless of the grade of injury. The clinical judgment of surgeon is important for deciding the length of observation [43]. Intensive care monitoring for at least 48-72 hours of hemodynamics and overall clinical condition is required for the rest of the cases. Other investigations and repeated clinical examinations and follow up investigations are done as indicated [44].

Thromboprophylaxis is indicated in patients with liver injury or other severe injuries who require hospitalization and are at a high risk for thromboembolism. At the same time, delay in the chemical thromboprophylaxis may be needed due to an increased risk of cerebral or bleeding from other sites. Success of pharmacologic prophylaxis is seen in patients in whom there are no other contraindications to pharmacologic prophylaxis and used when the hemoglobin gets stabilized with less than 1 g hemoglobin decrement over a 24-hour period of time [45].

6.2. Hepatic embolization

Hepatic embolization can be very useful way for prevention of bleeding. Success rates for embolization depends on many factors. Factors that determine the success includes institution policy, technique of embolization, access to arteries, skill of operator, and type of embolization material used. A properly carried out hepatic embolization has replaced the need for initial operative intervention from many sites. The highest success of hepatic embolization appears to be when used preemptively in patients who demonstrate extravasation of contrast on the initial abdominal CT scan and when patient is hemodynamically stable. The technical success of this technique ranges from 68% to 87%. The incidence of recurrent hemorrhage is found to be low in retrospective reviews. Patients who have no success with observational management can be treated with hepatic embolization. It can also be used adjunctively to manage patients with ongoing bleeding or rebleeding from the liver after surgical treatment for liver injury [22].

6.3. Benefits and risks of nonoperative management

One of the main advantages of nonoperative management is that it reduces the risks inherent to surgery and anesthesia procedures. However, one of the main disadvantages associated with NOM includes an increased risk of missed intra-abdominal injury, particularly hollow viscus injury, risks associated with embolization, and transfusion-related illness.

Blood transfusion is a life-saving measure during excessive bleeding and related complications. However, it is also associated with many complications. Commonly seen complications include intravascular volume overload (transfusion associated circulatory overload (TACO), transfusion-related acute lung injury (TRALI), immunologic and allergic reactions, as well as immunomodulation (transfusion-related immune modulation, TRIM), hypothermia, and coagulopathy. Hepatic embolization is also associated with additional risks. These includes risk of bleeding, complications at the arterial access site, necrosis of liver, abscess in the liver or subdiaphragmatic space, inadvertent embolization of other organs (e.g., bowel, pancreas) or lower extremities, arterial intimal dissection, contrast-induced allergic reactions, and contrast-induced renal toxicity and nephropathy. When embolization is performed following contrast CT scan, particularly in patients who with volume depletion, the risk of contrast-induced nephropathy is even greater. Repeated clinical monitoring and surgical intervention is a must if conservative treatment fails. Studies have shown statistically significant difference in terms of requirements for blood transfusion and intra-abdominal complications when comparing patients receiving operative and nonoperative treatment of liver injuries. However, it shows no difference in the length of hospital stay [46].

The underlying important requirement for use of conservative or NOM is that this should be under guidance of highly trained surgeons. This is because unexpected and difficult to manage complications can occur during observation, and surgeon should be able to convert this management to difficult surgical strategies [47].

6.4. Failure of nonoperative management

Failure of NOM is defined as the need for urgent surgical intervention and is generally related to hemodynamic instability and bleeding that becomes apparent by the need for ongoing fluid resuscitation or transfusion. Patients who become hemodynamically unstable, by definition, have failed NOM. The option here is almost limited to the life-saving emergency exploration laparotomy. Arterial embolization is less favored after NOM failure, mainly due to the time needed to set up the interventional radiology suite, the complexity of the embolization procedure, and the possible failure that will delay a definitive surgical intervention [48].

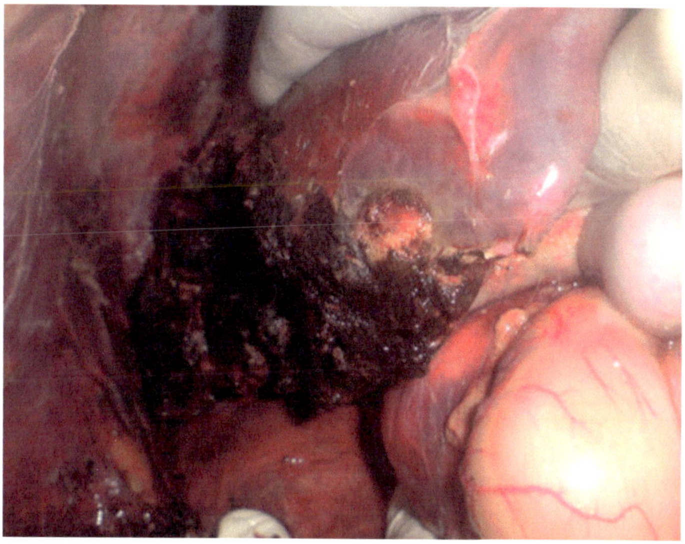

Figure 4. Patient with Grade IV liver injury, as shown in Figure 3C, who was hemodynamically unstable and showed extravasation of contrast and was unfit for angioembolization underwent laparotomy and resection of the fragmented right posterior liver segment.

A number of complications should be anticipated in NOM. One of the most common complications is biliary tree disruption with formation of biloma and/or persistent bile leak. Furthermore, hepatic necrosis can be seen following angioembolization for hepatic injury. It may also be seen following other procedures like laparotomy and hepatorrhaphy. Factors that may contribute to or indicate failure of NOM include advanced age of patient, delayed bleeding, sudden and severe hypotension, and active extravasation of contrast not controlled by angioembolization [35, 49, 50].

6.5. Surgical management

The operative management of liver injuries that require surgical intervention can be a challenge even for experienced surgeons (Table 7).

· Complex anatomical structure of the liver
· Large size
· High blood supply (vascularity), which is dual in nature
· Rich and difficult-to-access venous drainage

Table 7. Operative challenges in the management of liver injury

Operative intervention is most commonly preferred for penetrating abdominal or thoracic injuries with hemodynamically unstable patients. If the injury is a result of a high-velocity gunshot wound and if there is associated hollow viscus injury, it is always the preferred approach [51]. Hemodynamic status rather than grade of injury is more important indication for operative management in patients with blunt abdominal and chest injuries. As a general rule, a higher-grade injury usually has higher potential for failure of nonoperative management. Emergency laparotomy is also indicated in NOM if there is rebleeding, constant decline of hemoglobin, and increased transfusion requirement, as well as the failure of angioembolization of actively bleeding vessels [52].

Various surgical methods that are described include direct suture ligation of the parenchymal bleeding vessel, repair of venous injury under total vascular isolation and damage control surgery with utilization of preoperative, and/or postoperative angioembolization and perihepatic packing. Less preferred methods include anatomical resection of the liver, vascular ligation and use of the atriocaval shunt [53].

6.6. Damage control surgery

Damage control or damage limitation surgery is the concept originated from naval strategy, whereby a ship which has been damaged can be managed with minimal repairs to prevent it from sinking and definitive repairs can wait until it reaches port. One of the approaches includes perihepatic packing and closure of the abdominal incision using either a Bogata bag or a partial closure of proximal abdominal incision. With the similar approach, a minimum surgery is needed to stabilize the patient's condition, and in the meantime, the physiological derangement can be corrected. Damage control surgery is done with main objectives, including stopping any active surgical bleeding and controlling any contamination. The timing of reexploration depends upon many factors, including the correction of acidosis, coagulopathy, and hypothermia (i.e. trauma's lethal triad). The window considered safe during damage control surgery is 12-48 hours for reexploration and formal completion of the surgery [54, 55].

The algorithm for blunt liver trauma management is depicted in Figure 5.

7. Morbidity and mortality

Mortality rates for hepatic injury vary as per grade of the injury, associated injuries, and general condition of the patient. The outcome has improved over the years, and the major contributing factors are the new approaches in form of nonoperative management strategies, damage control, and use of perihepatic packing. Since mortality is rarely seen with Grade I and II injuries, the reduction seen was difficult to perceive. However, reduction in operative mortality has seen a great decline especially for higher-grade liver injuries (Grades III, IV, and V). The overall mortality rate may vary from 10% to 42% as per the higher grade of injuries [31].

Many studies have evaluated factors determining the mortality of hepatic injury treated by surgical management. Various factors have been found to have strong association with rate of

http://dx.doi.org/10.5772/61333

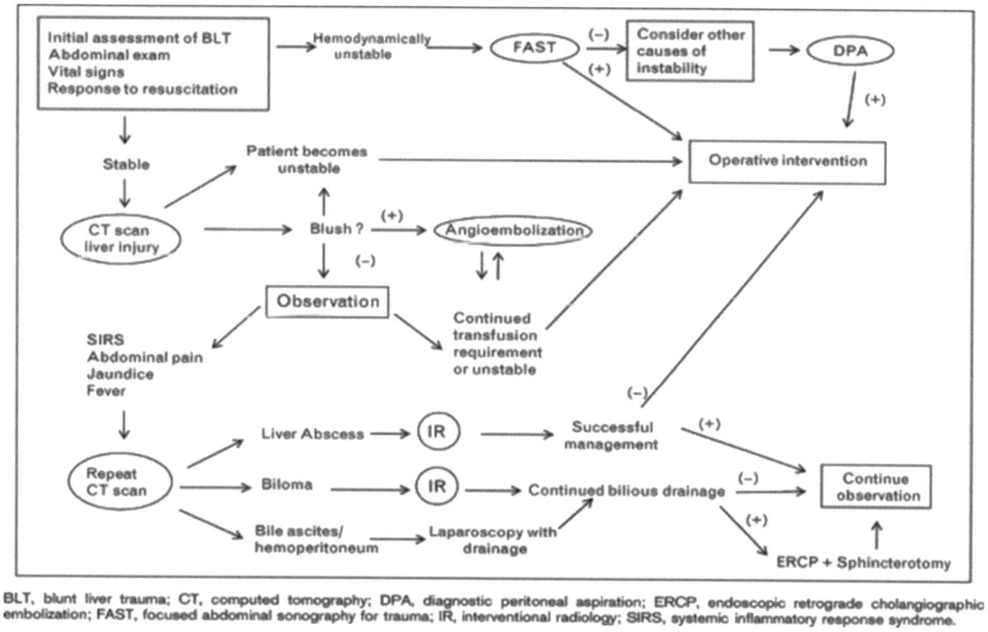

Figure 5. Algorithm For Nonoperative Management of Blunt Hepatic Trauma (adopted from Western Trauma Association critical decisions in trauma: nonoperative management of adult blunt hepatic trauma. J Trauma. 67:1144–1148, 2009).

mortality, which includes hemodynamic instability, coexisting musculoskeletal and chest injury, high levels of aspartate aminotransferase (AST), alanine aminotransferase (ALT), lactate dehydrogenase (LDH), long activated partial thromboplastin time (APTT), prothrombin time (PT), low fibrinogen levels, and platelet counts on admission. Not surprisingly, mortality is notably decreased when the liver trauma is managed by hepatobiliary surgeon if feasible [57].

8. Conclusion

i. Liver injury is a significant cause of morbidity and mortality in trauma patients, and being the largest solid organ within the abdominal cavity, it is easily injured.

ii. Chest X-ray and FAST are useful preliminary investigations in order to determine a correctible major injury. Diagnostic peritoneal lavage (DPL) may be preferred over FAST where the latter is not available.

iii. Further radiological assessment may aid diagnosis, but it is applicable if that is not delaying operative management of a patient in whom FAST is positive and patient is hemodynamically unstable.

iv. If FAST is positive and patient is hemodynamically stable, then CT scan remains the gold standard investigation as it delineates the extent of liver injury, identifies other associated injuries, and directs management.

v. For hemodynamically stable patients with liver injury, irrespective of grade of liver injury, the nonoperative management is preferred over definitive surgical intervention.

vi. Hepatic embolization may have better outcome for hemodynamically stable patients with liver injury who demonstrate pooling of intravenous contrast on initial or subsequent abdominal CT scan, rather than nonoperative management without embolization.

vii. Hepatic embolization requires specialized imaging facilities and an appropriately trained interventionist experienced with celiac artery catheterization. Failure of hepatic embolization to control bleeding indicates the need for surgery.

viii. Operative management involves initial control of hemorrhage and contamination followed by perihepatic packing and rapid closure, allowing for resuscitation to normal physiology in the intensive care unit and subsequent definitive reexploration.

ix. If the patient is hemodynamically unstable despite attempts to halt bleeding, techniques such as Pringle's maneuver (clamping of the hepatoduodenal ligament), simple suture and compression, hepatotomy and vascular ligation, or atriocaval shunt may be considered.

x. If these attempts also fail to achieve hemodynamic stability, transfer to a specialist liver surgery unit is advisable as there is substantial evidence to indicate that mortality is reduced when hepato-pancreato-biliary surgeons manage liver trauma.

Author details

Hanan Alghamdi

Address all correspondence to: hmalghamdi@uod.edu.sa; hananghamdi@yahoo.com

University of Dammam, King Fahd Hospital of the University, Saudi Arabia

References

[1] Mehta N, Babu S, Venugopal K. An experience with blunt abdominal trauma: evaluation, management and outcome. Clin Pract 2014 Jun 18;4(2):599.

[2] Deunk J, Brink M, Dekker H, et al. Predictors for the selection of patients for abdominal CT after blunt trauma: a proposal for a diagnostic algorithm. Ann Surg 2010, 251(3):512-20.

[3] Vukovic G, Lausevic Z. Diagnostics and treatment of liver injuries in polytrauma. HealthMed 2012;6:2796-801.

[4] Zargar M, Laal M. Liver trauma: operative and non operative management. Int J Collab Res Intern Med Public Health 2010;2(4):96-107.

[5] Petrowsky H, Raeder S, Zuercher L, Platz A, Simmen HP, Puhan MA, et al. A quarter century experience in liver trauma: a plea for early computed tomography and conservative management for all hemodynamically stable patients. World J Surg 2012;36:247-254.

[6] Stassen, N, Bhullar, et al. Nonoperative management of blunt hepatic injury: an Eastern Association for the Surgery of Trauma practice management guideline. J Trauma Acute Care Surg 2012; 73:S288.

[7] Tinkoff G, Esposito TJ, Reed J, et al. American Association for the Surgery of Trauma Organ Injury Scale I: spleen, liver, and kidney, validation based on the National Trauma Data Bank. J Am Coll Surg 2008; 207:646.

[8] Becker CD, Mentha G, Terrier F. Blunt abdominal trauma in adults: role of CT in the diagnosis and management of visceral injuries. Part 1: liver and spleen. Eur Radiol 1998; 8:553.

[9] Knudson MM, Mauli KI. Nonoperative management of solid organ injuries. Past, present & future. Surg Clin North Am 1999 Dec;79 (6):1357-71.

[10] Hassan R, Aziz AA. Computerized tomography (CT) imaging of injuries of blunt abdominal trauma: a pictorial assay. Malays J Med Sci 2010;17:29-39.

[11] Slotta JE, Justinger C, Kollmar O, Kollmar C, Schäfer T, Schilling MK. Liver injury following blunt abdominal trauma: a new mechanism-driven classification. Surg Today 2014 Feb;44(2):241-6.

[12] Bouillon B, Kanz KG, Lackner CK, Mutschler W, Sturm J. The importance of Advanced Trauma Life Support (ATLS) in the emergency room. Unfallchirurg Oct 2004;107 (10): 844-50.

[13] Hsu JM, Joseph AP, Tarlinton LJ, Macken L, Blome S. The accuracy of focused assessment with sonography in trauma (FAST) in blunt trauma patients: experience of an Australian major trauma service. Injury 2006;38:71-75.

[14] van der Vlies CH, Olthof DC, Gaakeer M. Changing patterns in diagnostic strategies and the treatment of blunt injury to solid abdominal organs. Int J Emerg Med 2011;4:47.

[15] Diercks DB, Mehrotra A, Nazarian DJ. Clinical policy: critical issues in the evaluation of adult patients presenting to the emergency department with acute blunt abdominal trauma. Ann Emerg Med 2011;4:57.

[16] Majid S, Gholamreza F, Mahmoud YM. New scoring system for intraabdominal injury diagnosis after blunt trauma. Chin J Traumatol 2014;17:19-24.

[17] Fang JF, Wong YC, Lin BC, et al. The CT risk factors for the need of operative treatment in initially hemodynamically stable patients after blunt hepatic trauma. J Trauma 2006; 61:547.

[18] Huber-Wagner S, Lefering R, Qvick LM, Körner M, Kay MV, Pfeifer KJ, et al. Effect of whole-body CT during trauma resuscitation on survival: a retrospective, multicentre study. Lancet 2009;373:1455-61.

[19] Ahmed N, Vernick JJ. Management of liver trauma in adults. J Emerg Trauma Shock 2011 Jan-Mar; 4(1): 114-19.

[20] Scalea TM, Rodriguez A, Chiu WC, Brenneman FD, Fallon WF, Jr, Kato K, et al. Focused Assessment with Sonography for Trauma (FAST): results from an international consensus conference. J Trauma 1999;46:466-72.

[21] Stengel D, Bauwens K, Rademacher G, Ekkernkamp A, Güthoff C. Emergency ultrasound-based algorithms for diagnosing blunt abdominal trauma. Cochrane Database Syst Rev 2013 Jul 31;7:CD004446.

[22] Letoublon C, Morra I, Chen Y, Monnin V, Voirin D, Arvieux C. Hepatic arterial embolization in the management of blunt hepatic trauma: indications and complications. J Trauma 2011 May;70(5):1032-6.

[23] Johnston JW, Gracias VH, Reilly PM. Hepatic angiography in the damage control population. J Trauma 2001;50:176.

[24] Koca B, Karabulut K, Ozbalci GS, Polat AK, Tarim IA, Gungor BB, et al. Is it possible to use transaminases for deciding on surgical or non-operative treatment for blunt liver trauma? Wien Klin Wochenschr 2015 Feb 27. [Epub ahead of print]

[25] Jansen JO, Yule SR, Loudon MA. Investigation of blunt abdominal trauma. BMJ 2008 Apr 26; 336(7650): 938-42.

[26] Tinkoff G, Esposito TJ, Reed J, et al. American Association for the Surgery of Trauma Organ Injury Scale I: spleen, liver, and kidney, validation based on the National Trauma Data Bank. J Am Coll Surg 2008; 207:646.

[27] Moore EE, Cogbill TH, Jurkovich GJ, Shackford SR, Malangoni MA, Champion HR. Organ injury scaling, Spleen, liver (1994 rev). J Trauma 1995;38:323.

[28] Yoon W, Jeong YY, Kim JK, Seo JJ, Lim HS, Shin SS, et al. CT in blunt liver trauma. Radiographics 2005 Jan-Feb;25(1):87-104.

[29] "Injury Scoring Scale." American Association for the Surgery of Trauma. Accessed from http://www.aast.org/library/traumatools/injuryscoringscales.aspx#liver (Accessed March 3, 2015).

[30] Pachter HL, Knudson MM, Esrig B, Ross S, Hoyt D, Cogbill T, et al. Status of nonoperative management of blunt hepatic injuries in 1195: a multicenter experience with 404 patients. J Trauma 1996, 40:31-8.

[31] Kozar RA, Feliciano DV, Moore EE, Moore FA, Cocanour CS, West MA, et al. Western Trauma Association/critical decisions in trauma: operative management of adult blunt hepatic trauma. J Trauma 2011 Jul;71(1):1-5.

[32] Petrowsky H, Raeder S, Zuercher L, et al. A quarter century experience in liver trauma: a plea for early computed tomography and conservative management for all hemodynamically stable patients. World J Surg 2012; 36:247.

[33] van der Wilden GM, Velmahos GC, Emhoff T, Brancato S, Adams C, Georgakis G, et al. Successful nonoperative management of the most severe blunt liver injuries: a multicenter study of the research consortium of new England centers for trauma. Arch Surg 2012;147:423-8.

[34] American College of Surgeons. Advanced Trauma Life Support Course Manual for Doctors. Chicago, IL: American College of Surgeons, 2008.

[35] Demetriades D, Hadjizacharia P, Constantinou C, Brown C, Inaba K, Rhee P, et al. Selective nonoperative management of penetrating abdominal solid organ injuries. Ann Surg 2006;244:620-8.

[36] Hommes M, Navsaria PH, Schipper IB, Krige JE, Kahn D, Nicol AJ. Management of blunt liver trauma in 134 severely injured patients. Injury 2014 Nov 26. pii: S0020-1383(14)00605-6. doi: 10.1016/j.injury.2014.11.019. [Epub ahead of print].

[37] Li M, Yu WK, Wang XB, Ji W, Li JS, Li N. Non-operative management of isolated liver trauma. Hepatobiliary Pancreat Dis Int 2014 Oct;13(5):545-50.

[38] Piper GL, Peitzman AB. Current management of hepatic trauma. Surg Clin North Am 2010; 90:775.

[39] Hurtuk M, Reed RL 2nd, Esposito TJ, et al. Trauma surgeons practice what they preach: the NTDB story on solid organ injury management. J Trauma 2006; 61:243.

[40] Coimbra R, Hoyt DB, Engelhart S, Fortlage D. Nonoperative management reduces the overall mortality of grades 3 and 4 blunt liver injuries. Int Surg 2006;91:251-7.

[41] Oyo-Ita A, Ugare UG, Ikpeme IA. Surgical versus non-surgical management of abdominal injury. Cochrane Database Syst Rev 2012 Nov 14;11:CD007383.

[42] Richardson JD. Changes in the management of injuries to the liver and spleen. J Am Coll Surg 2005; 200:648.

[43] Parks NA, Davis JW, Forman D, Lemaster D. Observation for nonoperative management of blunt liver injuries: how long is long enough? J Trauma 2011; 70:626.

[44] Raza M, Abbas Y, Devi V, Prasad KV, Rizk KN, Nair PP. Non operative management of abdominal trauma—a 10 years review. World J Emerg Surg 2013 Apr 5;8:14.

[45] Eberle BM, Schnüriger B, Inaba K, et al. Thromboembolic prophylaxis with low-molecular-weight heparin in patients with blunt solid abdominal organ injuries undergoing nonoperative management: current practice and outcomes. J Trauma 2011; 70:141.

[46] Meredith JW, Young JS, Bowling J. Nonoperative management of blunt hepatic trauma: the exception or the rule? J Trauma 1994;36:529-35.

[47] Gaspar B, Negoi I, Paun S, Hostiuc S, Ganescu R, Beuran M. Selective nonoperative management of abdominal injuries in polytrauma patients: a protocol only for experienced trauma centers. Maedica (Buchar) 2014 Jun;9(2):168-72.

[48] Polanco PM, Brown JB, Puyana JC, et al. The swinging pendulum: a national perspective of nonoperative management in severe blunt liver injury. J Trauma Acute Care Surg 2013; 75:590.

[49] Bala M, Gazalla SA, Faroja M, Bloom AI, Zamir G, Rivkind AI, et al. Complications of high grade liver injuries: management and outcome with focus on bile leaks. Scand J Trauma Resusc Emerg Med 2012;20:20.

[50] Giannopoulos GA, Katsoulis EI, Tzanakis NE, Panayotis AP, Digalakis M. Non-operative management of blunt abdominal trauma. Is it safe and feasible in a district general hospital? Scand J Trauma Resusc Emerg Med 2009,17:22-28.

[51] Marr JDF, Krige JEJ, Terblanche J. Analysis of 153 gunshot wounds of the liver. Br J Surg 2000;87:1030-4.

[52] David Richardson J, Franklin GA, Lukan JK, Carrillo EH, Spain DA, Miller FB, et al. Evolution in the management of hepatic trauma: a 25-year perspective. Ann Surg 2000;232:324-30.

[53] Duane TM, Como JJ, Bochicchio GV, Scalea TM. Re-evaluating the management and outcomes of severe blunt liver injury. J Trauma 2004;57:494-500.

[54] Krige JE, Bornman PC, Terblanche J. Liver trauma in 446 patients. S Afr J Surg 1997;35:10-5.

[55] Leppäniemi AK, Mentula PJ, Streng MH, Koivikko MP, Handolin LE. Severe hepatic trauma: nonoperative management, definitive repair, or damage control surgery? World J Surg 2011 Dec;35(12):2643-9.

[56] Kozar RA, Moore FA, Moore EE, West M, Cocanour CS, Davis J, et al. Western Trauma Association critical decisions in trauma: nonoperative management of adult blunt hepatic trauma. J Trauma. 2009;67:1144–1148.